T0259396

Perinatal and Neonatal Infections

Editors

JOSEPH B. CANTEY
ANDI L. SHANE

CLINICS IN PERINATOLOGY

www.perinatology.theclinics.com

Consulting Editor
LUCKY JAIN

June 2021 • Volume 48 • Number 2

ELSEVIER

1600 John F. Kennedy Boulevard • Suite 1800 • Philadelphia, Pennsylvania, 19103-2899

http://www.theclinics.com

CLINICS IN PERINATOLOGY Volume 48, Number 2
June 2021 ISSN 0095-5108, ISBN-13: 978-0-323-75705-8

Editor: Kerry Holland
Developmental Editor: Karen Solomon

Clinics in Perinatology (ISSN 0095-5108) is published quarterly by Elsevier Inc., 360 Park Avenue South, New York, NY 10010-1710. Months of issue are March, June, September, and December. Business and Editorial Offices: 1600 John F. Kennedy Blvd., Ste. 1800, Philadelphia, PA 19103-2899. Customer Service Office: 3251 Riverport Lane, Maryland Heights, MO 63043. Periodicals postage paid at New York, NY and additional mailing offices. Subscription prices are $321.00 per year (US individuals), $788.00 per year (US institutions), $365.00 per year (Canadian individuals), $835.00 per year (Canadian institutions), $435.00 per year (international individuals), $835.00 per year (international institutions), $100.00 per year (US and Canadian students), and $195.00 per year (International students). International air speed delivery is included in all Clinics subscription prices. All prices are subject to change without notice. **POSTMASTER:** Send address changes to *Clinics in Perinatology*, Elsevier Health Sciences Division, Subscription Customer Service, 3251 Riverport Lane, Maryland Heights, MO 63043. **Customer Service: Telephone: 1-800-654-2452** (U.S. and Canada); **1-314-447-8871** (outside U.S. and Canada). **Fax: 1-314-447-8029. E-mail: journalscustomerservice-usa@elsevier.com** (for print support); **journalsonlinesupport-usa@elsevier.com** (for online support).

Reprints. For copies of 100 or more, of articles in this publication, please contact the Commercial Reprints Department, Elsevier Inc., 360 Park Avenue South, New York, NY 10010-1710. Tel. 212-633-3874; Fax: 212-633-3820; E-mail: reprints@elsevier.com.

Clinics in Perinatology is also published in Spanish by McGraw-Hill Interamericana Editores S.A., P.O. Box 5-237, 06500 Mexico D.F., Mexico.

Clinics in Perinatology is covered in *MEDLINE/PubMed (Index Medicus) Current Contents, Excepta Medica, BIOSIS and ISI/BIOMED.*

Contributors

CONSULTING EDITOR

LUCKY JAIN, MD, MBA
George W. Brumley Jr Professor and Chairman, Emory University School of Medicine, Department of Pediatrics; Chief Academic Officer, Children's Healthcare of Atlanta; Executive Director, Emory + Children's Pediatric Institute, Atlanta, Georgia

EDITORS

JOSEPH B. CANTEY, MD, MPH
Associate Professor of Pediatrics, Division of Allergy, Immunology, and Infectious Diseases, Division of Neonatology, Department of Pediatrics, University of Texas Health San Antonio, San Antonio, Texas

ANDI L. SHANE, MD, MPH, MSc
Professor, Pediatric Infectious Diseases, Emory University School of Medicine, Children's Healthcare of Atlanta, Atlanta, Georgia

AUTHORS

IBUKUNOLUWA C. AKINBOYO, MD
Department of Pediatrics, Division of Pediatric Infectious Diseases, Duke University, Durham, North Carolina

RITU BANERJEE, MD, PhD
Vanderbilt University Medical Center, Nashville, Tennessee

MARIA E. BARBIAN, MD, FAAP
Assistant Professor in Pediatrics, Division of Neonatal-Perinatal Medicine, Emory University School of Medicine, Children's Healthcare of Atlanta, Atlanta, Georgia

ANDRES F. CAMACHO-GONZALEZ, MD, MSc
Associate Professor of Pediatrics, Division of Pediatric Infectious Diseases, Children's Healthcare of Atlanta, Emory University School of Medicine, Atlanta, Georgia

JOOEPH B. CANTEY, MD, MPH
Division of Allergy, Immunology, and Infectious Diseases, Division of Neonatology, Department of Pediatrics, University of Texas Health San Antonio, San Antonio, Texas

ALISON CHU, MD
Assistant Professor of Pediatrics, Division of Neonatology and Developmental Biology, Department of Pediatrics, Los Angeles, California

ANNABELLE DE ST. MAURICE, MD, MPH
Co-chief Infection Prevention Officer, Assistant Professor of Pediatrics, Division of Pediatric Infectious Diseases, Department of Pediatrics, Los Angeles, California

PATRICIA W. DENNING, MD, FAAP
Associate Professor in Pediatrics, Division of Neonatal-Perinatal Medicine, Emory University School of Medicine, Children's Healthcare of Atlanta, Director of Pediatrics, Emory University Hospital Midtown, Atlanta, Georgia

JENNIFER DUCHON, MDCM, MPH, FAAP
Associate Professor in Pediatrics, Division of Newborn Medicine, Jack and Lucy Department of Pediatrics, Icahn School of Medicine at Mount Sinai, New York, New York

MORVEN S. EDWARDS, MD
Professor of Pediatrics, Section of Infectious Diseases, Baylor College of Medicine, Houston, Texas

RACHEL L. EPSTEIN, MD, MSc
Assistant Professor, Department of Medicine, Section of Infectious Diseases, Boston University School of Medicine, Boston, Massachusetts

ELIZABETH ERVIN, MPH
Epidemiologist and Student, Post-Baccalaureate Premedical Program, University of Michigan, Ann Arbor, Michigan

CLAUDIA ESPINOSA, MD, MSc
Associate Professor, Department of Pediatrics, Division of Pediatric Infectious Diseases, Morsani College of Medicine, University of South Florida, Tampa, Florida

DONNA J. FISHER, MD
Associate Professor of Pediatrics, Medical Director of Hospital Epidemiology and Infection Prevention, University of Massachusetts Medical School-Baystate, Springfield, Massachusetts

DUSTIN D. FLANNERY, DO, MSCE
Assistant Professor, Department of Pediatrics, University of Pennsylvania Perelman School of Medicine, Division of Neonatology, Children's Hospital of Philadelphia, Philadelphia, Pennsylvania

SCOTT H. JAMES, MD
Department of Pediatrics, Division of Pediatric Infectious Diseases, The University of Alabama at Birmingham, Birmingham, Alabama

JULIA JOHNSON, MD, PhD
Division of Neonatology, Department of Pediatrics, Johns Hopkins School of Medicine, Johns Hopkins Children's Center, Baltimore, Maryland

SOPHIE KATZ, MD, MPH
Vanderbilt University Medical Center, Nashville, Tennessee

DAVID W. KIMBERLIN, MD
Department of Pediatrics, Division of Pediatric Infectious Diseases, The University of Alabama at Birmingham, Birmingham, Alabama

JOHN H. LEE, BS
Department of Pediatrics, University of Texas Health San Antonio, San Antonio, Texas

LAURA S. MADORE, MD
Assistant Professor of Pediatrics, Director of Neonatal Nutrition, University of Massachusetts Medical School-Baystate, Springfield, Massachusetts

ALEXANDRA K. MEDORO, MD
Department of Pediatrics, Divisions of Neonatology, and Pediatric Infectious Diseases, Nationwide Children's Hospital, The Ohio State University College of Medicine, Center for Perinatal Research, Abigail Wexner Research Institute at Nationwide Children's Hospital, Columbus, Ohio

SUSAN P. MONTGOMERY, DVM, MPH
Epidemiology Team Lead, Parasitic Diseases Branch, Division of Parasitic Diseases and Malaria, Center Global Health, Centers for Disease Control and Prevention, Atlanta, Georgia

SAGORI MUKHOPADHYAY, MD, MMSc
Division of Neonatology, Assistant Professor, Department of Pediatrics, Children's Hospital of Philadelphia, University of Pennsylvania Perelman School of Medicine, Philadelphia, Pennsylvania

PAUL PALUMBO, MD
Professor of Pediatrics and Medicine, Section of Infectious Diseases and International Health, Geisel School of Medicine at Dartmouth, Lebanon, New Hampshire

JESSICA ROBERTS, MD
Division of Neonatology, Assistant Professor, Department of Pediatrics, Emory University School of Medicine, Children's Healthcare of Atlanta, Atlanta, Georgia

PABLO J. SÁNCHEZ, MD
Professor, Department of Pediatrics, Divisions of Neonatology and Pediatric Infectious Diseases, Nationwide Children's Hospital, The Ohio State University College of Medicine, Center for Perinatal Research, Abigail Wexner Research Institute at Nationwide Children's Hospital, Columbus, Ohio

NICOLE L. SAMIES, DO
Department of Pediatrics, Division of Pediatric Infectious Diseases, The University of Alabama at Birmingham, Birmingham, Alabama

JOSHUA K. SCHAFFZIN, MD, PhD
Division of Infectious Diseases, Cincinnati Children's Hospital Medical Center, Department of Pediatrics, University of Cincinnati College of Medicine, Cincinnati, Ohio

HAYDEN SCHWENK, MD, MPH
Stanford University School of Medicine, Stanford, California

ELIZABETH SEWELL, MD, MPH
Division of Neonatology, Assistant Professor, Department of Pediatrics, Emory University School of Medicine, Children's Healthcare of Atlanta, Atlanta, Georgia

KELLY C. WADE, MD, PhD, MSCE
Professor of Clinical Pediatrics, Department of Pediatrics, University of Pennsylvania Perelman School of Medicine, Division of Neonatology, Children's Hospital of Philadelphia, Philadelphia, Pennsylvania

Contents

Neonatal sepsis is a major cause of morbidity and mortality in neonates and is challenging to diagnose. Infants manifest nonspecific clinical signs in response to sepsis; these signs may be caused by noninfectious conditions. Time to antibiotics affects neonatal sepsis outcome, so clinicians need to identify and treat neonates with sepsis expeditiously. Clinicians use serum biomarkers to measure inflammation and infection and assess the infant's risk of sepsis. However, current biomarkers lack sufficient sensitivity or specificity to be consider useful diagnostic tools. Continued research to identify novel biomarkers as well as novel ways of measuring them is sorely needed.

Necrotizing enterocolitis (NEC) is an inflammatory disease affecting premature infants. Intestinal microbial composition may play a key role in determining which infants are predisposed to NEC and when infants are at highest risk of developing NEC. It is unclear how to optimize antibiotic therapy in preterm infants to prevent NEC and how to optimize antibiotic regimens to treat neonates with NEC. This article discusses risk factors for NEC, how dysbiosis in preterm infants plays a role in the pathogenesis of NEC, and how probiotic and antibiotic therapy may be used to prevent and/or treat NEC and its sequelae.

Perinatal and neonatal infection and associated inflammatory response may adversely affect brain development and lead to neurodevelopmental impairment. Factors that predict the risk of infection and subsequent adverse outcomes have been identified but substantial gaps remain in identifying mechanisms and interventions that can alter outcomes. This article describes the current epidemiology of neonatal sepsis, the pathogenesis of brain injury with sepsis, and the reported long-term neurodevelopment outcomes among survivors.

PROGRAM OBJECTIVE

The goal of *Clinics in Perinatology* is to keep practicing perinatologists, neonatologists, obstetricians, practicing physicians and residents up to date with current clinical practice in perinatology by providing timely articles reviewing the state of the art in patient care.

TARGET AUDIENCE

Perinatologists, neonatologists, obstetricians, practicing physicians, residents and healthcare professionals who provide patient care utilizing findings from *Clinics in Perinatology*.

LEARNING OBJECTIVES

Upon completion of this activity, participants will be able to:

1. Review infection prevention in the nursery setting, antimicrobial stewardship, the role of human milk in infections, novel biomarkers for neonatal sepsis, and immunizations for neonates and young infants.
2. Discuss the diagnosis, management, and implications of neonatal infections on long-term neurodevelopment.
3. Recognize advances in treatment to combat neonatal pathogens.

ACCREDITATION

The Elsevier Office of Continuing Medical Education (EOCME) is accredited by the Accreditation Council for Continuing Medical Education (ACCME) to provide continuing medical education for physicians.

The EOCME designates this journal-based CME activity for a maximum of 13 *AMA PRA Category 1 Credit*(s)™. Physicians should claim only the credit commensurate with the extent of their participation in the activity.

All other health care professionals requesting continuing education credit for this enduring material will be issued a certificate of participation.

DISCLOSURE OF CONFLICTS OF INTEREST

The EOCME assesses conflict of interest with its instructors, faculty, planners, and other individuals who are in a position to control the content of CME activities. All relevant conflicts of interest that are identified are thoroughly vetted by EOCME for fair balance, scientific objectivity, and patient care recommendations. EOCME is committed to providing its learners with CME activities that promote improvements or quality in healthcare and not a specific proprietary business or a commercial interest.

The planning committee, staff, authors and editors listed below have identified no financial relationships or relationships to products or devices they or their spouse/life partner have with commercial interest related to the content of this CME activity:

Ibukunoluwa C. Akinboyo, MD; Ritu Banerjee, MD, PhD; Maria E. Barbian, MD, FAAP; Joseph B. Cantey, MD, MPH; Regina Chavous-Gibson, MSN, RN; Alison Chu, MD; Annabelle de St. Maurice, MD, MPH; Patricia W. Denning, MD, FAAP; Jennifer Duchon, MDCM, MPH, FAAP; Morven S. Edwards, MD; Rachel L. Epstein, MD, MSc; Elizabeth Ervin, MPH; Donna J. Fisher, MD; Dustin D. Flannery, DO, MSCE; Lucky Jain, MD, MBA; Scott H. James, MD; Julia Johnson, MD, PhD; Sophie Katz, MD, MPH; David W. Kimberlin, MD; John H. Lee, BS; Laura S. Madore, MD; Alexandra K. Medoro, MD; Susan P, Montgomery, DVM, MPH; Sagori Mukhopadhyay, MD, MMSc; Jessica Roberts, MD; Nicole L. Samies, DO; Pablo J. Sánchez, MD; Joshua K. Schaffzin, MD, PhD; Hayden Schwenk, MD, MPH; Elizabeth Sewell, MD, MPH; Andi L. Shane, MD, MPH, MSc; Jeyanthi Surendrakumar; Kelly C. Wade, MD, PhD, MSCE

The planning committee, staff, authors, and editors listed below have identified financial relationships or relationships to products or devices they or their spouse/life partner have with commercial interest related to the content of this CME activity:

Andres F. Camacho-Gonzalez, MD, MSc: research support from Gilead Sciences, Inc, Janssen Pharmaceuticals, Inc, and Merck & Co., Inc.

Claudia Espinosa, MD, MSc: research support from Gilead Sciences, Inc.

Paul Palumbo, MD: consultant/advisor for Gilead Sciences, Inc and Janssen Pharmaceuticals, Inc.

UNAPPROVED/OFF-LABEL USE DISCLOSURE

The EOCME requires CME faculty to disclose to the participants:

1. When products or procedures being discussed are off-label, unlabelled, experimental, and/or investigational (not US Food and Drug Administration [FDA] approved); and

2. Any limitations on the information presented, such as data that are preliminary or that represent ongoing research, interim analyses, and/or unsupported opinions. Faculty may discuss information about pharmaceutical agents that is outside of FDA-approved labelling. This information is intended solely for CME and is not intended to promote off-label use of these medications. If you have any questions, contact the medical affairs department of the manufacturer for the most recent prescribing information.

TO ENROLL
To enroll in the *Clinics in Perinatology* Continuing Medical Education program, call customer service at 1-800-654-2452 or sign up online at http://www.theclinics.com/home/cme. The CME program is available to subscribers for an additional annual fee of USD 265.00.

METHOD OF PARTICIPATION
In order to claim credit, participants must complete the following:
1. Complete enrolment as indicated above.
2. Read the activity.
3. Complete the CME Test and Evaluation. Participants must achieve a score of 70% on the test. All CME Tests and Evaluations must be completed online.

CME INQUIRIES/SPECIAL NEEDS
For all CME inquiries or special needs, please contact elsevierCME@elsevier.com.

CLINICS IN PERINATOLOGY

SERIES OF RELATED INTEREST

Pediatric Clinics of North America
https://www.pediatric.theclinics.com/
Obstetrics and Gynecology Clinics of North America
https://www.obgyn.theclinics.com/

THE CLINICS ARE AVAILABLE ONLINE!
Access your subscription at:
www.theclinics.com

Foreword

Neonates Have a Lot More at Stake When It Comes to Infections

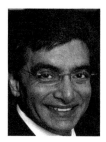

Lucky Jain, MD, MBA
Consulting Editor

For a variety of reasons, including of course COVID-19, the year 2020 will remain etched in our memories forever! Even though its impact on pediatric patients was not as severe, severe acute respiratory syndrome coronavirus 2 (SARS-CoV-2) virus disrupted lives and caused unparalleled misery and loss of life.[1,2] Studies are just beginning to emerge about COVID-19 long-haulers and multisystem inflammatory syndrome in children (MIS-C), reminding us that many of these infections leave a long trail of secondary effects even if the initial disease was mild.[3] The pathophysiologic mechanism of MIS-C remains unclear but may be linked to a postinfectious immune response. We in neonatal-perinatal medicine are burdened with one more worry: the potential impact of these pathogens on the growing brain.[4]

Indeed, cytomegalovirus and Zika virus infections have shown us that congenital and perinatally acquired infections can lead to severe long-term neurologic impairment.[5] Preterm newborns are particularly vulnerable to infection-induced neurologic injury, leading to cerebral palsy and mental disability. The mediators of such injury are varied and offer a window to potential interventions (**Fig. 1**).[6] Prevention efforts are critical since therapeutic options are limited and often ineffective against eliminating permanent sequelae. There is also the need for long-term follow-up of these patients since impairments such as hearing loss and cognitive delay can be missed during the critical period when interventions could be effective. Whether SARS-CoV-2 has any long-term effects on neonates who contracted the infection in the perinatal period will need to be studied closely. The same applies to infants and children with MIS-C.

All this to say that the importance of long-term follow-up of at-risk neonates cannot be overstated. In 2018, we dedicated an entire issue of the *Clinics in Perinatology* to "Long-Term Neurodevelopmental Outcomes of the NICU Graduate."[7] It was a remarkable issue edited by my good friend, Dr Ira Adams-Chapman, along with Dr Sara DeMauro. Sadly, Dr Adams-Chapman passed away in October 2020, leaving many

Clin Perinatol 48 (2021) xv–xvii
https://doi.org/10.1016/j.clp.2021.04.001
0095-5108/21/© 2021 Published by Elsevier Inc.

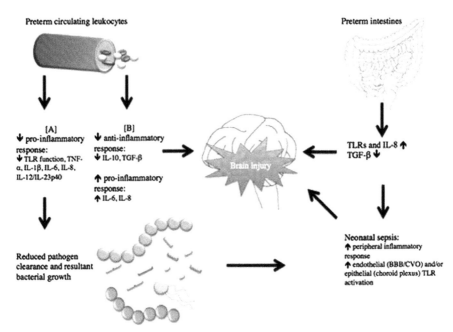

Fig. 1. Immature immune response places preterm infants at higher risks of developing infection-induced sepsis that may lead to brain injury. (*A, B*) Conflicting evidence. BBB, blood-brain barrier; CVO, circumventricular organs; IL, interleukin; TGF, transforming growth factor; TLR, toll-like receptor; TNF, tumor necrosis factor. (With permission from Jin C, Londono I, Mallard C, Lodygensky. New means to assess neonatal inflammatory brain injury. Journal of Neuroinflammation. 2015;12:180:1-14.)

who had worked with her closely, and those who were familiar with her work, in shock. Her many thoughtfully written articles remind us that newborn ailments and infections can lead to devastating permanent impairments and deserve close monitoring and interventions to promote optimal outcomes.[8]

In this issue of the *Clinics in Perinatology*, Drs Shane and Cantey have put together a classic series of articles dealing with common infections in the neonatal-perinatal period. They, like me, recall the many contributions of Dr Adams-Chapman and are dedicating this issue to her (**Fig. 2**). As always, I am grateful to the publishing staff

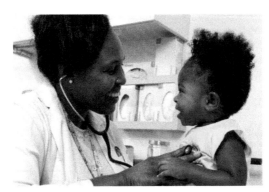

Fig. 2. Dr Ira Adams Chapman (1965-2020). (*Courtesy of* Department of Pediatrics, Emory University School of Medicine, Atlanta, GA; with permission.)

at Elsevier, including Kerry Holland and Karen Justine Solomon, for their support in bringing this important publication to you.

Lucky Jain, MD, MBA
Department of Pediatrics
Emory University School of Medicine
Children's Healthcare of Atlanta
1760 Haygood Drive, W409
Atlanta, GA 30322, USA

E-mail address:
ljain@emory.edu

REFERENCES

1. Berlin DA, Gulick RM, Martinez FJ. Severe COVID-19. N Engl J Med 2020;383: 2451–60.
2. HuB, Guo H, Zhou P, et al. Characteristics of SARS-CoV-2 and COVID 19. Nat Rev Microbiol 2021;19:141–54.
3. Rowley AH. Understanding SARS-CoV-2-related multisystem inflammatory syndrome in children. Nat Rev Immunol 2020;20:453–4.
4. Mwaniki MK, Atieno M, Lawn JE, et al. Long-term neurodevelopmental outcomes after intrauterine and neonatal insults: a systematic review. Lancet 2012;379: 445–52.
5. De Vries LS. Viral infections and the neonatal brain. Semin Pediatr Neurol 2020 32:100769.
6. Jin C, Londono I, Mallard C, et al. New means to assess neonatal inflammatory brain injury. J Neuroinflammation 2015;12:180.
7. Adams-Chapman I, De Mauro S. Long-term neurodevelopmental outcomes of the NICU graduate. Clin Perinatol 2018;45.
8. Adams-Chapman I. Necrotizing enterocolitis and neurodevelopmental outcome. Clin Perinatol 2018;45:453–66.

Preface

Neonatal-Perinatal Infections: An Update

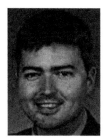
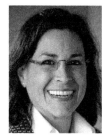

Joseph B. Cantey, MD, MPH   Andi L. Shane, MD, MPH, MSc

Editors

For as long as humankind has been birthing children, congenital and perinatal infections have been a major cause of morbidity and mortality among newborns. Our understanding of the complex mechanisms of maternal and infant immunity and infection continues to evolve, from the discovery that syphilis could be transmitted from infected women to their infants in the sixteenth century to the identification of severe acute respiratory syndrome coronavirus 2 in placental tissue in 2020. Our understanding of neonatal and perinatal infections has increased substantially since the publication of the 2015 issue devoted to this topic. In this brief time, neonates with congenital infections attributed to Chikungunya, Zika, and *Trypanosoma cruzi* have been recognized around the world as neonatologists and perinatologists collaborated across borders to diagnose and care for affected infants and their families. The resurgence of hepatitis C virus and congenital syphilis during the opioid epidemic and the seemingly eternal challenges of necrotizing enterocolitis, human immunodeficiency virus, and herpes simplex virus have continued to inspire targets for prevention. As always, neonatal infectious diseases are a shifting sea of challenge—and opportunity.

In this issue of *Clinics in Perinatology*, we are thrilled to have a distinguished slate of authors, who provide updates on these familiar and emerging pathogens and highlight advances that can be taken to the neonatal bedside. Infection prevention in the nursery setting, antimicrobial stewardship, the role of human milk in infections, novel biomarkers for neonatal sepsis, and immunizations for neonates and young infants are also explored in detail within this issue. In addition to a discussion of diagnosis and management, the implications of neonatal infections on long-term neurodevelopment are explored. The quest to combat neonatal pathogens continues, and readers will be well served to learn about the advances in our armamentarium.

The myriad of pathogens and the infants whom they infect each comprise two sides of a triangle in neonatal infectious diseases. The third side comprises the clinicians and

Clin Perinatol 48 (2021) xix–xx
https://doi.org/10.1016/j.clp.2021.03.014
0095-5108/21/© 2021 Published by Elsevier Inc.

researchers who dedicate their careers to the bench and bedside care and protection of neonates. To those who bend their time and thought toward these ever-changing and ever-challenging problems, we extend our thanks. To the authors who contributed to this issue during a global pandemic, we are exceedingly grateful. We would also like to thank Lucky Jain and the exceptional publishing staff at Elsevier, including Karen Solomon and Kerry Holland, for their support and patience.

The joy associated with the publication of this issue is lessened by the untimely death of one of our coauthors, friend and colleague, Ira S. Adams-Chapman, MD, MPH, to whom this issue is dedicated. Dr Adams-Chapman was a neonatologist and Director of the Developmental Progress Clinic at Emory University and Children's Healthcare of Atlanta in Georgia, where she cared for thousands of neonatal nursery graduates and their families, helping them to grow and thrive. A passionate clinician, researcher, and educator, she trained a generation of pediatricians and neonatologists while advocating for their needs as a member of the American Academy of Pediatrics Committee on the Fetus and Newborn. Her contributions to neurodevelopmental research, including her collaborations with colleagues at the Eunice Kennedy Shriver National Institute of Child Health and Human Development, are cited as key publications in the field of neurodevelopmental outcomes of premature neonates. Her loss is tempered by the impact that she has had on the care of preterm infants worldwide.

Joseph B. Cantey, MD, MPH
Division of Allergy, Immunology
and Infectious Diseases
Division of Neonatology
Department of Pediatrics
University of Texas Health San Antonio
7703 Floyd Curl Drive
San Antonio, TX 78229, USA

Andi L. Shane, MD, MPH, MSc
Chief, Division of Pediatric Infectious Disease
Marcus Professor of Hospital
Epidemiology and Infection Control
Emory University School of Medicine and
Children's Healthcare of Atlanta
Emory Children's Center
Room 504A
2015 Uppergate Drive NE
Atlanta, GA 30322, USA

E-mail addresses:
cantey@uthscsa.edu (J.B. Cantey)
ashane@emory.edu (A.L. Shane)

Biomarkers for the Diagnosis of Neonatal Sepsis

Joseph B. Cantey, MD, MPH[a],*, John H. Lee, BS[b]

KEYWORDS

- Biomarker • C-reactive protein • Complete blood count • Neonate • Procalcitonin
- Sepsis

KEY POINTS

- Early, accurate diagnosis of neonatal sepsis improves time to effective therapy for infants with sepsis while minimizing antibiotic exposure in uninfected infants.
- An ideal biomarker for neonatal sepsis should become abnormal before clinical signs develop and have near-perfect sensitivity and a rapid turnaround time.
- At present, no biomarker (including complete blood count with differential, C-reactive protein, and procalcitonin) has sufficient sensitivity to preclude the need for empiric antibiotic treatment of infants with suspected sepsis.
- Existing biomarkers have mediocre specificity, which has contributed to unnecessary antibiotic therapy for infants with culture-negative sepsis.
- Research efforts in partnership with biomedical engineers may identify novel biomarkers, including ones that can be detected via noninvasive sensors.

INTRODUCTION

Neonatal sepsis remains a substantial cause of morbidity and mortality in the nursery setting.[1] Sepsis in neonates and young infants is challenging to diagnose, because infants manifest nonspecific clinical signs in response to sepsis (eg, respiratory distress, hypotension, apnea) that could indicate noninfectious conditions. Furthermore, time to antibiotics affects neonatal sepsis outcome; therefore, there are both clinical and compliance motivations for identifying and treating neonates with sepsis expeditiously.[2,3] As a result, clinicians commonly use serum biomarkers to measure inflammation and infection and assess the infant's risk of sepsis. This article reviews the current state of neonatal sepsis diagnostics, highlights the uses and limitations of

[a] Department of Pediatrics, Division of Allergy, Immunology, and Infectious Diseases, University of Texas Health San Antonio, 7703 Floyd Curl Drive, San Antonio, TX 78229, USA; [b] Department of Pediatrics, University of Texas Health San Antonio, 7703 Floyd Curl Drive, San Antonio, TX 78229, USA
* Corresponding author.
E-mail address: cantey@uthscsa.edu

Clin Perinatol 48 (2021) 215–227
https://doi.org/10.1016/j.clp.2021.03.012
0095-5108/21/© 2021 Elsevier Inc. All rights reserved.

current biomarkers, and discusses the characteristics and development pathway of a theoretic ideal biomarker for neonatal sepsis.

DEFINITIONS

Neonatal sepsis has been loosely defined as an infection of a sterile site (eg, blood, urine, cerebrospinal fluid) and clinical signs of illness. Infection in the first 72 hours of life is defined as early-onset sepsis (EOS) and is generally associated with perinatal risk factors such as intrauterine infection and inflammation (ie, chorioamnionitis), prolonged rupture of membranes, and maternal group B *Streptococcus* colonization.[4,5] For infants cared for in the nursery or neonatal intensive care unit (NICU) setting, infection beyond age 72 hours is defined as late-onset sepsis (LOS) and is associated with health care–associated transmission.[6] Infections among infants aged more than 72 hours who have been discharged is generally associated with community-acquired pathogens and is referred to by a variety of names, including invasive bacterial infection, fever without a source, and serious bacterial infection.[7,8] However, a discussion of sepsis diagnostics for young infants presenting to care from the community with suspected sepsis is beyond the scope of this article.

Sepsis in adults is defined as life-threatening organ dysfunction as a result of a dysregulated response to infection.[9] Since the early 1990s, the diagnosis of sepsis has been based on a group of clinical findings designed to measure organ dysfunction systemic inflammatory response syndrome (SIRS). SIRS criteria have poor sensitivity and specificity for neonatal sepsis. Coggins and colleagues[10] evaluated SIRS criteria in a case-control study of infants with LOS in their NICU; the sensitivity and specificity of SIRS criteria were 42% and 74%, respectively. Concerningly, most septic infants who developed organ dysfunction did not meet SIRS criteria at the time cultures were obtained. The current diagnostic definition, the Third International Consensus Definitions for Sepsis and Septic Shock (Sepsis-3), mark an intentional shift away from SIRS.[9] The Sepsis-3 task force created the Sequential Organ Failure Assessment (SOFA). SOFA uses a variety of objective clinical components, including fraction of inspired oxygen; mean arterial pressure, including need for vasopressors; Glasgow coma scale score; need for mechanical ventilation; and bilirubin, platelet, and creatinine concentrations. The neonatal-specific SOFA score can be used to improve prediction of mortality in neonatal sepsis but is not intended as a diagnostic tool.[11,12] However, experts have called for specific consensus definitions of sepsis for preterm and term infants.[13]

CHALLENGES IN SEPSIS DIAGNOSTICS

The diagnosis of neonatal sepsis is difficult (**Fig. 1**). Distinguishing the individual components of sepsis from a dysregulated response to the infection is challenging. The 3 primary issues in neonatal sepsis diagnosis are (1) the myriad of clinical findings that mimic sepsis rather than represent it, and, as a direct result, (2) concern for falsely negative bacterial cultures, also known as culture-negative sepsis, and (3) the need to treat empirically for a minimum of 24 to 48 hours while cultures incubate. A further complication is that the initiation of antimicrobial therapy before cultures are obtained can sterilize subsequent cultures and decrease the opportunity for accurate diagnosis of sterile site infections.

Neonatal sepsis is rare; conditions that mimic sepsis are collectively common. For example, apnea, respiratory distress, and hypotension are all 10 to 100 times more common than EOS in very-low-birthweight (<1500 g) infants.[14] Transient tachypnea of the newborn, which also mimics EOS, is approximately 200 times more common

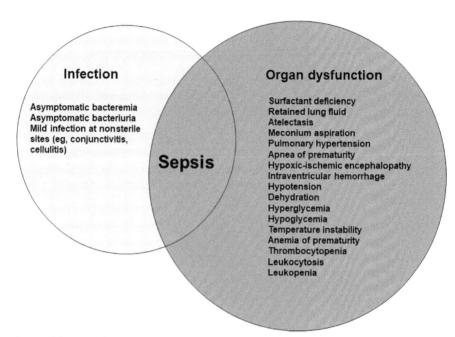

Fig. 1. Although a formal consensus definition of neonatal sepsis has not been developed, it is generally defined as an infection causing organ dysfunction because of a dysregulated response. As shown, there are many causes of organ dysfunction in infants, particularly those who are premature. Therefore, a careful evaluation for infection and organ dysfunction is indicated before assigning sepsis as the cause of these clinical signs.

than EOS (~60 per 1000 live births vs 0.3 per 1000 live births) and results in unnecessary evaluation and treatment of sepsis.[15,16] Respiratory distress syndrome affects most preterm infants, including virtually all infants less than 30 weeks' gestation, and is clinically and radiographically indistinguishable from pulmonary manifestations of EOS.[17] Clinicians appreciate the urgency of a neonatal sepsis diagnosis and institution of therapy, but identifying the 1 infant who is septic out of the many who have noninfectious presentations is challenging. Schulman and colleagues[18] evaluated antibiotic use in 116 California nurseries and found that the median number of infants treated for EOS for each proven case was 95 (range, 11–336). Antibiotic use for EOS did not correlate with the incidence of EOS at that center.[18] Similar studies in both well-baby nurseries and in NICUs have shown that antibiotic use does not correlate with infant or maternal risk factors.[19,20] Diagnostic subjectivity and inefficiency are major contributors to unnecessary antibiotic use in the nursery setting and have spurred efforts to develop objective sepsis biomarkers.[21]

Appropriately obtained bacterial cultures (usually blood culture alone for EOS and blood, urine, and cerebrospinal fluid for LOS) are the gold standard for the diagnosis of neonatal sepsis.[22] Cultures should be obtained before antibiotic therapy is initiated. Blood culture sensitivity is directly linked to volume; a weight-based approach is recommended by the American Academy of Pediatrics.[23,24] For most term neonates, this equates to 1 mL. The sensitivity of blood cultures approaches 100% if 1 mL of blood is obtained and the culture is processed correctly.[25–27] However, many clinicians caring for neonates with suspected sepsis incorrectly view the sensitivity of blood cultures as poor. In many situations, preanalytical issues such as inadequate blood volume or contamination are responsible for the absence of detection of a pathogen or detection of an organism that is not considered to be a pathogen. This problem results in the far-too-common practices of either providing prolonged antibiotic therapy to infants with sterile cultures for culture-negative sepsis or treating a contaminant organism as a true pathogen.[28–30] These practices are unnecessary at best and harmful at worst, leading to increased dysbiosis, adverse short-term and long-term outcomes, and antimicrobial resistance.[31] A full discussion of culture-negative sepsis is beyond the scope of this article, but it is an important contributor to the need for better sepsis biomarkers.

Although the sensitivity of a properly obtained blood culture is excellent to detect bacterial causes of neonatal sepsis, these cultures require incubation for hours to days to detect growth.[32] Most clinical microbiology laboratories incubate blood cultures for 3 to 7 days.[33] Identification of the causative bacteria for neonatal sepsis can be achieved in more than 99% of patients by 36 hours in LOS, and recent data suggest that as little as 24 hours may be sufficient to detect pathogens associated with EOS.[34–38] However, even if empiric antibiotics are discontinued after 24 hours of administration, infants are still exposed to at least 1 dose of aminoglycosides and/or multiple doses of β-lactams or vancomycin. Even a single dose of antibiotic is capable of causing significant dysbiosis that can persist for months and cause increased susceptibility to infection and autoimmune disease.[39–41]

These real and perceived limitations to culture-based approaches have fueled interest in developing rapid, accurate biomarkers for neonatal sepsis. Jörn-Hendrik Weitkamp[42] has described the ideal neonatal sepsis biomarker as needing near-perfect sensitivity and a rapid turnaround time. This combination would allow clinicians to delay the initiation of antibiotics for infants with a negative biomarker test. However, at present there is no test for neonatal sepsis that meets the criteria of an ideal biomarker.

CURRENT BIOMARKERS

The most frequently used laboratory parameters as neonatal sepsis biomarkers include complete blood counts (CBCs) with differential, C-reactive protein (CRP), and procalcitonin. However, numerous other assays have been investigated and are discussed briefly later. In general, the laboratory tests currently in use as sepsis biomarkers for neonates and young infants share common characteristics. Most have reasonably good sensitivity and therefore reasonable negative predictive value (NPV). However, specificity and positive predictive value (PPV) are generally poor. These characteristics mean that normal results can be reassuring, but abnormal results are less meaningful because many inflammatory conditions can affect these values in the absence of neonatal sepsis, including maternal preeclampsia, chorioamnionitis, hypoxic-ischemic injury, and in utero growth restriction.[43–47] The negative sequelae of relying on biomarkers with poor PPV to direct therapy may mean that uninfected neonates with sterile cultures are subject to prolonged antibiotic exposure, for culture-negative sepsis.[48,49] In addition, the excellent NPV must be interpreted within the context of the relative rarity of EOS and LOS, and therefore a low pretest probability. Schulman and colleagues[18] showed an incidence of 1.1% for EOS and ~5% for LOS in infants evaluated for sepsis. Using these low pretest probabilities, even a coin flip has excellent NPV (exceeding 95%).[50] The authors are reminded of the classic *Simpsons* episode[51] in which Lisa Simpson teaches her father about such specious reasoning. Lisa picks up a rock and facetiously claims that it keeps tigers away. Homer asks how, and a frustrated Lisa explains that it does not actually work, being just a rock, but there are no tigers in the neighborhood! Homer considers this for a moment, and then tries to buy the rock from his exasperated daughter.

In order to safely delay the initiation of antibiotic therapy from an infant with suspected sepsis, clinicians need a fast, accurate test with a negligible number of false-negatives, not a meaningful number of false-negatives buried in an avalanche of true-negatives. However, many current biomarkers perform well because of the low pretest probability of sepsis and are, in fact, little better than Lisa Simpson's rock.

COMPLETE BLOOD COUNT

White blood cells and their differential count is the oldest biomarker for neonatal sepsis, predating the widespread use of automated blood culture systems. The original description of vacuolization of the neutrophil as a specific finding in neonatal sepsis was published in 1966.[52] The use of the CBC as an adjunctive test for neonatal sepsis has become fairly widespread; a national survey published in 2017 found that 95% of nurseries use a CBC as part of their sepsis evaluations.[53] The exact use of CBCs varies widely; approaches include obtaining CBC at a single time point or serially, evaluating the total white blood cell count, neutrophil count, immature-to-total ratio, temporal trends, and evaluation of red blood cell and platelet size and morphology in addition to leukocytes.[54–56] Receiver-operator curves can be generated for these different values. Specific findings of sepsis (>75%) include low absolute leukocyte counts, severe neutropenia, and increased immature-to-total ratio ($\geq$25%). However, specificity comes at the cost of poor sensitivity for EOS and LOS, where the CBC has less than 50% sensitivity.[57] In a large retrospective cohort using the Pediatrix administrative database, the highest area under the curve (AUC) Hornik and colleagues[58] could generate using different combinations of CBC values was 0.686, and most infants with EOS had normal CBCs. The investigators concluded that the poor sensitivity of CBCs makes them poor diagnostic markers, and that the practice of obtaining a CBC as part of a sepsis evaluation is not supported.[58]

C-REACTIVE PROTEIN

CRP, an acute phase reactant made in the liver in response to inflammatory cytokines, has attracted widespread and prolonged interest as a neonatal sepsis biomarker. Studies evaluating the CRP for the diagnosis of EOS have consistently reported sensitivities of 50% to 70% with unacceptably high false-positives.[59,60] CRP levels increase naturally over the first 1 to 2 days of life to levels that approach abnormal.[61] A meta-analysis by Brown and colleagues[62] of 22 studies evaluating the accuracy of CRP to detect LOS showed that, at median specificity (74%), the sensitivity of CRP was 62%. Together, these data show that CRP is not a useful tool in the diagnosis of neonatal sepsis.

PROCALCITONIN

Current evidence does not support the use of procalcitonin rather than CRP, because both have significant limitations of sensitivity and specificity. Retrospective studies suggest a range of sensitivity and specificity for procalcitonin that is on par with or slightly superior to CBC and CRP, in the 65% to 85% range.[60,63–67] Meta-analysis of 39 studies comparing procalcitonin with CRP for EOS and LOS found a slightly superior sensitivity (77% vs 66%) and no difference in specificity (~80%–82%) for procalcitonin compared with CRP. In the neonatal procalcitonin intervention study (NeoPInS), which investigated antibiotic use, Stocker and colleagues[68] showed an AUC of 0.921 for procalcitonin at age 36 hours, which was slightly inferior to the AUC of CRP in the same study. Meta-analyses of 17 studies and 1086 neonates showed that, at the median sensitivity of 85%, the specificity of procalcitonin was 54%.[69] Despite initial excitement, the data do not support the use of procalcitonin as an ideal sepsis biomarker.

OTHERS

Numerous other serum biomarkers have been considered for the identification of neonatal sepsis.[70] These include, but are not limited to, interleukin-6,[71] presepsin,[72] cluster of differentiation (CD) 64,[73] CD11b,[74] serum amyloid A,[75] S100 protein A12,[76] lipopolysaccharide binding protein,[77] volatile organic compounds,[78] and soluble triggering receptor expressed on myeloid cell-1.[79] In addition, microbiome monitoring[80] and the application of mass spectroscopy to serum samples during sepsis evaluations[81] are novel approaches for biomarkers. Noninvasive biomarkers, such as heart rate characteristic (HRC) monitoring in preterm infants, have also been studied. In a randomized controlled trial of HRC monitoring for very-low-birthweight infants, Moorman and colleagues[82] saw a reduction in mortality following sepsis for infants receiving HRC monitoring compared with controls (10% vs 16.1%, absolute risk reduction of 6.1%, $P = .01$). A larger follow-up study showed a similar reduction in mortality among extremely low birthweight infants (<1000 g) receiving HRC monitoring.[83] This effect, presumably, is caused by HRC alerting clinicians about impending deterioration and improving time to sepsis evaluation and initiation of effective antimicrobial therapy.

Biosensing, in which a detector is used to directly sense the presence of 1 or more circulating biomolecules, is an exciting emerging field in sepsis diagnostics.[84] A variety of techniques, including electrochemical, optical, bioluminescent, and thermal, can be used to amplify and identify different circulating factors. Previous work has used biosensors to measure the biomarkers discussed earlier, such as CRP and interleukin-6.[85] However, more recent studies have turned toward direct identification of bacterial components such as lipopolysaccharide or bacterial ribosomal RNA.[86] Optical biosensors can measure a variety of physiologic changes via transcutaneous capture, including creatinine, bilirubin, or nitric oxide concentration.[87] If these technologies can be combined and optimized, it is possible that a wrist probe might be able to accurately detect an increased concentration in biomolecules caused by sepsis before clinical signs develop.

OPTIMAL CURRENT PRACTICE

In the absence of a fast, accurate sepsis biomarker with excellent sensitivity, how should clinicians approach infants with suspected sepsis? As endorsed by the American Academy of Pediatrics, the most effective current strategy for neonatal sepsis is the use of objective clinical risk factors to determine the pretest probability of sepsis, in combination with serial observation for equivocal or low-risk infants.[23] Several studies investigating the impact of observation-based instead of laboratory-based approaches have shown similar safety outcomes with reduced need for sepsis evaluations and antibiotic exposure. Cantoni and colleagues[88] performed a 2-year study in northeastern Italy that included 15,239 infants. In the first year, infants with 1 or more risk factors for EOS were evaluated with blood culture and CBC with differential. In the second year, infants were evaluated with serial physical examination alone and cultured only if clinical signs of illness developed. The investigators saw no difference in EOS incidence, time to antibiotic initiation, or mortality. However, they did see a 58% reduction in antibiotic use in the cohort evaluated during the second study year. A similar 4-year study from Norway evaluated a change in practice in which clinicians relied on serial physical examination and limited laboratory diagnostics and found a 60% reduction in antibiotic use with no change in EOS incidence.[89] The most common tool to help guide objective risk assessment in term and late-preterm infants is the Neonatal Sepsis Calculator,[90] which has been validated in numerous studies and has been shown to reduce sepsis evaluations and unnecessary antibiotic use.[91–93] In addition, instead of using 0.3 to 0.5 mL of blood on imperfect and generally unhelpful biomarkers, providers should add that blood to the culture bottle in order to optimize volume. This method improves the sensitivity of the gold standard test and minimizes confusing or inaccurate biomarker results.

FUTURE RESEARCH

Imagine for a moment a future in which the ideal biomarker has been identified. This mythological test, the SeptiCheck (Cantey Fantasy Industries, San Antonio, TX) is a rapid point-of-care test that requires 0.3 mL of blood and results in a qualitative yes/no result within 10 minutes. It has 99.3% sensitivity and 99% specificity for neonatal sepsis. Infants with suspected sepsis who have a negative SeptiCheck can be observed closely; infants whose SeptiCheck is positive, which occurs infrequently because sepsis is rare and the excellent specificity of the test minimizes false-positives, cultures are obtained and the infant is started on empiric antibiotic therapy pending cultures. Sepsis evaluations and unnecessary antibiotic exposure plummet, and morbidity and mortality from proven sepsis decrease with faster time to initiation of antibiotic therapy.

How do clinicians get there from here? First and foremost, clinicians and researchers must not be discouraged by the middling utility of current sepsis biomarkers, but instead should continue the search for biomarkers that are informative. Translational studies that enroll neonates before they develop clinical illness will be needed to identify biomarkers with early, predictive kinetics: a test that becomes abnormal before clinical illness, peaks concomitantly with sepsis, and decreases with disease resolution. Novel approaches such as microbiome monitoring, mass spectroscopy, and others should be applied to well and sick neonates to generate novel biomarker targets for formal hypothesis testing. In addition, continued partnerships with engineers will be critical. The ideal biomarker, if it exists, cannot be found without collaboration with biomedical, electrical, chemical, and computer science engineers. The ultimate goal for clinicians is not to shorten antibiotic duration for infants with suspected sepsis but to have a rapid, sensitive test that supports initiation of antibiotics only when needed. Until that day comes, clinicians should reconsider how laboratory parameters can be optimally used in combination with the prenatal history and physical examination applying diagnostic and antimicrobial stewardship

CLINICS CARE POINTS

- Early diagnosis of neonatal sepsis improves time to effective therapy, but current biomarkers are insufficiently sensitive or specific to be clinically useful.

- There is currently no consensus definition of neonatal sepsis, and extrapolation of sepsis criteria from older children or adults is highly inaccurate.

- The most evidence-based clinical role for current biomarkers (complete blood count, C-reactive protein, or procalcitonin) is to help providers discontinue empiric antibiotics at 24-48 hours when cultures are sterile.

- Abnormal biomarkers are not an indication to continue antibiotic therapy in a well-appearing infant whose cultures are sterile.

- Management guided by serial examination and objective risk factors is non-inferior to biomarker-based management and can reduce unnecessary blood draws and antibiotic exposure.

Best practices

What is the current practice for diagnosing neonatal sepsis?

- Neonatal sepsis is frequently suspected when infants have clinical signs consistent with sepsis, or for well-appearing infants with risk factors for sepsis.
- Bacterial cultures of blood (and urine, cerebrospinal fluid, or other sterile sites for late-onset sepsis) are the reference standard for neonatal sepsis.
- Serum biomarkers (e.g., complete blood count with differential, C-reactive protein, procalcitonin) are frequently obtained to help make the diagnosis of neonatal sepsis.
- Current biomarkers are insufficiently sensitive or specific to be consistently useful in the diagnosis of neonatal sepsis.
- The ideal biomarker would have near-perfect sensitivity, rapid turnaround time, and the ability to identify sepsis before clinical signs develop.
- Continued collaboration between clinicians, informaticists, and biomedical engineers is essential to develop novel biomarkers that meet these criteria.

What changes in current practice are likely to improve outcomes?

- Providing education for clinicians regarding the limitations of current sepsis biomarkers
- Re-emphasizing the importance of culture- or molecular-based technologies in the diagnosis of neonatal sepsis

Major recommendations

- The systematic use of current sepsis biomarkers should be discouraged; instead, that blood volume should be added to the blood culture to optimize sensitivity of the reference standard.
- Nurseries should have process improvement methods in place to ensure that adequate ($\geq$1 mL) blood volume is inoculated into culture media.
- Perform collaborative, exploratory studies that incorporate novel approaches such as mass spectrometry and other biomedical engineering approaches, aimed at identifying novel biomarkers that can be adapted for clinical use.

Rating for strength of the evidence: Quality of evidence moderate, strength of recommendation moderate.

DISCLOSURE

The authors have nothing to disclose.

REFERENCES

1. Shane AL, Sanchez PJ, Stoll BJ. Neonatal sepsis. Lancet 2017;390:1770–80.

2. Weinberger J, Rhee C, Klompas M. A critical analysis of the literature on time-to-antibiotics in suspected sepsis. J Infect Dis 2020;222:S110–8.

3. Weiss SL, Peters MJ, Alhazzani W, et al. Surviving sepsis campaign international guidelines for the management of septic Shock and sepsis-associated organ dysfunction in children. Pediatr Crit Care Med 2020;21:e52–106.

4. Simonsen KA, Anderson-Berry AL, Delair SF, et al. Early-onset neonatal sepsis. Clin Microbiol Rev 2014;27:21–47.

5. Stoll BJ, Puopolo KM, Hansen NI, et al. Early-onset neonatal sepsis 2015 to 2017, the rise of Escherichia coli, and the need for novel prevention strategies. JAMA Pediatr 2020;174:e200593.

6. Greenberg RG, Kandefer S, Do BT, et al. Late-onset sepsis in extremely premature infants: 2000-2011. Pediatr Infect Dis J 2017;36:774–9.

7. Aronson PL, Shabanova V, Shapiro ED, et al. A prediction model to identify Febrile infants </=60 Days at low risk of invasive bacterial infection. Pediatrics 2019;144.

8. Aronson PL, Wang ME, Shapiro ED, et al. Risk stratification of Febrile infants ≤60 Days old without routine lumbar puncture. Pediatrics 2018;142:e20183604.

9. Singer M, Deutschman CS, Seymour CW, et al. The Third international consensus definitions for sepsis and septic Shock (Sepsis-3). JAMA 2016;315:801–10.

10. Coggins S, Harris MC, Grundmeier R, et al. Performance of pediatric systemic inflammatory response syndrome and organ dysfunction criteria in late-onset sepsis in a quaternary neonatal intensive care unit: a case-control study. J Pediatr 2020;219:133–9.e131.

11. Kurul S, Simons SHP, Ramakers CRB, et al. Association of inflammatory biomarkers with subsequent clinical course in suspected late onset sepsis in preterm neonates. Crit Care 2021;25:12.

12. Wynn JL, Polin RA. A neonatal sequential organ failure assessment score predicts mortality to late-onset sepsis in preterm very low birth weight infants. Pediatr Res 2020;88:85–90.

13. Wynn JL, Wong HR, Shanley TP, et al. Time for a neonatal-specific consensus definition for sepsis. Pediatr Crit Care Med 2014;15:523–8.

14. Dempsey EM, Barrington KJ. Diagnostic criteria and therapeutic interventions for the hypotensive very low birth weight infant. J Perinatol 2006;26:677–81.

15. Weintraub AS, Cadet CT, Perez R, et al. Antibiotic use in newborns with transient tachypnea of the newborn. Neonatology 2013;103:235–40.

16. Morrison JJ, Rennie JM, Milton PJ. Neonatal respiratory morbidity and mode of delivery at term: influence of timing of elective caesarean section. Br J Obstet Gynaecol 1995;102:101–6.

17. Leonidas JC, Hall RT, Beatty EC, et al. Radiographic findings in early onset neonatal group b streptococcal septicemia. Pediatrics 1977;59(Suppl):1006–11.

18. Schulman J, Benitz WE, Profit J, et al. Newborn antibiotic exposures and association with proven bloodstream infection. Pediatrics 2019;144:e20191105.

19. Cordero L, Ayers LW. Duration of empiric antibiotics for suspected early-onset sepsis in extremely low birth weight infants. Infect Control Hosp Epidemiol 2003;24:662–6.

20. Spitzer AR, Kirkby S, Kornhauser M. Practice variation in suspected neonatal sepsis: a costly problem in neonatal intensive care. J Perinatol 2005;25:265–9.

21. Cantey JB. The spartacus problem: diagnostic inefficiency of neonatal sepsis. Pediatrics 2019;144:e20192576.

22. Cantey JB, Patel SJ. Antimicrobial stewardship in the NICU. Infect Dis Clin North Am 2014;28:247–61.

23. Puopolo KM, Benitz WE, Zaoutis TE, et al. Management of neonates born at ≥35 0/7 Weeks' gestation with suspected or proven early-onset bacterial sepsis. Pediatrics 2018;142:e20182894.

24. Puopolo KM, Benitz WE, Zaoutis TE, et al. Management of neonates born at ≤34 6/7 Weeks' gestation with suspected or proven early-onset bacterial sepsis. Pediatrics 2018;142:e20182896.

25. Schelonka RL, Chai MK, Yoder BA, et al. Volume of blood required to detect common neonatal pathogens. J Pediatr 1996;129:275–8.

26. De SK, Shetty N, Kelsey M. How to use... blood cultures. Arch Dis Child Educ Pract Ed 2014;99:144–51.

27. Connell TG, Rele M, Cowley D, et al. How reliable is a negative blood culture result? Volume of blood submitted for culture in routine practice in a children's hospital. Pediatrics 2007;119:891–6.

28. Klingenberg C, Kornelisse RF, Buonocore G, et al. Culture-negative early-onset neonatal sepsis - at the crossroad between efficient sepsis care and antimicrobial stewardship. Front Pediatr 2018;6:285.

29. Greenberg RG, Chowdhury D, Hansen NI, et al. Prolonged duration of early antibiotic therapy in extremely premature infants. Pediatr Res 2019;85:994–1000.

30. Cantey JB, Sanchez PJ. Prolonged antibiotic therapy for "culture-negative" sepsis in preterm infants: it's time to stop! J Pediatr 2011;159:707–8.

31. Cantey JB, Baird SD. Ending the culture of culture-negative sepsis in the neonatal ICU. Pediatrics 2017;140:e20170044.

32. Kirn TJ, Weinstein MP. Update on blood cultures: how to obtain, process, report, and interpret. Clin Microbiol Infect 2013;19:513–20.

33. Bourbeau PP, Foltzer M. Routine incubation of BacT/ALERT FA and FN blood culture bottles for more than 3 days may not be necessary. J Clin Microbiol 2005;43:2506–9.

34. Kumar Y, Qunibi M, Neal TJ, et al. Time to positivity of neonatal blood cultures. Arch Dis Child Fetal Neonatal Ed 2001;85:F182–6.

35. Lefebvre CE, Renaud C, Chartrand C. Time to positivity of blood cultures in infants 0 to 90 Days old presenting to the emergency department: is 36 hours enough? J Pediatr Infect Dis Soc 2017;6:28–32.

36. Theodosiou AA, Mashumba F, Flatt A. Excluding clinically significant bacteremia by 24 hours in otherwise well Febrile children younger than 16 years: a study of more than 50,000 blood cultures. Pediatr Infect Dis J 2019;38:e203–8.

37. Kuzniewicz MW, Mukhopadhyay S, Li S, et al. Time to positivity of neonatal blood cultures for early-onset sepsis. Pediatr Infect Dis J 2020;39:634–40.

38. Marks L, de Waal K, Ferguson JK. Time to positive blood culture in early onset neonatal sepsis: a retrospective clinical study and review of the literature. J Paediatr Child Health 2020;56:1371–5.

39. Niu X, Daniel S, Kumar D, et al. Transient neonatal antibiotic exposure increases susceptibility to late-onset sepsis driven by microbiota-dependent suppression of type 3 innate lymphoid cells. Sci Rep 2020;10:12974.

40. Singer JR, Blosser EG, Zindl CL, et al. Preventing dysbiosis of the neonatal mouse intestinal microbiome protects against late-onset sepsis. Nat Med 2019;25:1772–82.

41. Ng KM, Aranda-Diaz A, Tropini C, et al. Recovery of the gut microbiota after antibiotics depends on host diet, community context, and environmental reservoirs. Cell Host Microbe 2020;28:628.

42. Weitkamp JH. The role of biomarkers in suspected neonatal sepsis. Clin Infect Dis 2020.

43. Marins LR, Anizelli LB, Romanowski MD, et al. How does preeclampsia affect neonates? Highlights in the disease's immunity. J Matern Fetal Neonatal Med 2019;32:1205–12.

44. Amarilyo G, Oren A, Mimouni FB, et al. Increased cord serum inflammatory markers in small-for-gestational-age neonates. J Perinatol 2011;31:30–2.
45. Zanardo V, Peruzzetto C, Trevisanuto D, et al. Relationship between the neonatal white blood cell count and histologic chorioamnionitis in preterm newborns. J Matern Fetal Neonatal Med 2012;25:2769–72.
46. Rath S, Narasimhan R, Lumsden C. C-reactive protein (CRP) responses in neonates with hypoxic ischaemic encephalopathy. Arch Dis Child Fetal Neonatal Ed 2014;99:F172.
47. Howman RA, Charles AK, Jacques A, et al. Inflammatory and haematological markers in the maternal, umbilical cord and infant circulation in histological chorioamnionitis. PLoS One 2012;7:e51836.
48. Gyllensvard J, Ingemansson F, Hentz E, et al. C-reactive protein- and clinical symptoms-guided strategy in term neonates with early-onset sepsis reduced antibiotic use and hospital stay: a quality improvement initiative. BMC Pediatr 2020;20:531.
49. Cantey JB, Wozniak PS, Sanchez PJ. Prospective surveillance of antibiotic use in the neonatal intensive care unit: results from the SCOUT study. Pediatr Infect Dis J 2015;34:267–72.
50. Cantey JB, Bultmann CR. C-reactive protein testing in late-onset neonatal sepsis: hazardous Waste. JAMA Pediatr 2020;174:235–6.
51. Much apu about nothing. in Dietter S: the Simpsons. 1996.
52. Zieve PD, Haghshenass M, Blanks M, et al. Vacuolization of the neutrophil. An aid in the diagnosis of septicemia. Arch Intern Med 1966;118:356–7.
53. Mukhopadhyay S, Taylor JA, Von Kohorn I, et al. Variation in sepsis evaluation across a national network of nurseries. Pediatrics 2017;139:e20162845.
54. Mikhael M, Brown LS, Rosenfeld CR. Serial neutrophil values facilitate predicting the absence of neonatal early-onset sepsis. J Pediatr 2014;164:522–8, e521-523.
55. Weinberg AG, Rosenfeld CR, Manroe BL, et al. Neonatal blood cell count in health and disease. II. Values for lymphocytes, monocytes, and eosinophils. J Pediatr 1985;106:462–6.
56. Cornbleet PJ. Clinical utility of the band count. Clin Lab Med 2002;22:101–36.
57. Newman TB, Puopolo KM, Wi S, et al. Interpreting complete blood counts soon after birth in newborns at risk for sepsis. Pediatrics 2010;126:903–9.
58. Hornik CP, Benjamin DK, Becker KC, et al. Use of the complete blood cell count in early-onset neonatal sepsis. Pediatr Infect Dis J 2012;31:799–802.
59. Yochpaz S, Friedman N, Zirkin S, et al. C-reactive protein in early-onset neonatal sepsis - a cutoff point for CRP value as a predictor of early-onset neonatal sepsis in term and late preterm infants early after birth? J Matern Fetal Neonatal Med 2020;1–6.
60. Eschborn S, Weitkamp JH. Procalcitonin versus C-reactive protein: review of kinetics and performance for diagnosis of neonatal sepsis. J Perinatol 2019;39: 893–903.
61. Macallister K, Smith-Collins A, Gillet H, et al. Serial C-reactive protein measurements in newborn infants without evidence of early-onset infection. Neonatology 2019;116:85–91.
62. Brown JVE, Meader N, Wright K, et al. Assessment of C-reactive protein diagnostic test accuracy for late-onset infection in newborn infants: a systematic review and meta-analysis. JAMA Pediatr 2020;174:260–8.
63. Liu C, Fang C, Xie L. Diagnostic utility of procalcitonin as a biomarker for late-onset neonatal sepsis. Transl Pediatr 2020;9:237–42.

64. Frerot A, Baud O, Colella M, et al. Cord blood procalcitonin level and early-onset sepsis in extremely preterm infants. Eur J Clin Microbiol Infect Dis 2019;38: 1651–7.

65. Mohsen AH, Kamel BA. Predictive values for procalcitonin in the diagnosis of neonatal sepsis. Electron Physician 2015;7:1190–5.

66. Morad EA, Rabie RA, Almalky MA, et al. Evaluation of procalcitonin, C-reactive protein, and interleukin-6 as early markers for diagnosis of neonatal sepsis. Int J Microbiol 2020;2020:8889086.

67. Stocker M, van Herk W, El Helou S, et al. C-reactive protein, procalcitonin, and white blood count to rule out neonatal early-onset sepsis within 36 hours: a secondary analysis of the neonatal procalcitonin intervention study. Clin Infect Dis 2020.

68. Stocker M, van Herk W, El Helou S, et al. Procalcitonin-guided decision making for duration of antibiotic therapy in neonates with suspected early-onset sepsis: a multicentre, randomised controlled trial (NeoPIns). Lancet 2017;390:871–81.

69. Pontrelli G, De Crescenzo F, Buzzetti R, et al. Accuracy of serum procalcitonin for the diagnosis of sepsis in neonates and children with systemic inflammatory syndrome: a meta-analysis. BMC Infect Dis 2017;17:302.

70. Hincu MA, Zonda GI, Stanciu GD, et al. Relevance of biomarkers currently in use or research for practical diagnosis approach of neonatal early-onset sepsis. Children (Basel) 2020;7:309.

71. Chiesa C, Pacifico L, Natale F, et al. Fetal and early neonatal interleukin-6 response. Cytokine 2015;76:1–12.

72. Parri N, Trippella G, Lisi C, et al. Accuracy of presepsin in neonatal sepsis: systematic review and meta-analysis. Expert Rev Anti Infect Ther 2019;17:223–32.

73. Dai J, Jiang W, Min Z, et al. Neutrophil CD64 as a diagnostic marker for neonatal sepsis: meta-analysis. Adv Clin Exp Med 2017;26:327–32.

74. Qiu X, Li J, Yang X, et al. Is neutrophil CD11b a special marker for the early diagnosis of sepsis in neonates? A systematic review and meta-analysis. BMJ Open 2019;9:e025222.

75. Bourika V, Hantzi E, Michos A, et al. Clinical value of serum amyloid-A protein, high-density lipoprotein cholesterol and apolipoprotein-A1 in the diagnosis and follow-up of neonatal sepsis. Pediatr Infect Dis J 2020;39:749–55.

76. Tosson AMS, Glaser K, Weinhage T, et al. Evaluation of the S100 protein A12 as a biomarker of neonatal sepsis. J Matern Fetal Neonatal Med 2020;33:2768–74.

77. Mussap M, Noto A, Fravega M, et al. Soluble CD14 subtype presepsin (sCD14-ST) and lipopolysaccharide binding protein (LBP) in neonatal sepsis: new clinical and analytical perspectives for two old biomarkers. J Matern Fetal Neonatal Med 2011;24(Suppl 2):12–4.

78. Berkhout DJC, Niemarkt HJ, Andriessen P, et al. Preclinical detection of non-catheter related late-onset sepsis in preterm infants by Fecal volatile compounds analysis: a prospective, multi-center cohort study. Pediatr Infect Dis J 2020;39: 330–5.

79. Bellos I, Fitrou G, Daskalakis G, et al. Soluble TREM-1 as a predictive factor of neonatal sepsis: a meta-analysis. Inflamm Res 2018;67:571–8.

80. Agudelo-Ochoa GM, Valdes-Duque BE, Giraldo-Giraldo NA, et al. Gut microbiota profiles in critically ill patients, potential biomarkers and risk variables for sepsis. Gut Microbes 2020;12:1707610.

81. Chatziioannou AC, Wolters JC, Sarafidis K, et al. Targeted LC-MS/MS for the evaluation of proteomics biomarkers in the blood of neonates with necrotizing enterocolitis and late-onset sepsis. Anal Bioanal Chem 2018;410:7163–75.

82. Moorman JR, Carlo WA, Kattwinkel J, et al. Mortality reduction by heart rate characteristic monitoring in very low birth weight neonates: a randomized trial. J Pediatr 2011;159:900–906 e901.
83. Schelonka RL, Carlo WA, Bauer CR, et al. Mortality and neurodevelopmental outcomes in the heart rate characteristics monitoring randomized controlled trial. J Pediatr 2020;219:48–53.
84. Balayan S, Chauhan N, Chandra R, et al. Recent advances in developing biosensing based platforms for neonatal sepsis. Biosens Bioelectron 2020;169: 112552.
85. Sun LP, Huang Y, Huang T, et al. Optical microfiber reader for enzyme-linked immunosorbent assay. Anal Chem 2019;91:14141–8.
86. Kurundu Hewage EMK, Spear D, Umstead TM, et al. An electrochemical biosensor for rapid detection of pediatric bloodstream infections. SLAS Technol 2017;22:616–25.
87. Doulou S, Leventogiannis K, Tsilika M, et al. A novel optical biosensor for the early diagnosis of sepsis and severe Covid-19: the PROUD study. BMC Infect Dis 2020;20:860.
88. Cantoni L, Ronfani L, Da Riol R, et al. Physical examination instead of laboratory tests for most infants born to mothers colonized with group B Streptococcus: support for the Centers for Disease Control and Prevention's 2010 recommendations. J Pediatr 2013;163:568–73.
89. Vatne A, Klingenberg C, Oymar K, et al. Reduced antibiotic exposure by serial physical examinations in term neonates at risk of early-onset sepsis. Pediatr Infect Dis J 2020;39:438–43.
90. Permanente K. Neonatal early-onset sepsis calculator. Kaiser Permanente Division of Research; 2021.
91. Kuzniewicz MW, Puopolo KM, Fischer A, et al. A quantitative, risk-based approach to the management of neonatal early-onset sepsis. JAMA Pediatr 2017;171:365–71.
92. Benitz WE, Achten NB. Technical assessment of the neonatal early-onset sepsis risk calculator. Lancet Infect Dis 2020.
93. Deshmukh M, Mehta S, Patole S. Sepsis calculator for neonatal early onset sepsis - a systematic review and meta-analysis. J Matern Fetal Neonatal Med 2019; 34(11):1832–40.

Necrotizing Enterocolitis

Jennifer Duchon, MDCM, MPH[a], Maria E. Barbian, MD[b],
Patricia W. Denning, MD[c],*

KEYWORDS

- Necrotizing enterocolitis • NEC • Prematurity • Probiotics • Intestinal immaturity
- Intestinal inflammation • Antibiotic use in newborns

KEY POINTS

- Necrotizing enterocolitis (NEC) is an inflammatory disease of the gut primarily affecting premature infants.
- Age at diagnosis is inversely proportional to gestational age at birth, reflecting the accrual of risk factors such as dysbiosis and the developmental immune state of the intestine.
- Measures focused on preventing the development of dysbiosis, including administration of probiotics, protocolized feedings focused on mother's own milk, avoiding acid blockers, and judicious use of antimicrobials, remain the primary tools to prevent NEC.
- More sophisticated risk assessment techniques (genomics) and diagnostic techniques (stool microbiome analyses or serum/urine metabolomic analyses) may help differentiate infants with or at risk for impending NEC.

INTRODUCTION

Necrotizing enterocolitis (NEC) is a devastating intestinal disorder characterized by intestinal inflammation and necrosis.[1] This disease is one of the most common gastrointestinal emergencies in newborn infants and primarily affects premature infants who have survived the early neonatal period.[1] NEC was first described more than a century ago. In the 1940s to 1950s, a series of cases of necrotizing enterocolitis were published.[2,3] Since then, many clinicians and scientists have devoted their research to understanding the pathogenesis of NEC, developing therapies and interventions to prevent this disease, and to advancing management strategies.

[a] Division of Newborn Medicine, Jack and Lucy Department of Pediatrics, Icahn School of Medicine at Mount Sinai, 1000 10th Avenue, New York, NY 10019, USA; [b] Division of Neonatal-Perinatal Medicine, Emory University School of Medicine and Children's Healthcare of Atlanta, 2015 Uppergate Drive Northeast, 3rd Floor, Atlanta, GA 30322, USA; [c] Division of Neonatal-Perinatal Medicine, Emory University School of Medicine, Children's Healthcare of Atlanta, Emory University Hospital Midtown, 550 Peachtree Street, 3rd Floor MOT, Atlanta, GA 30308, USA
* Corresponding author.
E-mail address: pllin@emory.edu

Clin Perinatol 48 (2021) 229–250
https://doi.org/10.1016/j.clp.2021.03.002
0095-5108/21/© 2021 Elsevier Inc. All rights reserved.
perinatology.theclinics.com

Necrotizing Enterocolitis: a Final Common Pathway of Multiple Disorders?

A key challenge in delineating risk factors for NEC is that the clinical presentation of an inflammatory bowel disease of the newborn may represent a final common pathway of multiple differing causes.[4,5] At present, clinical diagnosis of NEC relies on nonspecific indicators of intestinal inflammation, such as feeding intolerance, abdominal distention, bloody stools, serum markers of infection/inflammation, and radiographic findings that may not be as specific as originally thought. As more becomes known about clinical NEC, it is becoming increasingly recognized that NEC in full term infants,[4] has a different disease trigger than preterm infants; and preterm infants who develop devastating NEC totalis (NEC involving necrosis of >80% the intestine) have different causal pathways to disease than those infants with indolent NEC.[5–8] For this reason, definitive risk factor assessments may be confounded by the fact that clinical NEC may represent multiple disease entities.

How to delineate or define these multiple disease entities is a challenge to investigators, leading to difficulty in the ability to truly capture a numerator across centers. Kim and colleagues[5] elegantly describe these challenges in terms of aligning the need of researchers to define NEC in order to strengthen their understanding of risk factors and pathogenesis with the need of clinicians to appropriately treat the patient in front of them.

Through decades of research, understanding of the complex factors involved in the development of NEC has improved. However, despite these advances, the pathophysiology of NEC is still not fully understood. Part of this challenge may be the heterogeneous nature of this clinical entity. For the purposes of simplification, this article focuses on preterm NEC but acknowledges that this may still represent a clinical diagnosis with multiple causes.

Necrotizing Enterocolitis: a Developmental Disease

One consistent feature of NEC is the strong inverse relationship between gestational age at birth and time of disease onset. NEC in full-term infants typically develops within the first few days of life, whereas NEC in preterm infants of less than 29 weeks' gestational age has symptom onset at several weeks of life, typically at 30 to 32 weeks postmenstrual age.[9] A recent white paper from the International Neonatal Consortium (INC) suggests considering an alternative diagnosis in preterm infants who develop pneumoperitoneum at less than 10 days of life.[10,11] This recommendation is meant to help standardize inclusion into research studies, including clinical trials and risk factor analyses.

EPIDEMIOLOGY

NEC occurs in approximately 5% of infants admitted to neonatal intensive care units (NICUs), with an incidence of 9% of infants born at 22 to 29 weeks' gestational age.[6] There is a wide range of disease incidence between hospitals in North America, as well as internationally, with individual institutions reporting up to a 20% incidence.[6,12] Prematurity is the primary risk factor for this disease, and preterm infants bear much of the disease burden, comprising 70% to 90% of total NEC cases. Term or near-term infants with underlying abnormalities of the intestinal tract or prenatal, perinatal, and/or postnatal compromise of intestinal blood flow such as those relating to maternal drug use, asphyxia, or structural congenital heart lesions are also at risk.[7] Neither the incidence nor the outcome of NEC have seen significant improvements over time, unlike other neonatal conditions, such as early-onset and late-onset neonatal sepsis, although some networks with strong quality-improvement initiatives report better outcomes.[13]

Gender does not influence NEC incidence. Male sex, although not an independent risk factor for NEC development, is linked to an increase in mortality. Both black race and Hispanic ethnicity are described as risk factors for both the development of and a higher mortality from NEC, although this may be cofounded by socioeconomic status and comorbid conditions of pregnancy.[14,15]

PATHOPHYSIOLOGY

NEC is a complicated disease, in part because its pathogenesis is multifactorial, with a likely unique combination of individual factors. At present, it is known that the main factors involved in the pathogenesis of NEC include prematurity, microbial dysbiosis (abnormal intestinal microbiota), feeding, and impaired intestinal oxygen delivery.[16] Of these, prematurity is the strongest risk factor. Premature infants are particularly vulnerable to developing NEC because they have immature host defenses,[17] including immature intestinal motility and digestion, immature intestinal barrier function, and immature intestinal immunity regulation[1,16] (**Fig. 1**). This article will focus on reviewing the role of immature intestinal immunity and microbial dysbiosis in the pathogenesis of NEC.

Immature Intestinal Immunity

The adaptive immune system normally plays an important role in regulating the innate immune system. However, at birth, all infants have immature adaptive immune systems.[17] During pregnancy, maternal transfer of immunoglobulin G (IgG) through the placenta and after birth, through human milk, helps to protect newborns until their own adaptive immune systems develop.[18] In infants who are born prematurely, the placental transfer of IgG is significantly diminished. If preterm infants do not receive human milk, the disparity in IgG levels is even greater,[19] increasing their risk for the development of inflammatory disorders such as NEC.

One of the key factors in the pathogenesis of NEC is an abnormally upregulated inflammatory response to environmental stimuli.[1,20,21] Inflammation is typically a closely regulated host response that recruits leukocytes to defend against potential

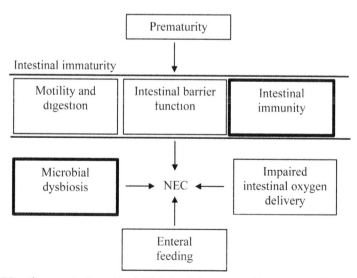

Fig. 1. NEC pathogenesis. *From* Lin, P. W. & Stoll, B. J. Necrotising enterocolitis. Lancet 368, 1271-1283 (2006). Reprinted with permission of Elsevier.

pathogens. Although regulated inflammation is necessary for long-term survival, an exaggerated inflammatory response can result in damage to surrounding tissue, propagating a proinflammatory response and causing further tissue damage.[1] Typically, tissue injury triggers an inflammatory response that results in the release of neutrophil-derived oxidants and proteases, damaging the intestinal barrier.[1] Once the intestinal barrier is compromised, opportunistic organisms can breach the epithelial barrier, resulting in more inflammation and worsening tissue damage.[1]

Tissue affected by NEC has features of mucosal edema, coagulation necrosis, and hemorrhage. These features are likely the result of an exaggerated inflammatory response that may be triggered by environmental stressors such as formula feeding and hypoxia. Following these environmental triggers, there is excessive inflammatory signaling in response to normal bacterial colonization[22] or, at times, pathogenic bacteria. Thus, an exaggerated inflammatory response triggers an inflammatory cascade that ultimately results in irreversible tissue damage.

The inflammatory mediators that are implicated in the pathogenesis of NEC include platelet activating factor (PAF), tumor necrosis factor alpha, and interleukins (IL-1, IL-6, IL-8, IL-10, IL-12, and IL-18).[1] In addition, NEC is associated with an increased expression of toll-like receptor 4 (TLR4), a receptor for lipopolysaccharide (LPS),[23,24] a bacterial endotoxin.[25] Further investigations of TLR4 have revealed its important role in host-microbe interactions and how these interactions lead to the development of NEC. Mice deficient in TLR4 were protected from developing NEC.[26] In addition, in both mice and humans that developed NEC, the expression of TLR4 was higher than in mice that did not have NEC.[25,27] Once TLR4 is activated, there is induction of apoptosis in enterocytes and reduction in mucosal repair and enterocyte proliferation.[28,29] These events lead to mucosal breakdown and bacterial translocation, resulting in a classic picture of sepsis seen with NEC.[30] Mouse NEC models have also revealed that upregulation of TLR4 occurs when the intestinal mucosa is exposed to environmental stressors such as LPS or hypoxia.[25] In addition, preterm infants have been found to have higher levels of TLR4 compared with term infants.[31] Thus, preterm infants have higher expression of TLR4 and, when faced with common environmental stressors, such as hypoxia, expression of TLR4 is upregulated. When TLR4 binds to LPS, activation of the transcription factor nuclear factor-kB (NF-κB) occurs, releasing proinflammatory cytokines[32] and triggering a massive inflammatory response.

Microbial Dysbiosis

The development of NEC has been associated with use of antibiotics[33–36] and acid suppressors,[37] all of which can alter an infant's gut microbiome. Certain bacterial species have been linked to presentations of NEC.[38] In addition, several case-control studies have shown that early microbial dysbiosis, with an abundance of Gammaproteobacteria, precedes NEC in many preterm infants.[39] Longitudinal stool colonization studies also note specific changes to infants' microbiomes before the development of NEC (including a bloom of Gammaproteobacteria).[40–44] Furthermore, in vitro studies support the idea that pathogenic stimuli, from bacteria in the Gammaproteobacteria family such as *Salmonella* spp and *Escherichia coli*, trigger exaggerated inflammatory responses in immature intestinal epithelial cells.[20,21,45] Thus, although bacteria are involved in the pathogenesis of NEC, there is no single organism associated with NEC. Rather, in many infants, there are shifts in their microbiomes that precede the onset of NEC.[39–44] These findings support the role of microbial dysbiosis as a major contributor to NEC.[46]

The intestinal microbiome plays a critical role in intestinal health through regulation of genes involved in barrier function, digestion, and angiogenesis,[47] and in education of the host immune system. Commensal bacteria can dampen inflammatory signaling[48] by inhibition of the NF-κB signaling, while also competing with pathogenic bacteria.[49–53] Given the important role of the microbiome in intestinal health and immune development, when microbial dysbiosis occurs, premature infants are at an increased risk of developing NEC. However, premature infants are especially susceptible to microbial dysbiosis because of their frequent exposure to antibiotics and organisms in the health care environment.[54] When microbial dysbiosis occurs, pathogenic bacteria may trigger an inflammatory response in the host through established host-bacterial interactions. First, a family of pattern recognition receptors transmits signals from microbial-associated molecular patterns to induce proinflammatory responses in host cells.[48,49,55–61] Thus, the combination of a proinflammatory state with microbial dysbiosis results in an overgrowth of pathogenic bacteria. A paucity of microbiome-mediated dampening of host inflammatory signaling places preterm infants at risk of developing NEC.

ADVANCES IN PREVENTIVE/THERAPEUTIC OPTIONS
Optimizing the Microbiome to Prevent Necrotizing Enterocolitis

In 2009, a sentinel multicenter retrospective cohort study conducted by participating sites in the National Institute of Child Health and Human Development (NICHD) network described prior and prolonged antimicrobial use in the initial days of neonatal life as a risk factor for preterm NEC.[33] Prolonged antimicrobial use creates dysbiosis, which in turn is a necessary component of preterm NEC. The link between intestinal dysbiosis, altered microbiota with an unfavorable colonization balance between commensal and pathogenic bacteria, and the development of NEC is now well supported. Microbiologic data from deep genomic sequencing techniques have shown differential stool composition in infants near the time of NEC onset, with a predominance of Gammaproteobacteria such as Enterobacter and E coli species and an overall decrease in bacterial diversity.[62] Longitudinal data collected from stool have also shown a relationship between days of antimicrobial usage and decreased bacterial diversity in infants who develop NEC.[39,40,62]

Subsequent clinical studies, primarily observational cohort studies, yield varying results when assessing the association between prior antimicrobial receipt and the risk for NEC in preterm infants.[36,63,64] One explanation is that, if antimicrobial therapy adversely affects colonization of the neonatal intestine by selecting for an unfavorable balance between commensal and pathogenic bacteria, the effect of exposure may take weeks to develop. It can be hypothesized that the biologically active ingredient, pathogenic bacteria, have yet to emerge as the dominant colonizing species or that the intestine is relatively sterile from recent antimicrobial use.

Although therapies for either the prevention or treatment of NEC are limited, researchers have identified interventions that decrease the risk of NEC by supporting the infant's microbiome through the use of feeding guidelines, human milk,[65] probiotics,[46] avoiding acid-blockade therapy,[66] and antimicrobial stewardship.

Standardized feeding protocols

A standardized feeding protocol provides preterm infants with a consistent approach to the initiation of feeds, duration of trophic feeds, advancement and fortification of feeds, criteria to stop or halt feeds, identification and handling of feeding intolerance, and preferred nutritional product.[67] In 2005, a meta-analysis of 6 observational studies evaluating the implementation of a standard feeding protocol for infants with a birthweight less than 2500 g reduced the incidence of NEC by 87%.[68] Additional studies of the implementation of feeding protocols consistently show an unchanged to a decreased rate of NEC,[69–74] fewer days of parenteral nutrition,[69,73] improved weight gain,[69,71,73] and in 1 study a reduction in late-onset sepsis.[71] Importantly, no study showed an increase in the rate of NEC or other adverse events[67] when a standardized feeding protocol was implemented. In 2017, a meta-analysis of 9 observational studies (N = 4755 infants) found a 67% reduction in the odds of NEC (odds ratio [OR], 0.33; 95% confidence interval [CI], 0.17–0.65) among infants weighing less than 1500 g when standardized feeding protocols were implemented.[67] The details of the feeding protocols seem to be less important than reducing variation in clinical management among clinicians.[68,75] Based on this evidence, implementation of a standardized feeding protocol, such as American Society for Parenteral and Enteral Nutrition[76] or the California Perinatal Quality Collaborative[71,77] guidelines, should be strongly considered because these may decrease the incidence of NEC, or decrease days of parenteral nutrition, without adverse effects.

Human milk

In 1990, a prospective multicenter study including 926 preterm infants evaluated the effect of human milk versus formula feeding on the development of NEC.[78] Among infants who were exclusively formula fed, NEC was 6-10 more common than among infants who exclusively received human milk and 3 times more common than among infants who received a combination of human milk and formula.[78] In 2012, the American Academy of Pediatrics endorsed human milk as the preferential nutritional source for preterm infants, because of noted reductions in the rates of sepsis, NEC, retinopathy of prematurity, and mortality with improved feeding tolerance, neurodevelopmental outcomes, and immune function.[79] In 2014, a meta-analysis evaluated 11 randomized or quasi–randomized controlled trials comparing the growth and development of preterm infants receiving formula versus donor human milk (DHM).[80] Of the 11 trials, only 4 used fortified DHM. Although the formula-fed infants had better growth, there were no differences in neurodevelopmental outcomes or postdischarge growth rates; however, formula feeding increased the risk of NEC with risk ratio 2.77 (95% CI, 1.4–5.46).[80]

Investigators have also evaluated the benefit of an exclusive human milk diet in preterm infants. Preterm infants require fortification of human milk or formula for optimal growth and development. Fortification can be accomplished by adding bovine-based fortifier or DHM-based fortifier to human milk. Some refer to a diet that includes mother's own milk or DHM and DHM-based fortifier as an exclusive human milk diet. Four studies have evaluated the difference in NEC (defined as Bell stage II or greater) between the 2 types of fortified diets.[81–84] A meta-analysis of the 4 studies with infants weighing less than 1250 g at birth (N = 1164) revealed that infants fed with DHM-based fortifier had approximately 64% lower odds of NEC compared with those fed with bovine-based fortifiers (OR, 0.36; 95% CI, 0.13–1.00).[67] In addition, the highest amount of protection from DHM-based fortifier was shown in NICUs with high rates of NEC.[67] Importantly, there have been no reports of adverse effects from an exclusive human milk diet, but growth should be monitored closely.[85] Thus, human milk has strong, established benefits to preterm infants, and the use of human milk is of upmost importance.

Human milk contains antimicrobial and antiinflammatory factors that protect newborn infants from infectious and inflammatory diseases.[86,87] Many components of human milk provide protection for and promote maturation of the newborn intestine[88] (**Table 1**). Human milk contains oligosaccharides, which are nondigestible and promote the growth of gut microbiome.[89–91] The caseins in human milk help to protect the intestinal barrier by stimulating mucin production through augmentation in the number of goblet cells and Paneth cells in the gut and through upregulation of the MUC2 gene.[92] The triglycerides in human milk have been shown to have antiviral, antibacterial, and antiprotozoal properties.[93–95] In addition, human milk contains bioactive proteins, such as lactoferrin and lysozyme.[17] Lactoferrin has antibacterial, antifungal, and antiviral activity,[96–98] whereas lysozyme has antibacterial properties.[99] Together, these 2 proteins can eliminate gram-negative bacteria.[100] In 2015, a meta-analysis reported that lactoferrin supplementation with or without probiotics may reduce the incidence of necrotizing enterocolitis and late-onset sepsis in preterm infants.[101] Human milk also contains PAF acetylhydrolase, which inactivates PAF, a key inflammatory mediator in the pathogenesis of NEC.[102,103]

Table 1
Beneficial components of human milk

Component	Mechanism	Role in NEC
Oligosaccharides	Promote growth of commensal bacteria	May reduce NEC risk by promoting healthy microbiome
Caseins	Increase number of Paneth cells and goblet cells	Promote protection of epithelial barrier
Triglycerides	Increase number of Paneth cells and goblet cells May reduce adherence of bacteria to intestinal epithelia	—
Lysozyme	Antibacterial activity	—
Lactoferrin	Antibacterial, antifungal, and antiviral activity Reduces bioavailability of iron to pathogens	Lactoferrin supplementation may reduce risk of NEC
PAF acetylhydrolase	Inactivates PAF	Inactivates important mediator of NEC
IL-10	Antiinflammatory properties	IL-10 supplementation protective in NEC animal models High levels of IL-10 in human milk associated with decreased risk of NEC
TGF-β	Regulates inflammation and wound healing	—
IGF	Promotes proliferation of intestinal epithelial cells Reduces apoptosis of intestinal epithelial cells	IGF supplementation reduces NEC in animal models
EGF	Promotes proliferation of intestinal epithelial cells Increases expression of tight junction proteins Increases mucin production Inhibits TLR4 Promotes antiinflammatory macrophages	Decreased expression of EGF associated with increased NEC risk EGF supplementation reduces NEC in animal models EGF supplementation promotes intestinal mucosa in humans

Abbreviations: EGF, epidermal growth factor; IGF, insulinlike growth factor; TGF, transforming growth factor.

Adapted from Denning, T. L., Bhatia, A. M., Kane, A. F., Patel, R. M. & Denning, P. W. Pathogenesis of NEC: Role of the innate and adaptive immune response. Semin Perinatol 41, 15-28.

Human milk also contains the cytokines transforming growth factor beta (TGF-β) and IL-10.[104,105] There are both mouse and human studies that stress the important role of IL-10, an antiinflammatory cytokine, in protecting premature infants from developing NEC.[17] In mice deficient in IL-10[106,107] and preterm human infants with genetic defects in IL-10 receptor,[108] there is an increased risk of developing colitis. In addition, animal models of NEC show that human milk increases levels of IL-10 and decreases NEC severity.[109] TGF-β regulates the inflammatory response,[110] promotes wound healing,[111,112] and stimulates production of IgA in the gut.[113]

Human milk contains growth factors such as epidermal growth factor (EGF) and insulinlike growth factor (IGF). IGF is thought to promote the proliferation of, and prevent apoptosis of, intestinal epithelial cells.[87] EGF promotes the healing, proliferation, and differentiation of intestinal epithelial cells.[114] EGF also promotes a healthy intestinal barrier by increasing the production of mucus by increasing the number of goblet cells and their production of MUC2, and by improving intestinal barrier function by increasing expression of tight junction proteins.[115,116] EGF also has antiinflammatory effects through promotion of antiinflammatory macrophages and reduction of proinflammatory macrophages.[117] EGF is present in amniotic fluid and colostrum. The human milk from women with preterm infants has 50% to 80% more EGF than milk from women who deliver infants at term gestation.[118] In addition, EGF is a powerful inhibitor of TLR4.[119] In animal models of NEC, EGF supplementation reduces the incidence of NEC.[120–125]

Avoiding acid-blockade therapy

Acid-blockade therapy is known to negatively alter the intestinal microbiome in preterm infants.[126] Not only does H2-blocker therapy reduce microbial diversity, it increases the relative abundance of bacterial species associated with NEC development (Proteobacteria). In preterm infants, inhibitors of gastric acid have been shown to increase the risk of NEC.[66,127,128] Interestingly, small early clinical studies have also shown a benefit of enteral hydrochloric acid (HCl) supplementation in NEC reduction.[37] Although HCl therapy is not currently recommended for the prevention of NEC in preterm infants, acid-blockade therapy should be avoided.

Probiotics

Probiotics are live microbes that, when administered, provide a health benefit. There have been many in vitro and in vivo studies that have shown the mechanisms through which probiotics and commensal bacteria protect the immature gut. Probiotics upregulate cytoprotective genes,[47] downregulate proinflammatory genes,[49,129–131] produce short-chain fatty acids,[132,133] support barrier function and maturation,[134,135] compete with other microbiomes,[136] and regulate innate and adaptive immune pathways.[25,26] In addition, probiotic bacterial DNA has been found to inhibit TLR4 signaling through activation of TLR9.[27,137]

The beneficial impact of probiotics on the incidence of NEC in premature infants has been shown in animal studies, implementation cohort studies, and more than 35 randomized controlled trials.[138] Although these evaluations have notable heterogeneity with respect to probiotic strain selection, dose, and age of initiation, including bacterial strains and doses of probiotic administered,[139,140] the meta-analysis of these studies shows a reduction of NEC when probiotics are administered to preterm infants (relative risk, 0.53; 95% CI, 0.42–0.66).[46] Although multiple randomized control trials support the use of probiotics to prevent NEC, many clinicians are apprehensive about administering probiotics to premature infants.[140] Concerns about the safety of probiotics, the lack of federal regulation in the production of probiotics, and paucity of data on long-term effects are some of the common concerns.[138] Thus, despite the evidence supporting the use of probiotic supplementation to decrease NEC risk, there is variability in clinical practice.

Prebiotics are potentially another supplement that can optimize the preterm intestinal microbiome. Prebiotics are nondigestible products that promote the growth of desirable commensal bacteria. Studies are limited but suggest that prebiotics can improve the stool microbiome composition of preterm infants, reduce incidence of late-onset sepsis, and decrease the time to reach full feeds. To date, prebiotic supplementation has not been shown to reduce NEC incidence in preterm infants.[91,141]

Antimicrobial stewardship

Preterm infants, particularly extremely low birth weight infants, often receive empiric antimicrobial treatment for the first few days of life.[33,142] A large retrospective cohort study evaluating the association between duration of initial antibiotic course and the development of NEC or death in extremely low birthweight infants with negative blood culture results reported that the odds of NEC or death increased with each day of empiric antimicrobials.[33] In 2011, a study including infants who were less than or equal to 32 weeks' gestational age and less than or equal to 1500 g birth at birth with negative blood culture results evaluated the association between prolonged initial antibiotic therapy and late-onset sepsis, death, or NEC.[35] Prolonged empiric antimicrobial administration was associated with an increased OR of late-onset sepsis (OR, 2.45; 95% CI, 1.28–4.67) and the combination of late-onset sepsis, NEC, or death (OR, 2.66; 95% CI, 1.12–6.3).[35] Alexander and colleagues[36] performed a retrospective, 2:1 control-case analysis to determine whether duration of antibiotic exposure is an independent risk factor for NEC. Among infants with negative cultures, exposure to more than 10 days of antibiotics led to a close to 3-fold increase in the risk of developing NEC.[36] Thus, all 3 of these studies found increased odds of NEC or death after 4 days of empiric antimicrobials when blood cultures were negative.[33,35,36] This association may be caused by the effect of antibiotics on the gut microbiome, resulting in diminished diversity, facilitating the growth of pathogenic bacteria, potentially triggering inflammatory responses in the gut. In addition, a study from 2006 suggested that the use of cefotaxime instead of gentamicin for the first 3 days after birth was associated with higher mortality risk.[143] Based on the evidence from these studies, it is prudent not only to restrict empiric antimicrobials to 48 hours of administration if blood cultures are negative and the infant is clinically stable but also to use narrow-spectrum agents if clinically feasible.

Treatment During Necrotizing Enterocolitis

Supportive therapy

Nearly all reviews of NEC point out the lack of therapy for the disease itself once the process of bowel necrosis has begun. Treatment consists of allowing the bowel the greatest chance of recovery, which generally consist of rest, supporting hemodynamics, and optimizing nutritional status.

Enteral feeds are discontinued and a suction tube is placed for gastric decompression to decrease the stress of substrate and swallowed air in the inflamed intestine. Infants who depend on noninvasive respiratory support may be intubated if there is concern for exacerbating bowel distention or if abdominal distention impedes lung function.

Medical therapy

Antimicrobial therapy is almost universally prescribed to manage NEC and is primarily geared toward preventing bacteremia and other complications, such as infectious peritonitis or intraabdominal abscess caused by translocation of organisms through a compromised intestinal barrier.[144] No evidence-based antimicrobial regimen exists, either for selection of antimicrobial or for duration of therapy.[145–147] Most regimens consist of broad-spectrum coverage for enteric gram-negative and anaerobic organisms (ie, ampicillin with an aminoglycoside ± clindamycin or metronidazole, or piperacillin/tazobactam ± an aminoglycoside). Use of vancomycin may be indicated if the infant is known to be colonized with methicillin-resistant *Staphylococcus aureus* (MRSA), or if the rates of hospital-associated MRSA are of concern. Regimens may also be targeted to cover organisms that were associated with a previous infection in the host or to cover organisms more commonly associated with infections in the NICU, hospital, or community. Although studies exist linking the addition of anaerobic therapy with later stricture formation,[145,148,149] a large multicenter cohort study noted that this association is most likely a consequence of survival bias.[149] Duration of therapy ranges from 7 to 14 days for medically managed NEC and may be longer for disease requiring surgical intervention. Because there are limited evidence-based recommendations for resumption of feeding or cessation of antimicrobials, short courses of both may be indicated when evidence of intestinal inflammation has remitted.[150]

Stem cell therapy has been considered as a treatment of NEC in preclinical studies. Exosomes, small extracellular vesicles of stem cells, are thought to mediate the paracrine pathways, including the inflammatory cascade, angiogenesis, fibrosis, and cell death and repair.[151–154] Amniotic fluid stem cells and human milk–derived exosomes may be especially advantageous as therapy for NEC.[152,155]

Surgical therapy

Weighing the risks and benefits of operating on a severely ill neonate is challenging, especially because demarcating unsalvageable bowel from bowel that could potentially recover is not always a clear-cut surgical decision. Pneumoperitoneum is an absolute indication for urgent surgical intervention, and relative indications for surgical exploration include refractory thrombocytopenia, acidosis, or shock, indicating necrotic bowel. Other radiographic findings, such as a fixed loop or portal venous air, are indicators for surgical intervention. The optimal time to operate is after the bowel has irrevocably necrosed but before perforation, which is difficult to predict.[4] Some clinicians think that earlier surgical intervention may alleviate the inflammatory state that is responsible for poor neurodevelopmental outcomes.[156] Surgical management options include primary peritoneal drain and/or exploratory laparotomy. Studies have failed to show consistent benefits of one approach rather than the other.[4,157] Poorer neurodevelopmental outcomes are noted in infants managed with drain compared with those managed with laparotomy, but this may reflect underlying clinical conditions that precluded laparotomy.[158] Regardless, extremely low birthweight infants who had surgically managed NEC fare worse with respect to both short-term and long-term outcomes than those who only required medical therapy.[159,160]

Treating the Sequelae of Necrotizing Enterocolitis

One challenging sequela of surgical NEC is short bowel syndrome (SBS), where anatomic and functional loss of intestine occurs because of extensive surgical resection, leading to a constellation of symptoms that includes malabsorption and prolonged need for total parental nutrition (TPN). Severe SBS is common after extensive ileal resections and loss of greater than 50% of small intestine length and is associated with impaired resorption of vitamin B_{12}, bile salts, fatty acids, and fluid.[161] With aggressive rehabilitation, most infants regain intestinal autonomy, including those living with 10% to 30% of predicted small bowel length.[162] Fish oil and lipid mixtures reduce TPN-related liver failure, and autologous intestinal reconstruction surgery[162] combined with medical intestinal rehabilitation reduces the necessity for small bowel or multivisceral transplant.[163]

The administration of glucagonlike peptide-2 (GLP-2), a regulator of growth and function in the intestinal mucosa that in the short term slows intestinal motility and increases mesenteric blood flow, over time may lead to an increase in intestinal surface area.[164] Teduglutide, a long-acting GLP-2 ligand, used successfully in adults and older children with SBS is under limited investigation for use in neonates with SBS.[165]

Derangements in the intestinal microbiome in SBS after NEC are expected,[166] but prebiotics and probiotics have not been validated for improving overall progress toward intestinal autonomy. Early, small randomized controlled trials showed a beneficial effect of oral antibiotics on the risk of NEC,[167–170] and some clinicians still recommend antimicrobials such as metronidazole to minimize dysbiosis by suppressing bacterial overgrowth. However, treatment of dysbiosis both before NEC and in SBS is discouraged because of concerns about antimicrobial resistance (such as vancomycin-resistant enterococcus, and aminoglycoside resistant gram-negative organisms) from selective pressure on the microbiome.

Most intriguing is the concept of creating an autologous artificial intestine; this combines a bioscaffold composed of components of tissue such as collagen, or synthetic polymers coated with a biologic matrix, or scaffolds of decellularized tissues such as intestinal submucosa. These artificial intestines may be seeded with growth factors such as vascular endothelial growth factor (VEGF) that recruit an endogenous blood supply, and implantation of stem cells, as described for the treatment of NEC.[171,172]

On the Horizon: New Diagnostic and Detection Modalities

Early diagnosis, or ideally early identification, of at infants at high risk for NEC is key to mitigating the disease process. Biomarkers, defined by the US Food and Drug Administration–National Institutes of Health Biomarker Working Group, are a "defined characteristic that is, measured as an indicator of normal biological processes, pathogenic processes, or response to an exposure or intervention."[173] Biomarkers can be used for diagnosing or excluding NEC, risk assessment of the probability of NEC, or prognostication of disease progression.[174,175] Reliable, noninvasive biomarkers that are detectable early in the disease course, facilitating mitigation, would be beneficial in surveillance efforts.

Genomics

Candidate single nucleotide polymorphisms (SNPs) with a relationship to NEC are typically searched for based on preclinical or translational research hypotheses. These candidate genes have shown variable results despite biological plausibility, such as TLR4 or VEGF genetic variations, and mutations in genes for proinflammatory substances (PAF, NF-κB). Genome-wide approaches study millions of SNPs at a time in a candidate population in an agnostic manner. These techniques, such as genome-wide association study (GWAS) or whole-exome sequencing, have the advantage of increased objectivity to the choice of SNP but have been criticized as overly exploratory.[176] Using GWAS, a stringent definition of NEC, and a large validation set, clusters of SNPs on chromosome 8 were associated with proven surgical NEC. However, all genomic studies can be influenced by epigenetics and require a careful validation set.[177]

Metabolomics/volatile organic compounds

Ample evidence has been presented posing dysbiosis as a necessary precedent to NEC.[39,178] Given the time-dependent nature of colonization, aberrant or otherwise, it is unclear whether there is a critical mass or distribution of organisms that fit the component cause of dysbiosis into the causal pie, leading to disease.

An area of active research is using metabolomics to look for stool, serum, or urine biomarkers that may indicate changes in the microbiome that could herald NEC development. At present, no single biomarker for NEC has been identified in these studies. However, ongoing research may identify a panel of biomarkers that may lead to early diagnosis or prognostic indicators.[179–181]

Promising work has assessed volatile organic compounds (VOCs) as an early signal of NEC. This approach has the advantage of being noninvasive with no need for specimen collection, although present pattern recognition may not give an early enough signal of disease.[182–184] If VOC analysis were coupled with machine learning techniques in a prospective manner, a sensitive, noninvasive early detection system could be developed.

SUMMARY

NEC is an inflammatory bowel disease primarily affecting premature infants. The clinical presentation of NEC may represent a spectrum of disease with varying causal mechanisms. This article focuses mainly on preterm NEC, which typically presents at 30 to 32 weeks' corrected gestational age. Recent evidence indicates that immature intestinal immunity and intestinal dysbiosis play key roles in NEC pathogenesis. Management includes supportive measures and surgical intervention when medical management is not successful. Synergistic approaches to optimize the intestinal microbiome of the preterm infant with human milk feedings, adherence to feeding guidelines, probiotic supplementation, avoiding gastric acid blockade therapy, and antimicrobial stewardship contribute to preventive efforts. Minimal evidence regarding the duration of bowel rest and the optimal antimicrobial therapy in the management of NEC represent areas for further investigation. Improving understanding of risk factors, including diagnostic and prognostic biomarkers and innovative therapies for NEC and its sequelae, would be beneficial in reducing the burden of disease and improving neonatal outcomes.

Best practices

Current practice:

- To prevent NEC:
  - Feeding guidelines
  - Human milk feeds

- To manage NEC:
  - Bowel rest
  - Antimicrobials

Changes in practice that may improve outcome (if not already implemented in the NICU):

- Feeding guidelines

- Avoiding gastric acid blocker therapy

- Probiotics

- Antimicrobial stewardship

On the horizon:

- Better identification of at-risk infants:
  - Genomic identifiers

- Early diagnosis of precursors to NEC:
  - Stool microbiome analyses
  - Metabolomics/VOC analyses
- Innovative therapies:
  - For NEC:
    - Stem cell therapy
    - Exosomes
    - GLP-2
  - For SBS:
    - Autologous artificial transplant

DISCLOSURE

Dr Denning receives 5-P01 HL086773 and CHOA Friends Grant. Dr Barbian receives Marshall Klaus Perinatal Research Award, American Academy of Pediatrics and Warshaw Fellow Research Award Emory University and Children's Healthcare of Atlanta Pediatric Institute.

REFERENCES

1. Lin PW, Stoll BJ. Necrotising enterocolitis. Lancet 2006;368:1271–83.
2. Schmid KO. A specially severe form of enteritis in newborn, enterocolitis ulcerosa necroticans. I. Pathological anatomy. Osterr Z Kinderheilkd Kinderfuersorge 1952;8:114–35 [in Undetermined language].
3. Stiennon OA. Pneumatosis intestinals in the newborn. AMA Am J Dis Child 1951; 81:651–63.
4. Knell J, Han SM, Jaksic T, et al. Current status of necrotizing enterocolitis. Curr Probl Surg 2019;56:11–38.
5. Kim JH, Sampath V, Canvasser J. Challenges in diagnosing necrotizing enterocolitis. Pediatr Res 2020;88:16–20.
6. Stoll BJ, et al. Trends in care practices, morbidity, and mortality of extremely preterm neonates, 1993-2012. JAMA 2015;314:1039–51.
7. Christensen RD, Lambert DK, Baer VL, et al. Necrotizing enterocolitis in term infants. Clin Perinatol 2013;40:69–78.
8. Thompson A, et al. Risk factors for necrotizing enterocolitis totalis: a case-control study. J Perinatol 2011;31:730 8.
9. Gordon PV, Clark R, Swanson JR, et al. Can a national dataset generate a nomogram for necrotizing enterocolitis onset? J Perinatol 2014;34:732–5.
10. Caplan MS, et al. Necrotizing enterocolitis: using regulatory science and drug development to improve outcomes. J Pediatr 2019;212:208–15.e1.
11. Gordon PV, Swanson JR, MacQueen BC, et al. A critical question for NEC researchers: can we create a consensus definition of NEC that facilitates research progress? Semin Perinatol 2017;41:7–14.
12. Yee WH, et al. Incidence and timing of presentation of necrotizing enterocolitis in preterm infants. Pediatrics 2012;129:e298–304.
13. Horbar JD, et al. Variation in performance of neonatal intensive care units in the United States. JAMA Pediatr 2017;171:e164396.
14. Guner YS, et al. State-based analysis of necrotizing enterocolitis outcomes. J Surg Res 2009;157:21–9.

15. Carter BM, Holditch-Davis D. Risk factors for necrotizing enterocolitis in preterm infants: how race, gender, and health status contribute. Adv Neonatal Care 2008;8:285–90.
16. Patel RM, Denning PW. Intestinal microbiota and its relationship with necrotizing enterocolitis. Pediatr Res 2015;78:232–8.
17. Denning TL, Bhatia AM, Kane AF, et al. Pathogenesis of NEC: role of the innate and adaptive immune response. Semin Perinatol 2017;41:15–28.
18. Madani G, Heiner DC. Antibody transmission from mother to fetus. Curr Opin Immunol 1989;1:1157–64.
19. Cheng MM, et al. Development of serum IgA and IgM levels in breast-fed and formula-fed infants during the first week of life. Early Hum Dev 2012;88:743–5.
20. Nanthakumar NN, Fusunyan RD, Sanderson I, et al. Inflammation in the developing human intestine: a possible pathophysiologic contribution to necrotizing enterocolitis. Proc Natl Acad Sci U S A 2000;97:6043–8.
21. Claud EC, et al. Developmentally regulated IkappaB expression in intestinal epithelium and susceptibility to flagellin-induced inflammation. Proc Natl Acad Sci U S A 2004;101:7404–8.
22. Luig M, Lui K, Nsw & Group AN. Epidemiology of necrotizing enterocolitis–Part I: changing regional trends in extremely preterm infants over 14 years. J Paediatr Child Health 2005;41:169–73.
23. Akira S, Takeda K, Kaisho T. Toll-like receptors: critical proteins linking innate and acquired immunity. Nat Immunol 2001;2:675–80.
24. Lemaitre B, Nicolas E, Michaut L, et al. The dorsoventral regulatory gene cassette spatzle/Toll/cactus controls the potent antifungal response in Drosophila adults. Cell 1996;86:973–83.
25. Leaphart CL, et al. A critical role for TLR4 in the pathogenesis of necrotizing enterocolitis by modulating intestinal injury and repair. J Immunol 2007;179:4808–20.
26. Jilling T, et al. The roles of bacteria and TLR4 in rat and murine models of necrotizing enterocolitis. J Immunol 2006;177:3273–82.
27. Gribar SC, et al. Reciprocal expression and signaling of TLR4 and TLR9 in the pathogenesis and treatment of necrotizing enterocolitis. J Immunol 2009;182:636–46.
28. Good M, et al. Amniotic fluid inhibits Toll-like receptor 4 signaling in the fetal and neonatal intestinal epithelium. Proc Natl Acad Sci U S A 2012;109:11330–5.
29. Neal MD, et al. A critical role for TLR4 induction of autophagy in the regulation of enterocyte migration and the pathogenesis of necrotizing enterocolitis. J Immunol 2013;190:3541–51.
30. Hackam D, Caplan M. Necrotizing enterocolitis: pathophysiology from a historical context. Semin Pediatr Surg 2018;27:11–8.
31. Nino DF, Sodhi CP, Hackam DJ. Necrotizing enterocolitis: new insights into pathogenesis and mechanisms. Nat Rev Gastroenterol Hepatol 2016;13:590–600.
32. Palsson-McDermott EM, O'Neill LA. Signal transduction by the lipopolysaccharide receptor, Toll-like receptor-4. Immunology 2004;113:153–62.
33. Cotten CM, et al. Prolonged duration of initial empirical antibiotic treatment is associated with increased rates of necrotizing enterocolitis and death for extremely low birth weight infants. Pediatrics 2009;123:58–66.
34. Kenyon S, Boulvain M, Neilson JP. Antibiotics for preterm rupture of membranes. Cochrane Database Syst Rev 2010:CD001058. https://doi.org/10.1002/14651858.CD001058.pub2.

35. Kuppala VS, Meinzen-Derr J, Morrow AL, et al. Prolonged initial empirical antibiotic treatment is associated with adverse outcomes in premature infants. J Pediatr 2011;159:720–5.
36. Alexander VN, Northrup V, Bizzarro MJ. Antibiotic exposure in the newborn intensive care unit and the risk of necrotizing enterocolitis. J Pediatr 2011;159: 392–7.
37. Carrion V, Egan EA. Prevention of neonatal necrotizing enterocolitis. J Pediatr Gastroenterol Nutr 1990;11:317–23.
38. Coggins SA, Wynn JL, Weitkamp JH. Infectious causes of necrotizing enterocolitis. Clin Perinatol 2015;42:133–54, ix.
39. Pammi M, et al. Intestinal dysbiosis in preterm infants preceding necrotizing enterocolitis: a systematic review and meta-analysis. Microbiome 2017;5:31.
40. Warner BB, et al. Gut bacteria dysbiosis and necrotising enterocolitis in very low birthweight infants: a prospective case-control study. Lancet 2016;387:1928–36.
41. Wang Y, et al. 16S rRNA gene-based analysis of fecal microbiota from preterm infants with and without necrotizing enterocolitis. ISME J 2009;3:944–54.
42. Morrow AL, et al. Early microbial and metabolomic signatures predict later onset of necrotizing enterocolitis in preterm infants. Microbiome 2013;1:13.
43. Mai V, et al. Fecal microbiota in premature infants prior to necrotizing enterocolitis. PLoS One 2011;6:e20647.
44. de la Cochetiere MF, et al. Early intestinal bacterial colonization and necrotizing enterocolitis in premature infants: the putative role of Clostridium. Pediatr Res 2004;56:366–70.
45. Claud EC, Savidge T, Walker WA. Modulation of human intestinal epithelial cell IL-8 secretion by human milk factors. Pediatr Res 2003;53:419–25.
46. Patel RM, Underwood MA. Probiotics and necrotizing enterocolitis. Semin Pediatr Surg 2018;27:39–46.
47. Hooper LV, et al. Molecular analysis of commensal host-microbial relationships in the intestine. Science 2001;291:881–4.
48. Collier-Hyams LS, Neish AS. Innate immune relationship between commensal flora and the mammalian intestinal epithelium. Cell Mol Life Sci 2005;62: 1339–48.
49. Neish AS, et al. Prokaryotic regulation of epithelial responses by inhibition of IkappaB-alpha ubiquitination. Science 2000;289:1560–3.
50. Wallace TD, Bradley S, Buckley ND, et al. Interactions of lactic acid bacteria with human intestinal epithelial cells: effects on cytokine production. J Food Prot 2003;66:466–72.
51. Madsen KL, Doyle JS, Jewell LD, et al. Lactobacillus species prevents colitis in interleukin 10 gene-deficient mice. Gastroenterology 1999;116:1107–14.
52. Kelly D, et al. Commensal anaerobic gut bacteria attenuate inflammation by regulating nuclear-cytoplasmic shuttling of PPAR-gamma and RelA. Nat Immunol 2004;5:104–12.
53. Collier-Hyams LS, Sloane V, Batten BC, et al. Cutting edge: bacterial modulation of epithelial signaling via changes in neddylation of cullin-1. J Immunol 2005; 175:4194–8.
54. Stoll BJ, et al. Early-onset sepsis in very low birth weight neonates: a report from the National Institute of Child Health and Human Development Neonatal Research Network. J Pediatr 1996;129:72–80.
55. Neish AS. The gut microflora and intestinal epithelial cells: a continuing dialogue. Microbes Infect 2002;4:309–17.

56. Neish AS. Molecular aspects of intestinal epithelial cell-bacterial interactions that determine the development of intestinal inflammation. Inflamm Bowel Dis 2004;10:159–68.
57. Neish AS. Bacterial inhibition of eukaryotic pro-inflammatory pathways. Immunol Res 2004;29:175–86.
58. Young AN, et al. Beta defensin-1, parvalbumin, and vimentin: a panel of diagnostic immunohistochemical markers for renal tumors derived from gene expression profiling studies using cDNA microarrays. Am J Surg Pathol 2003; 27:199–205.
59. Zeng H, et al. Flagellin is the major proinflammatory determinant of enteropathogenic Salmonella. J Immunol 2003;171:3668–74.
60. Collier-Hyams LS, et al. Cutting edge: Salmonella AvrA effector inhibits the key proinflammatory, anti-apoptotic NF-kappa B pathway. J Immunol 2002;169: 2846–50.
61. Lin PW, et al. Paneth cell cryptdins act in vitro as apical paracrine regulators of the innate inflammatory response. J Biol Chem 2004;279:19902–7.
62. Greenwood C, et al. Early empiric antibiotic use in preterm infants is associated with lower bacterial diversity and higher relative abundance of Enterobacter. J Pediatr 2014;165:23–9.
63. Li Y, et al. Early use of antibiotics is associated with a lower incidence of necrotizing enterocolitis in preterm, very low birth weight infants: the NEOMUNE-NeoNutriNet cohort study. J Pediatr 2020;227:128–34.e2.
64. Greenberg RG, et al. Prolonged duration of early antibiotic therapy in extremely premature infants. Pediatr Res 2019;85:994–1000.
65. Sisk PM, Lovelady CA, Dillard RG, et al. Early human milk feeding is associated with a lower risk of necrotizing enterocolitis in very low birth weight infants. J Perinatol 2007;27:428–33.
66. Guillet R, et al. Association of H2-blocker therapy and higher incidence of necrotizing enterocolitis in very low birth weight infants. Pediatrics 2006;117: e137–42.
67. Gephart SM, et al. NEC-zero recommendations from scoping review of evidence to prevent and foster timely recognition of necrotizing enterocolitis. Matern Health Neonatol Perinatol 2017;3:23.
68. Patole SK, de Klerk N. Impact of standardised feeding regimens on incidence of neonatal necrotising enterocolitis: a systematic review and meta-analysis of observational studies. Arch Dis Child Fetal Neonatal Ed 2005;90:F147–51.
69. Hanson C, Sundermeier J, Dugick L, et al. Implementation, process, and outcomes of nutrition best practices for infants <1500 g. Nutr Clin Pract 2011;26: 614–24.
70. Smith JR. Early enteral feeding for the very low birth weight infant: the development and impact of a research-based guideline. Neonatal Netw 2005;24:9–19.
71. McCallie KR, et al. Improved outcomes with a standardized feeding protocol for very low birth weight infants. J Perinatol 2011;31(Suppl 1):S61–7.
72. Viswanathan S, et al. Standardized slow enteral feeding protocol and the incidence of necrotizing enterocolitis in extremely low birth weight infants. JPEN J Parenter Enteral Nutr 2015;39:644–54.
73. Butler TJ, Szekely LJ, Grow JL. A standardized nutrition approach for very low birth weight neonates improves outcomes, reduces cost and is not associated with increased rates of necrotizing enterocolitis, sepsis or mortality. J Perinatol 2013;33:851–7.

74. Loomis T, Byham-Gray L, Ziegler J, et al. Impact of standardized feeding guidelines on enteral nutrition administration, growth outcomes, metabolic bone disease, and cholestasis in the NICU. J Pediatr Gastroenterol Nutr 2014;59:93–8.
75. Patole S, McGlone L, Muller R. Virtual elimination of necrotising enterocolitis for 5 years - reasons? Med Hypotheses 2003;61:617–22.
76. Dutta S, et al. Guidelines for feeding very low birth weight infants. Nutrients 2015;7:423–42.
77. Collaborative CPQ. CPQCC Nutrition Toolkit Appendices. 2008. Available at: https://www.cpqcc.org/qi-tool-kits/nutritional-support-vlbw-infant.
78. Lucas A, Cole TJ. Breast milk and neonatal necrotising enterocolitis. Lancet 1990;336:1519–23.
79. Section on B. Breastfeeding and the use of human milk. Pediatrics 2012;129: e827–41.
80. Quigley M, McGuire W. Formula versus donor breast milk for feeding preterm or low birth weight infants. Cochrane Database Syst Rev 2014:CD002971. https://doi.org/10.1002/14651858.CD002971.pub3.
81. Sullivan S, et al. An exclusively human milk-based diet is associated with a lower rate of necrotizing enterocolitis than a diet of human milk and bovine milk-based products. J Pediatr 2010;156:562–7.e1.
82. Cristofalo EA, et al. Randomized trial of exclusive human milk versus preterm formula diets in extremely premature infants. J Pediatr 2013;163:1592–5.e1.
83. Herrmann K, Carroll K. An exclusively human milk diet reduces necrotizing enterocolitis. Breastfeed Med 2014;9:184–90.
84. Assad M, Elliott MJ, Abraham JH. Decreased cost and improved feeding tolerance in VLBW infants fed an exclusive human milk diet. J Perinatol 2016;36: 216–20.
85. Hair AB, Hawthorne KM, Chetta KE, et al. Human milk feeding supports adequate growth in infants </= 1250 grams birth weight. BMC Res Notes 2013;6:459.
86. Jakaitis BM, Denning PW. Human breast milk and the gastrointestinal innate immune system. Clin Perinatol 2014;41:423–35.
87. Chatterton DE, Nguyen DN, Bering SB, et al. Anti-inflammatory mechanisms of bioactive milk proteins in the intestine of newborns. Int J Biochem Cell Biol 2013; 45:1730–47.
88. Goldman AS. Modulation of the gastrointestinal tract of infants by human milk. Interfaces and interactions. An evolutionary perspective. J Nutr 2000;130: 426S–31S.
89. Newburg DS. Neonatal protection by an innate immune system of human milk consisting of oligosaccharides and glycans. J Anim Sci 2009;87:26–34.
90. Underwood MA, et al. Human milk oligosaccharides in premature infants: absorption, excretion, and influence on the intestinal microbiota. Pediatr Res 2015;78:670–7.
91. Srinivasjois R, Rao S, Patole S. Prebiotic supplementation in preterm neonates: updated systematic review and meta-analysis of randomised controlled trials. Clin Nutr 2013;32:958–65.
92. Plaisancie P, et al. A novel bioactive peptide from yoghurts modulates expression of the gel-forming MUC2 mucin as well as population of goblet cells and Paneth cells along the small intestine. J Nutr Biochem 2013;24:213–21.
93. Lawrence RM, Pane CA. Human breast milk: current concepts of immunology and infectious diseases. Curr Probl Pediatr Adolesc Health Care 2007;37:7–36.

94. Thormar H, Isaacs CE, Brown HR, et al. Inactivation of enveloped viruses and killing of cells by fatty acids and monoglycerides. Antimicrob Agents Chemother 1987;31:27–31.
95. Newburg DS, Walker WA. Protection of the neonate by the innate immune system of developing gut and of human milk. Pediatr Res 2007;61:2–8.
96. Manzoni P, et al. Bovine lactoferrin supplementation for prevention of late-onset sepsis in very low-birth-weight neonates: a randomized trial. JAMA 2009;302: 1421–8.
97. Manzoni P, et al. Bovine lactoferrin prevents invasive fungal infections in very low birth weight infants: a randomized controlled trial. Pediatrics 2012;129:116–23.
98. Valenti P, Antonini G. Lactoferrin: an important host defence against microbial and viral attack. Cell Mol Life Sci 2005;62:2576–87.
99. Lonnerdal B. Bioactive proteins in breast milk. J Paediatr Child Health 2013; 49(Suppl 1):1–7.
100. Ellison RT 3rd, Giehl TJ. Killing of gram-negative bacteria by lactoferrin and lysozyme. J Clin Invest 1991;88:1080–91.
101. Pammi M, Abrams SA. Oral lactoferrin for the prevention of sepsis and necrotizing enterocolitis in preterm infants. Cochrane Database Syst Rev 2015:CD007137. https://doi.org/10.1002/14651858.CD007137.pub4.
102. Furukawa M, Narahara H, Yasuda K, et al. Presence of platelet-activating factor-acetylhydrolase in milk. J Lipid Res 1993;34:1603–9.
103. Moya FR, et al. Platelet-activating factor acetylhydrolase in term and preterm human milk: a preliminary report. J Pediatr Gastroenterol Nutr 1994;19:236–9.
104. Hawkes JS, Bryan DL, James MJ, et al. Cytokines (IL-1beta, IL-6, TNF-alpha, TGF-beta1, and TGF-beta2) and prostaglandin E2 in human milk during the first three months postpartum. Pediatr Res 1999;46:194–9.
105. Namachivayam K, et al. Preterm human milk contains a large pool of latent TGF-beta, which can be activated by exogenous neuraminidase. Am J Physiol Gastrointest Liver Physiol 2013;304:G1055–65.
106. Emami CN, et al. Role of interleukin-10 in the pathogenesis of necrotizing enterocolitis. Am J Surg 2012;203:428–35.
107. Kuhn R, Lohler J, Rennick D, et al. Interleukin-10-deficient mice develop chronic enterocolitis. Cell 1993;75:263–74.
108. Glocker EO, et al. Inflammatory bowel disease and mutations affecting the interleukin-10 receptor. N Engl J Med 2009;361:2033–45.
109. Dvorak B, et al. Maternal milk reduces severity of necrotizing enterocolitis and increases intestinal IL-10 in a neonatal rat model. Pediatr Res 2003;53:426–33.
110. Maheshwari A, et al. TGF-beta2 suppresses macrophage cytokine production and mucosal inflammatory responses in the developing intestine. Gastroenterology 2011;140:242–53.
111. Penttila IA. Milk-derived transforming growth factor-beta and the infant immune response. J Pediatr 2010;156:S21–5.
112. Yuen DE, Stratford AF. Vitamin A activation of transforming growth factor-beta1 enhances porcine ileum wound healing in vitro. Pediatr Res 2004;55:935–9.
113. Ogawa J, et al. Role of transforming growth factor-beta in breast milk for initiation of IgA production in newborn infants. Early Hum Dev 2004;77:67–75.
114. Su Y, Yang J, Besner GE. HB-EGF promotes intestinal restitution by affecting integrin-extracellular matrix interactions and intercellular adhesions. Growth Factors 2013;31:39–55.
115. Coursodon CF, Dvorak B. Epidermal growth factor and necrotizing enterocolitis. Curr Opin Pediatr 2012;24:160–4.

116. Clark JA, et al. Intestinal barrier failure during experimental necrotizing entero-colitis: protective effect of EGF treatment. Am J Physiol Gastrointest Liver Physiol 2006;291:G938–49.

117. Wei J, Besner GE. M1 to M2 macrophage polarization in heparin-binding epidermal growth factor-like growth factor therapy for necrotizing enterocolitis. J Surg Res 2015;197:126–38.

118. Dvorak B, Fituch CC, Williams CS, et al. Increased epidermal growth factor levels in human milk of mothers with extremely premature infants. Pediatr Res 2003;54:15–9.

119. Good M, et al. Breast milk protects against the development of necrotizing enterocolitis through inhibition of Toll-like receptor 4 in the intestinal epithelium via activation of the epidermal growth factor receptor. Mucosal Immunol 2015; 8:1166–79.

120. Dvorak B, et al. Comparison of epidermal growth factor and heparin-binding epidermal growth factor-like growth factor for prevention of experimental necrotizing enterocolitis. J Pediatr Gastroenterol Nutr 2008;47:11–8.

121. Dvorak B, et al. Epidermal growth factor reduces the development of necrotizing enterocolitis in a neonatal rat model. Am J Physiol Gastrointest Liver Physiol 2002;282:G156–64.

122. Wei J, Zhou Y, Besner GE. Heparin-binding EGF-like growth factor and enteric neural stem cell transplantation in the prevention of experimental necrotizing enterocolitis in mice. Pediatr Res 2015;78:29–37.

123. Yang J, et al. Heparin-binding epidermal growth factor-like growth factor and mesenchymal stem cells act synergistically to prevent experimental necrotizing enterocolitis. J Am Coll Surg 2012;215:534–45.

124. Chen CL, et al. Heparin-binding EGF-like growth factor protects intestinal stem cells from injury in a rat model of necrotizing enterocolitis. Lab Invest 2012;92:331–44.

125. Yu X, Radulescu A, Zorko N, et al. Heparin-binding EGF-like growth factor in-creases intestinal microvascular blood flow in necrotizing enterocolitis. Gastro-enterology 2009;137:221–30.

126. Gupta RW, et al. Histamine-2 receptor blockers alter the fecal microbiota in pre-mature infants. J Pediatr Gastroenterol Nutr 2013;56:397–400.

127. More K, Athalye-Jape G, Rao S, et al. Association of inhibitors of gastric acid secretion and higher incidence of necrotizing enterocolitis in preterm very low-birth-weight infants. Am J Perinatol 2013. https://doi.org/10.1055/s-0033-1333071.

128. Terrin G, et al. Ranitidine is associated with infections, necrotizing enterocolitis, and fatal outcome in newborns. Pediatrics 2012;129:e40–5.

129. Lin PW, et al. Lactobacillus rhamnosus blocks inflammatory signaling in vivo via reactive oxygen species generation. Free Radic Biol Med 2009;47:1205–11.

130. Wickramasinghe S, Pacheco AR, Lemay DG, et al. Bifidobacteria grown on hu-man milk oligosaccharides downregulate the expression of inflammation-related genes in Caco-2 cells. BMC Microbiol 2015;15:172.

131. Underwood MA, et al. Bifidobacterium longum subsp. infantis in experimental necrotizing enterocolitis: alterations in inflammation, innate immune response, and the microbiota. Pediatr Res 2014;76:326–33.

132. Kumar A, et al. The bacterial fermentation product butyrate influences epithelial signaling via reactive oxygen species-mediated changes in cullin-1 neddyla-tion. J Immunol 2009;182:538–46.

133. Rivera-Chavez F, Lopez CA, Baumler AJ. Oxygen as a driver of gut dysbiosis. Free Radic Biol Med 2017;105:93–101.

134. Bron PA, et al. Can probiotics modulate human disease by impacting intestinal barrier function? Br J Nutr 2017;117:93–107.

135. Patel RM, et al. Probiotic bacteria induce maturation of intestinal claudin 3 expression and barrier function. Am J Pathol 2012;180:626–35.

136. Martinez FA, Balciunas EM, Converti A, et al. Bacteriocin production by Bifido-bacterium spp. A review. Biotechnol Adv 2013;31:482–8.

137. Good M, et al. Lactobacillus rhamnosus HN001 decreases the severity of necro-tizing enterocolitis in neonatal mice and preterm piglets: evidence in mice for a role of TLR9. Am J Physiol Gastrointest Liver Physiol 2014;306:G1021–32.

138. Barbian ME, Buckle R, Denning PW, et al. To start or not: factors to consider when implementing routine probiotic use in the NICU. Early Hum Dev 2019; 135:66–71.

139. Sawh SC, Deshpande S, Jansen S, et al. Prevention of necrotizing enterocolitis with probiotics: a systematic review and meta-analysis. PeerJ 2016;4:e2429.

140. Patel RM, Denning PW. Therapeutic use of prebiotics, probiotics, and postbiot-ics to prevent necrotizing enterocolitis: what is the current evidence? Clin Peri-natol 2013;40:11–25.

141. Chi C, Buys N, Li C, et al. Effects of prebiotics on sepsis, necrotizing enteroco-litis, mortality, feeding intolerance, time to full enteral feeding, length of hospital stay, and stool frequency in preterm infants: a meta-analysis. Eur J Clin Nutr 2019;73:657–70.

142. Clark RH, Bloom BT, Spitzer AR, et al. Reported medication use in the neonatal intensive care unit: data from a large national data set. Pediatrics 2006;117: 1979–87.

143. Clark RH, Bloom BT, Spitzer AR, et al. Empiric use of ampicillin and cefotaxime, compared with ampicillin and gentamicin, for neonates at risk for sepsis is asso-ciated with an increased risk of neonatal death. Pediatrics 2006;117:67–74.

144. Heida FH, et al. Bloodstream infections during the onset of necrotizing entero-colitis and their relation with the pro-inflammatory response, gut wall integrity and severity of disease in NEC. J Pediatr Surg 2015;50:1837–41.

145. Shah D, Sinn JK. Antibiotic regimens for the empirical treatment of newborn in-fants with necrotising enterocolitis. Cochrane Database Syst Rev 2012:CD007448. https://doi.org/10.1002/14651858.CD007448.pub2.

146. Valpacos M, et al. Diagnosis and management of necrotizing enterocolitis: an international survey of neonatologists and pediatric surgeons. Neonatology 2018;113:170–6.

147. Zani A, et al. International survey on the management of necrotizing enteroco-litis. Eur J Pediatr Surg 2015;25:27–33.

148. Faix RG, Polley TZ, Grasela TH. A randomized, controlled trial of parenteral clin-damycin in neonatal necrotizing enterocolitis. J Pediatr 1988;112:271–7.

149. Autmizguine J, et al. Anaerobic antimicrobial therapy after necrotizing enteroco-litis in VLBW infants. Pediatrics 2015;135:e117–25.

150. Patel EU, Wilson DA, Brennan EA, et al. Earlier re-initiation of enteral feeding af-ter necrotizing enterocolitis decreases recurrence or stricture: a systematic re-view and meta-analysis. J Perinatol 2020;40:1679–87.

151. Nitkin CR, et al. Stem cell therapy for preventing neonatal diseases in the 21st century: current understanding and challenges. Pediatr Res 2020;87:265–76.

152. Villamor-Martinez E, Hundscheid T, Kramer BW, et al. Stem cells as therapy for necrotizing enterocolitis: a systematic review and meta-analysis of preclinical studies. Front Pediatr 2020;8:578984.
153. McCulloh CJ, Olson JK, Zhou Y, et al. Stem cells and necrotizing enterocolitis: a direct comparison of the efficacy of multiple types of stem cells. J Pediatr Surg 2017;52:999–1005.
154. Li B, et al. Intestinal epithelial tight junctions and permeability can be rescued through the regulation of endoplasmic reticulum stress by amniotic fluid stem cells during necrotizing enterocolitis. FASEB J 2021;35:e21265.
155. Li B, et al. Bovine milk-derived exosomes enhance goblet cell activity and prevent the development of experimental necrotizing enterocolitis. PLoS One 2019; 14:e0211431.
156. Hackam DJ, Sodhi CP, Good M. New insights into necrotizing enterocolitis: from laboratory observation to personalized prevention and treatment. J Pediatr Surg 2019;54:398–404.
157. Rao SC, Basani L, Simmer K, et al. Peritoneal drainage versus laparotomy as initial surgical treatment for perforated necrotizing enterocolitis or spontaneous intestinal perforation in preterm low birth weight infants. Cochrane Database Syst Rev 2011:CD006182. https://doi.org/10.1002/14651858.CD006182.pub2.
158. Moschopoulos C, et al. The neurodevelopmental perspective of surgical necrotizing enterocolitis: the role of the gut-brain axis. Mediators Inflamm 2018;2018: 7456857.
159. Hong CR, et al. Growth morbidity in extremely low birth weight survivors of necrotizing enterocolitis at discharge and two-year follow-up. J Pediatr Surg 2018;53:1197–202.
160. Shah TA, et al. Hospital and neurodevelopmental outcomes of extremely low-birth-weight infants with necrotizing enterocolitis and spontaneous intestinal perforation. J Perinatol 2012;32:552–8.
161. Mutanen A, Wales PW. Etiology and prognosis of pediatric short bowel syndrome. Semin Pediatr Surg 2018;27:209–17.
162. Fallon EM, et al. Neonates with short bowel syndrome: an optimistic future for parenteral nutrition independence. JAMA Surg 2014;149:663–70.
163. Frongia G, et al. Comparison of LILT and STEP procedures in children with short bowel syndrome – a systematic review of the literature. J Pediatr Surg 2013;48: 1794–805.
164. Sigalet DL. Advances in glucagon like peptide-2 therapy. physiology, current indications and future directions. Semin Pediatr Surg 2018;27:237–41.
165. Sigalet DL, et al. A safety and pharmacokinetic dosing study of glucagon-like peptide 2 in infants with intestinal failure. J Pediatr Surg 2017;52:749–54.
166. Olieman J, Kastelijn W. Nutritional feeding strategies in pediatric intestinal failure. Nutrients 2020;12. https://doi.org/10.3390/nu12010177.
167. Grylack LJ, Scanlon JW. Oral gentamicin therapy in the prevention of neonatal necrotizing enterocolitis. A controlled double-blind trial. Am J Dis Child 1978; 132:1192–4.
168. Rowley MP, Dahlenburg GW. Gentamicin in prophylaxis of neonatal necrotising enterocolitis. Lancet 1978;2:532.
169. Ng PC, Dear PR, Thomas DF. Oral vancomycin in prevention of necrotising enterocolitis. Arch Dis Child 1988;63:1390–3.
170. Siu YK, et al. Double blind, randomised, placebo controlled study of oral vancomycin in prevention of necrotising enterocolitis in preterm, very low birthweight infants. Arch Dis Child Fetal Neonatal Ed 1998;79:F105–9.

171. Martin LY, et al. Tissue engineering for the treatment of short bowel syndrome in children. Pediatr Res 2018;83:249–57.
172. Kovler ML, Hackam DJ. Generating an artificial intestine for the treatment of short bowel syndrome. Gastroenterol Clin North Am 2019;48:585–605.
173. Cagney DN, et al. The FDA NIH Biomarkers, EndpointS, and other Tools (BEST) resource in neuro-oncology. Neuro Oncol 2018;20:1162–72.
174. Goldstein GP, Sylvester KG. Biomarker discovery and utility in necrotizing enterocolitis. Clin Perinatol 2019;46:1–17.
175. Gephart SM, et al. Changing the paradigm of defining, detecting, and diagnosing NEC: perspectives on Bell's stages and biomarkers for NEC. Semin Pediatr Surg 2018;27:3–10.
176. Cuna A, George L, Sampath V. Genetic predisposition to necrotizing enterocolitis in premature infants: current knowledge, challenges, and future directions. Semin Fetal Neonatal Med 2018;23:387–93.
177. Jilling T, et al. Surgical necrotizing enterocolitis in extremely premature neonates is associated with genetic variations in an intergenic region of chromosome 8. Pediatr Res 2018;83:943–53.
178. Fundora JB, Guha P, Shores DR, et al. Intestinal dysbiosis and necrotizing enterocolitis: assessment for causality using Bradford Hill criteria. Pediatr Res 2020;87:235–48.
179. Thomaidou A, et al. A pilot case-control study of urine metabolomics in preterm neonates with necrotizing enterocolitis. J Chromatogr B Analyt Technol Biomed Life Sci 2019;1117:10–21.
180. Stewart CJ, et al. Metabolomic and proteomic analysis of serum from preterm infants with necrotising entercolitis and late-onset sepsis. Pediatr Res 2016; 79:425–31.
181. Agakidou E, Agakidis C, Gika H, et al. Emerging biomarkers for prediction and early diagnosis of necrotizing enterocolitis in the era of metabolomics and proteomics. Front Pediatr 2020;8:602255.
182. Berkhout DJC, et al. Detection of sepsis in preterm infants by fecal volatile organic compounds analysis: a proof of principle study. J Pediatr Gastroenterol Nutr 2017;65:e47–52.
183. Probert C, et al. Faecal volatile organic compounds in preterm babies at risk of necrotising enterocolitis: the DOVE study. Arch Dis Child Fetal Neonatal Ed 2020;105:474–9.
184. de Meij TG, et al. Early detection of necrotizing enterocolitis by fecal volatile organic compounds analysis. J Pediatr 2015;167:562–7.e1.

Association of Infection in Neonates and Long-Term Neurodevelopmental Outcome

Elizabeth Sewell, MD, MPH[a], Jessica Roberts, MD[b],
Sagori Mukhopadhyay, MD, MMSc[c],*

KEYWORDS

- Neonate • Sepsis • Preterm • Bacteremia • Bacterial meningitis
- Necrotizing enterocolitis neurodevelopment • Cerebral palsy

KEY POINTS

- Neonatal bacterial sepsis remains a leading cause of neonatal mortality that is inversely proportional to gestational age.
- Systemic infection and inflammation can adversely affect early-life brain development, resulting in long-term neurologic impairments among surviving infants.
- Although most studies report an increased risk of neurologic impairment in preterm infants with neonatal infection, robust long-term outcomes beyond early childhood, especially in full term infants, are lacking.
- Strategies to prevent infection, early management, close follow-up, and early intervention among affected children remain foundational to improving outcomes.

INTRODUCTION

Parents, neonatal providers, and researchers identified survival, sepsis prevention, and intact long-term neurodevelopmental function as core outcomes for neonates who require intensive care soon after birth.[1] These outcomes are related; sepsis during initial hospitalization increases risk for both in-hospital mortality and for adverse childhood neurodevelopmental outcomes.[2–6] For infants admitted to the neonatal intensive care unit (NICU), technologies that are lifesaving can also increase the risk

[a] Division of Neonatology, Department of Pediatrics, Emory University School of Medicine & Children's Healthcare of Atlanta, 2015 Uppergate Drive, Office #318, Atlanta, GA 30322, USA; [b] Division of Neonatology, Department of Pediatrics, Emory University School of Medicine & Children's Healthcare of Atlanta, 2015 Uppergate Drive, Atlanta, GA 30322, USA; [c] Division of Neonatology, Department of Pediatrics, Children's Hospital of Philadelphia, Perelman School of Medicine, University of Pennsylvania, 800 Spruce Street, 2nd Floor Cathcart Building, Newborn Medicine, Philadelphia, PA, USA
* Corresponding author.
E-mail address: Mukhopadhs@email.chop.edu

Clin Perinatol 48 (2021) 251–261
https://doi.org/10.1016/j.clp.2021.03.001
0095-5108/21/© 2021 Elsevier Inc. All rights reserved.

for unintended consequences, including bacterial infection.[7] Improvements in preventive efforts have reduced the overall incidence of infection.[8,9] However, evolving microbiology with changes in resistance patterns,[10,11] and increasing vulnerability of high-risk infants admitted to NICUs,[12] highlight the need for ongoing surveillance, better application of known therapies, and discovery of new interventions.[13]

EPIDEMIOLOGY OF NEONATAL BACTERIAL INFECTIONS

Bacterial infection, defined as blood or cerebrospinal fluid (CSF) culture-confirmed infection, is described as early-onset (<72 hours after birth) and late-onset infection (≥72 hours after birth until the end of neonatal period at 28 days for term infants and usually until discharge among those continuously hospitalized) in neonates.[9,13,14] This temporal distinction reflects the differing pathogenesis,[15,16] microbiology,[17,18] and preventive strategies.[8,19,20] Meningitis is often associated with bacteremia in early-onset sepsis (EOS),[17] but later may occur in a third of cases without associated bacteremia.[21] Necrotizing enterocolitis (NEC) frequently occurs in the late-onset period[22] and may be associated with bacteremia.[23] Although few studies directly compare neurodevelopmental outcome among infants with early versus late infection, both presentations are associated with increased risk of mortality and neurodevelopmental impairment (NDI).[2,3,24]

Early-Onset Sepsis

Based on cases reported in 2005 to 2014 to the Centers for Disease Control and Prevention,[14] EOS incidence is estimated at 0.77 per 1000 live births (LBs) with a stable trend over the years of surveillance.[9] Among the 1484 cases identified, group B *Streptococcus* (GBS) was the leading cause of EOS, followed by *Escherichia coli* and viridans group streptococci. Incidence of all-cause EOS is significantly higher in preterm infants, where *E coli* is the most commonly detected pathogen.[9] Case fatality is substantially higher in preterm infants as well, with 165 out of 1484 (11%) deaths among EOS cases and 125 out of 165 (76%) of these occurring in very-low-birth-weight (VLBW; ie, birth weight <1500 g) infants. Multivariate modeling revealed a significantly increased risk for mortality with VLBW status (adjusted odds ratio [OR], 3.88; 95% confidence interval [CI], 1.47–10.22) and meningitis (adjusted OR, 3.53; 95% CI, 1.74–7.16).[9] Although more infants with *E coli* infection died (23%) compared with GBS (7%), the difference was not significant when adjusting for gestational age.[9] Similar incidence rates for EOS were reported in full-term infants in a multicenter study of academic centers that provide care for high-risk deliveries.[17] However, incidence of all-cause EOS and *E coli* infection among VLBW infants increased from 11.00 to 15.05 per 1000 LB (*P* = 0.03), and from 5.07 to 8.68 per 1000 LB (*P* = 0.008), respectively.[17]

Late-Onset Sepsis

Unlike EOS, estimates for incidence of late-onset sepsis (LOS) often represent center-specific data with few nationally representative data sources.[18,25–28] LOS epidemiology is also often reported separately for high-risk infants with prolonged admissions after birth[18,25] and community-associated LOS,[27,29] with few studies that capture rates across all groups.[30] Because many high-risk infants receive routine follow-up for underlying complications of prematurity, birth anomalies, or neonatal depression at birth, information for long-term outcomes associated with LOS is enriched for high-risk infants and may be difficult to generalize to all neonates with LOS.

Late-onset sepsis among infants with prolonged admission after birth

Incidence of LOS is inversely proportional to gestational age[25] and directly proportional to the length of stay,[26] making VLBW infants one of the highest-risk populations for LOS. A reduction in incidence of LOS from 21.9% (2005) to 10.1% (2014) was reported for VLBW infants admitted to NICUs across the United States.[8] Among extremely preterm infants (<28 weeks) admitted to 12 academic sites, LOS rates also decreased but were higher overall at 41% (2000–2005) and 34% (2006–2011) with an unchanged mortality (18%).[18] The microbiology of LOS included gram-positive bacteria (>75% cases), most frequently coagulase-negative *Staphylococcus* species (CoNS) and *Staphylococcus aureus*; gram-negative bacteria (17%), most frequently *E coli*; and fungal organisms, most commonly of *Candida* species. Among late preterm infants (34–36 weeks) and term infants (≥37 weeks) without anomalies who required admission to an NICU, a cumulative rate of LOS was reported at 6.30 episodes per 1000 NICU admissions for late preterm and 2.7 episodes per 1000 NICU admissions for term infants, with a distribution of pathogens in both groups similar to those reported in extremely preterm infants.[26,28] Compared with the higher mortality reported among preterm infants,[18] mortality among term infants with LOS was lower at 4%, but was substantially higher than the less than 1% mortality among term infants without late-onset infection.[28]

Late-onset sepsis among infants not continuously admitted after birth

Data from an integrated health care system have been used to report the incidence of LOS among term infants without underlying medical conditions.[27,31] Among 224,553 full-term deliveries, 6232 (3%) infants were evaluated and 13% of those were found to have a serious bacterial infection, defined as bacteremia, urinary tract infection (UTI), or meningitis. UTI episodes were the most frequent, followed by bacteremia and meningitis, although the investigators recognized potential for ascertainment bias with changing testing patterns with neonatal age.[27] The estimated incidence rate reported per 1000 full-term LBs was 3.46 (95% CI, 3.34–3.60) for UTI, 0.57 (95% CI, 0.55–0.59) for bacteremia, and 0.07 (95% CI, 0.069–0.074) for meningitis. The microbiology of community-acquired LOS, as opposed to that of health care–associated LOS among neonates readmitted to the hospital, is dominated by gram-negative bacteria, specifically *E coli*, with a lower proportion attributed to CoNS.[18,27,29]

PATHOGENESIS OF INFECTION AND BRAIN INJURY

The association of perinatal and postnatal infection with neonatal brain injury has been described, particularly with the manifestation of cystic periventricular leukomalacia (PVL).[32] With advances in neuroimaging techniques, there has been increased recognition of the incidence and importance of noncystic, diffuse white matter injury.[33] Although the association of fetal and neonatal infection and brain injury has been established, the degree, timing, and mechanism of involvement are still being debated.

The process of neonatal brain injury in the setting of infection is best described with neonatal meningitis, where there is direct penetration of bacteria across the blood-brain barrier to infiltrate the central nervous system.[34] Interestingly, infection without direct bacterial invasion of the central nervous system can also lead to brain injury and NDI.[34] Although the exact mechanism of how this occurs is still incompletely understood, the immaturity of the blood-brain barrier in preterm infants and the inflammation generated by pathogens can activate a local inflammatory response and/or cause direct cytotoxic injury.[34]

One mechanism that has been suggested is that inflammation associated with infection and hypoxic-ischemic injury occur upstream of the site of infection, instigating the cascade of events leading to brain injury.[33] These events can happen in isolation or combination, and one has the potential to potentiate the effects of the other.[33] In this proposed pathway, infection and hypoxia/ischemia lead to proinflammatory microglial activation, which leads to release of inflammatory cytokines such as tumor necrosis factor-alpha and interleukin-1β, release of reactive oxygen and nitrogen species, and an increase in glutamate levels with subsequent excitotoxicity.[33] In addition, other types of microglia important to normal development may be converted to a proinflammatory state.[35] The combination of these factors results in oligodendroglial injury and/or subsequent inhibition of maturation and myelination, axonal damage, and neuronal loss.[36]

PERINATAL INFLAMMATION AND NEURODEVELOPMENTAL OUTCOMES

Many studies have investigated the relationship of clinical and histologic chorioamnionitis at the time of delivery and NDI in newborns.[37–41] Most of these studies have focused on preterm infants and on cerebral palsy (CP) as an outcome, and few report evidence for confirmed infection in newborns.[40,41] In clinical practice, a diagnosis of chorioamnionitis increases the risk of culture-confirmed EOS, but most infants delivered to mothers with chorioamnionitis are not infected.[42] However, immune activation and inflammation (with or without infection) in chorioamnionitis can result in injury to the developing brain that may lead to long-term sequelae.[39]

A meta-analysis of studies published through September 2016 reviewed the association of chorioamnionitis and CP, and found differing results by study design: studies that investigated the risk of CP among infants with chorioamnionitis versus those that investigated the incidence of chorioamnionitis among infants with CP.[37] Among preterm infants, an increased risk of CP was associated with histologic chorioamnionitis, but not with clinical chorioamnionitis. In contrast, an increased incidence of clinical chorioamnionitis was found among patients with CP for all birth gestations, whereas the incidence of histologic chorioamnionitis was increased only in term infants. The difference in associations between studies that look forward from exposure to backwards from outcome may be caused by a second factor on the causal pathway, which may be prematurity itself[37] or a genetic predisposition (eg, polymorphism in the interleukin-6 gene).[43]

Neurologic deficits other than CP have been predominantly reported in preterm infants. In a 10-year prospective cohort study of infants less than 28 weeks' gestational age, investigators found higher adjusted odds for CP, autism, and epilepsy among infants with histologic chorioamnionitis.[39] No effect on cognitive function was noted. In contrast, a study of infants born at 24 to 32 weeks' gestation found an association of histologic chorioamnionitis with motor or cognitive function at 2 years of age that was not significant after adjusting for key postnatal variables such as LOS.[41] The role of study design, bias in selection, and varying study definitions has been proposed as an explanation for the inconsistency of findings across publications on the impact of chorioamnionitis on neurodevelopmental outcome.[37,38]

NEURODEVELOPMENTAL OUTCOMES AFTER NEONATAL INFECTIONS
Early-Onset Sepsis

Adverse outcomes have been reported among survivors of EOS, with 6.3% of episodes resulting in survival with an oxygen requirement, hearing loss, or seizures.[9] In contrast with studies on chorioamnionitis, few studies report the long-term neurologic outcomes among infants with culture-confirmed EOS in the absence of meningitis. Published studies often focus on preterm infants and report an association of EOS with increased risk of mortality and abnormal cranial imaging.[3,24,44]

In a cohort of 7354 infants born less than 26 weeks in gestation, EOS occurred in 153 infants, and 41% of the infants with EOS died before 2 years of age.[3] Infants with EOS have an increased adjusted relative risk of death or NDI at 2 years of age of 1.23 (95% CI, 1.10–1.37), compared with infants without EOS. Impairments in both cognitive and motor scores were noted.[3] In a 5-year follow-up study of 2665 infants born at less than 28 weeks' gestation, investigators found an increased risk of CP in survivors of EOS without an increased risk for impaired cognitive outcomes.[24]

Meningitis

Meningitis, both early and late onset, has been associated with poor neurodevelopmental outcome. Since the late 1990s, neonatal mortality caused by meningitis has remained stable at 10%.[44–50] Along with increasing rates of survival, up to half of surviving neonates are estimated to have NDI.[4,49,51–54] The rate of moderate or severe NDI in surviving infants ranges from 15% to 25%.[44,51–53,55–58] In a survey of physicians, 5-year-old survivors of neonatal bacterial meningitis had a 4-fold to16-fold increase in serious disability compared with hospital-matched and physician-matched controls without meningitis.[51] Infants surviving bacterial meningitis have an increased risk of CP, cognitive impairment, behavioral problems, and speech, auditory and visual impairment; neurologic complications such as hydrocephalus and seizures are also common.[4,51,53,58,59]

Preterm infants with meningitis are at significantly increased risk of death and NDI.[47–50,60] The mortalities from GBS and E coli meningitis seem to be approximately equal.[4,45,50,58] The risk for poor outcome is not affected by pathogen[4,53,58]; seizures and delayed time to CSF sterilization are associated with worse outcomes.[44,61,62]

Late-Onset Sepsis

Systemic infection associated with LOS is often associated with hemodynamic instability, inflammatory response, multisystem organ failure, and worse short-term and long-term outcomes, particularly for premature infants.[4,63] Neuroimaging may offer insight into mechanisms of brain injury and adverse neurodevelopmental outcomes.[32,64,65] An association between PVL and culture-confirmed infections (blood, CSF, or tracheal) in preterm infants less than 34 weeks' gestation was noted to increase with recurrent infectious episodes.[65] Similarly, repeated culture-confirmed infectious episodes showed progressive white matter injury with serial MRI studies.[64]

In a large cohort study, extremely-low-birth-weight (ELBW; ie, <1000 g) infants across 4 different categories of infection (culture-negative clinical infection only, culture-confirmed sepsis only, both culture-confirmed sepsis and an episode of NEC, and culture-confirmed meningitis ± sepsis) had higher likelihood of NDI at 18 to 22 months, including CP, lower mental developmental index score, lower psychomotor developmental index scores, and visual impairment, compared with infants without any diagnoses of/treatment of infection.[4] Hearing impairment was associated with sepsis and sepsis/NEC. This study also found an association between neonatal infection and poor head growth, which has been associated with impaired cognitive functioning and academic performance.[4,66] Similarly, in a multicenter Swiss study of preterm infants born 24 to 27 weeks' gestation, culture-confirmed sepsis was associated with CP and NDI at 2 years of age compared with infants with culture-negative suspected sepsis and those without any sepsis events.[67] These associations did not hold for culture-negative suspected sepsis cases, a group that included some infants with NEC. With longer follow-up, at 5 years, Mitha and colleagues[24] examined outcomes of infants born at 22 to 32 weeks' gestation. A higher risk of CP was found with LOS, alone and in combination with EOS, although it did not correlate with severe cognitive impairment.

Candidiasis, with or without bacteremia, has been associated with significant mortality and NDI.[68] In a multicenter study, infants with gram-negative, fungal, and combination (multiple episodes with different pathogens or a single polymicrobial episode) infection had a higher incidence of hearing impairment than those with no infections and those with CoNS infections.[4] Other studies have reported an increased risk of CP[67] and cognitive delay[69] in infants with LOS CoNS infection.

Necrotizing Enterocolitis

NEC often affects infants with other complications of prematurity that are also associated with poorer neurodevelopmental outcomes.[70,71] This pathologic milieu raises concern about the impact on the developing preterm brain,[63] and several investigators have reported associations that vary with severity of disease, degree of systemic illness, and management. The pathophysiology of NEC-associated NDI likely is multifactorial, akin to the pathophysiology of NEC itself.[70]

In a systematic review of 11 observational studies (1989–2006), ELBW infants with NEC had a higher risk of NDI, including CP, cognitive impairment, and severe visual impairment, than those without NEC (OR, 1.82; 95%CI, 1.46–2.27).[72] This risk was higher in those requiring surgery. The largest study in this review, a multicenter retrospective analysis of ELBW infants from Neonatal Research Network sites,[73] found that infants with NEC managed by surgery had an increased risk for cystic PVL, low Mental Development Index (<70), low Physical Development Index (<70), and NDI at 18-month to 22-month follow-up assessment compared with infants who had medically managed NEC. This association was also reported in a systematic review, in which the overall OR for NDI was 2.3 times higher among infants with surgically managed NEC.[74,75] Comparisons of outcomes in patients with NEC-associated and non–NEC-associated intestinal perforations have yielded varied results, some with similar risk of NDI and others with more NDI in those with NEC-associated perforations.[76,77] Other factors associated with NEC and its management might also affect neurodevelopmental outcomes, including the method of surgical intervention.[78]

Psychomotor impairment was found to be statistically associated with surgical NEC among infants born between 23 and 27 weeks; those who also had late-onset bacteremia were at increased risk for CP and microcephaly.[79] However, medical NEC, with or without late-onset bacteremia, did not increase risk for NDI.

SUMMARY

Efforts to improve sepsis-related NDI outcomes among neonates include a multistep approach consisting of (1) strategies to prevent neonatal infection, (2) early diagnosis and appropriate treatment of infection, (3) judicious follow-up and early intervention for at-risk infants, and (4) improved interventions to optimize functional rehabilitation of children with sequelae, including adequate seizure management, timely neurosurgical and orthopedic interventions, if indicated, and multidisciplinary support for deficits in motor, cognitive, and behavioral development.

Challenges in describing the impact of infection on NDI include the inconsistency in definitions of exposure outcomes. Interventions that target host responses may have greater impact on long-term outcomes but are sparsely studied in the neonatal population. Rigorous studies with long-term developmental follow-up that include objective definitions of infection and consistent outcome measurements are needed to provide prognostic information.

CLINICS CARE POINTS

- Comparing long-term impairment in neonates with infection is limited because of few prospective follow-up studies in term neonates and a lack of standard definitions for infections and outcomes.

- Establishing follow-up that coordinates developmental assessment, neurologic testing, and early intervention may facilitate early identification and initiation of rehabilitation efforts.

- Novel interventions to target inflammatory pathways mediating injury may improve outcomes in infants with infection beyond survival.

DISCLOSURE

Dr Mukhopadhyay is supported by the Eunice Kennedy Shriver National Institute of Child Health and Human Development of the National Institutes of Health (K23HD088753).

REFERENCES

1. Webbe JWH, Duffy JMN, Afonso E, et al. Core outcomes in neonatology: development of a core outcome set for neonatal research. Arch Dis Child Fetal Neonatal Ed 2020;105:425–31.
2. Mukhopadhyay S, Puopolo KM, Hansen NI, et al. Neurodevelopmental outcomes following neonatal late-onset sepsis and blood culture-negative conditions. In: Archives of disease in childhood: fetal and neonatal Edition. 2020.
3. Mukhopadhyay S, Puopolo KM, Hansen NI, et al. Impact of early-onset sepsis and antibiotic use on death or survival with neurodevelopmental impairment at 2 years of age among extremely preterm infants. J Pediatr 2020;221:39–46.e5.
4. Stoll BJ, Hansen NI, Adams-Chapman I, et al. Neurodevelopmental and growth impairment among extremely low-birth-weight infants with neonatal infection. JAMA 2004;292:2357–65.
5. Adams-Chapman I. Long-term impact of infection on the preterm neonate. Semin perinatology 2012;36:462–70.
6. Bassler D, Stoll BJ, Schmidt B, et al. Using a count of neonatal morbidities to predict poor outcome in extremely low birth weight infants: added role of neonatal infection. Pediatrics 2009;123:313–8.
7. Stoll BJ, Hansen N, Fanaroff AA, et al. Late-onset sepsis in very low birth weight neonates: the experience of the NICHD Neonatal Research Network. Pediatrics 2002;110:285–91.
8. Horbar JD, Edwards EM, Greenberg LT, et al. Variation in performance of neonatal intensive care units in the United States. JAMA Pediatr 2017;171: e164396.
9. Schrag SJ, Farley MM, Petit S, et al. Epidemiology of invasive early-onset neonatal sepsis, 2005 to 2014. Pediatrics (Evanston) 2016;138:e20162013.
10. Mukhopadhyay S, Wade KC, Puopolo KM. Drugs for the prevention and treatment of sepsis in the newborn. Clin Perinatol 2019;46:327–47.

11. Bizzarro MJ, Dembry L-, Baltimore RS, et al. Changing patterns in neonatal Escherichia coli sepsis and ampicillin resistance in the era of intrapartum antibiotic prophylaxis. Pediatrics (Evanston) 2008;121:689–96.
12. Patel RM, Rysavy MA, Bell EF, et al. Survival of infants born at periviable gestational ages. Clin Perinatol 2017;44:287–303.
13. Adams M, Bassler D. Practice variations and rates of late onset sepsis and necrotizing enterocolitis in very preterm born infants, a review. Transl Pediatr 2019;8: 212–26.
14. Weston EJ, Pondo T, Lewis MM, et al. The Burden of invasive early-onset neonatal sepsis in the United States, 2005–2008. Pediatr Infect Dis J 2011;30:937–41.
15. Benirschke K. Routes and types of infection in the fetus and the newborn. AMA Am J Dis Child 1960;99:714–21.
16. Stoll BJ, Hansen N, Fanaroff AA, et al. Late-onset sepsis in very low birth weight neonates: the experience of the NICHD neonatal research Network. Pediatrics (Evanston). 2002;110:285–91.
17. Stoll BJ, Puopolo KM, Hansen NI, et al. Early-onset neonatal sepsis 2015 to 2017, the rise of Escherichia coli, and the need for Novel prevention strategies. JAMA Pediatr 2020;174:e200593.
18. Greenberg RG, Kandefer S, Do BT, et al. Late-onset sepsis in extremely premature infants: 2000-2011. Pediatr Infect Dis J 2017;36:774–9.
19. Sinha A, Murthy V, Nath P, et al. Prevention of late onset sepsis and central-line associated blood Stream infection in preterm infants. Pediatr Infect Dis J 2016; 35:401–6.
20. Verani JR, McGee L, Schrag SJ. Prevention of perinatal group B streptococcal disease: revised guidelines from CDC, 2010. MMWR Recomm Rep 2010; 59:1–31.
21. Stoll BJ, Hansen N, Fanaroff AA, et al. To tap or not to tap: high likelihood of meningitis without sepsis among very low birth weight infants. Pediatrics (Evanston) 2004;113:1181–6.
22. Kliegman RM, Fanaroff AA. Necrotizing enterocolitis. N Engl J Med 1984;310: 1093–103.
23. Bizzarro MJ, Ehrenkranz RA, Gallagher PG. Concurrent bloodstream infections in infants with necrotizing enterocolitis. J Pediatr 2014;164:61–6.
24. Mitha A, Foix-L'Helias L, Arnaud C, et al. Neonatal infection and 5-year neurodevelopmental outcome of very preterm infants. Pediatrics (Evanston) 2013;132: e372–80.
25. Gowda H, Norton R, White A, et al. Late-onset neonatal sepsis—a 10-year review from North Queensland, Australia. Pediatr Infect Dis J 2017;36:883–8.
26. Cohen-Wolkowiez M, Moran C, Benjamin DK, et al. Early and late onset sepsis in late preterm infants. Pediatr Infect Dis J 2009;28:1052–6.
27. Greenhow T, Hung Y, Herz A, et al. The changing epidemiology of serious bacterial infections in young infants. Pediatr Infect Dis J 2014;33:595–9.
28. Testoni D, Hayashi M, Cohen-Wolkowiez M, et al. Late-onset bloodstream infections in hospitalized term infants. Pediatr Infect Dis J 2014;33:920–3.
29. Biondi E, Evans R, Mischler M, et al. Epidemiology of bacteremia in febrile infants in the United States. Pediatrics (Evanston) 2013;132:990–6.
30. Berardi A, Sforza F, Baroni L, et al. Epidemiology and complications of late-onset sepsis: an Italian area-based study. PLoS One 2019;14:e0225407.
31. Greenhow TL, Hung Y, Herz AM. Changing epidemiology of bacteremia in infants aged 1 week to 3 months. Pediatrics 2012;129:590.

32. Shah DK, Doyle LW, Anderson PJ, et al. Adverse neurodevelopment in preterm infants with postnatal sepsis or necrotizing enterocolitis is mediated by white matter abnormalities on magnetic resonance imaging at term. J Pediatr 2008;153: 170–5.e1.

33. Volpe JJ, Kinney HC, Jensen FE, et al. The developing oligodendrocyte: key cellular target in brain injury in the premature infant. Int J Dev Neurosci 2011; 29:423–40.

34. Volpe JJ, Inder TE, Darras BT, et al. Volpe's Neurology of the newborn. 6th edition. Philadelphia: Elsevier; 2017.

35. Volpe JJ. Microglia: newly discovered complexity could lead to targeted therapy for neonatal white matter injury and dysmaturation, vol. 12. *NPM.* IOS Press J Neonatal Perinatal Med; 2019. p. 239.

36. Volpe JJ. Brain injury in premature infants: a complex amalgam of destructive and developmental disturbances. Lancet Neurol 2009;8:110–24.

37. Shi Z, Ma L, Luo K, et al. Chorioamnionitis in the development of cerebral palsy: a meta-analysis and systematic review. Pediatrics 2017;139.

38. Maisonneuve E, Ancel P-, Foix-L'Hélias L, et al. Impact of clinical and/or histological chorioamnionitis on neurodevelopmental outcomes in preterm infants: a literature review. J Gynecol Obstet Hum Reprod 2017;46:307–16.

39. Venkatesh KK, Leviton A, Hecht JL, et al. Histologic chorioamnionitis and risk of neurodevelopmental impairment at age 10 years among extremely preterm infants born before 28 weeks of gestation. Am J Obstet Gynecol 2020;223: 745.e1–10.

40. Wu YW, Escobar GJ, Grether JK, et al. Chorioamnionitis and cerebral palsy in term and near-term infants. JAMA 2003;290:2677–84.

41. Bierstone D, Wagenaar N, Gano DL, et al. Association of histologic chorioamnionitis with perinatal brain injury and early childhood neurodevelopmental outcomes among preterm neonates. JAMA Pediatr 2018;172:534–41.

42. Mukhopadhyay S, Eichenwald EC, Puopolo KM. Neonatal early-onset sepsis evaluations among well-appearing infants: projected impact of changes in CDC GBS guidelines. J Perinatol 2012;33:198–205.

43. Wu YW, Croen LA, Torres AR, et al. Interleukin-6 genotype and risk for cerebral palsy in term and near-term infants. Ann Neurol 2009;66:663–70.

44. Klinger G, Chin C-, Beyene J, et al. Predicting the outcome of neonatal bacterial meningitis. Pediatrics (Evanston) 2000;106:477–82.

45. Holt DE, Halket S, de Louvois J, et al. Neonatal meningitis in england and wales: 10 years on. Arch Dis Child Fetal Neonatal Ed 2001;84:85.

46. Thigpen MC, Whitney CG, Messonnier NE, et al. Bacterial meningitis in the United States, 1998–2007. N Engl J Med 2011;364:2016–25.

47. Okike I, Ladhani S, Johnson A, et al. Clinical characteristics and risk factors for poor outcome in infants less than 90 Days of age with bacterial meningitis in the United Kingdom and Ireland. Pediatr Infect Dis J 2018;37:837–43.

48. Okike IO, Johnson AP, Henderson KL, et al. Incidence, etiology, and outcome of bacterial meningitis in infants aged. Clin Infect Dis 2014;59:150.

49. Ouchenir L, Renaud C, Khan S, et al. The epidemiology, management, and outcomes of bacterial meningitis in infants. Pediatrics (Evanston) 2017;140: e20170476.

50. Gaschignard J, Levy C, Romain O, et al. Neonatal bacterial meningitis. Pediatr Infect Dis J 2011;30:212–7.

51. De Louvois J, Halket S, Harvey D. Neonatal meningitis in England and Wales: sequelae at 5 years of age. Eur J Pediatr 2005;164:730.

52. Libster R, Edwards KM, Levent F, et al. Long-term outcomes of group B streptococcal meningitis. Pediatrics 2012;130:8.

53. Stevens JP, Eames M, Kent A, et al. Long term outcome of neonatal meningitis. Arch Dis Child Fetal Neonatal Ed 2003;88:179.

54. Heath PT, Okike IO. Neonatal bacterial meningitis: an update. Paediatrics Child Health 2010;20:526–30.

55. Harvey D, Holt DE, Bedford H. Bacterial meningitis in the newborn: a prospective study of mortality and morbidity. Semin Perinatol 1999;23:218–25.

56. de Louvois J, Blackbourn J, Hurley R, et al. Infantile meningitis in England and Wales: a two year study. Arch Dis Child 1991;66:603–7.

57. Kohli-Lynch M, Russell NJ, Seale AC, et al. Neurodevelopmental impairment in children after group B streptococcal disease worldwide: systematic review and meta-analyses. Clin Infect Dis 2017;65:S190–9.

58. Doctor BA, Newman N, Minich NM, et al. Clinical outcomes of neonatal meningitis in very-low-birth-weight infants. Clin Pediatr 2001;40:473–80.

59. Kadambari S, Trotter C, Heath PT, et al. Group B Streptococcal disease in England (1998 - 2017): a population based observational study 2020. Clin Infect Dis 2020. September 29:ciaa1485. doi: 10.1093/cid/ciaa1485. Epub ahead of print. PMID: 32989454.

60. Basmaci R, Bonacorsi S, Bidet P, et al. Escherichia coli meningitis features in 325 children from 2001 to 2013 in France. Clin Infect Dis 2015;61:779–86.

61. Greenberg RG, Benjamin DK, Cohen-Wolkowiez M, et al. Repeat lumbar punctures in infants with meningitis in the neonatal intensive care unit. J Perinatol 2010;31:425–9.

62. Levent F, Baker C, Rench M, et al. Early outcomes of group B streptococcal meningitis in the 21st century. Pediatr Infect Dis J 2010;29:1009–12.

63. Adams-Chapman I, Stoll BJ. Neonatal infection and long-term neurodevelopmental outcome in the preterm infant. Curr Opin Infect Dis 2006;19:290–7.

64. Glass TJA, Chau V, Grunau RE, et al. Multiple postnatal infections in newborns born preterm predict delayed maturation of motor pathways at term-equivalent age with poorer motor outcomes at 3 years. J Pediatr 2018;196:91–7.e1.

65. Graham EM, Holcroft CJ, Rai KK, et al. Neonatal cerebral white matter injury in preterm infants is associated with culture positive infections and only rarely with metabolic acidosis. Am J Obstet Gynecol 2004;191:1305–10.

66. Hack M, Breslau N, Weissman B, et al. Effect of very low birth weight and subnormal head size on cognitive abilities at school age. N Engl J Med 1991;325:231–7.

67. Schlapbach LJ, Aebischer M, Adams M, et al. Impact of sepsis on neurodevelopmental outcome in a Swiss National Cohort of extremely premature infants. Pediatrics 2011;128:348.

68. Benjamin DK, Stoll BJ, Fanaroff AA, et al. Neonatal candidiasis among extremely low birth weight infants: risk factors, mortality rates, and neurodevelopmental outcomes at 18 to 22 months. Pediatrics 2006;117:84–92.

69. Alshaikh B, Yee W, Lodha A, et al. Coagulase-negative staphylococcus sepsis in preterm infants and long-term neurodevelopmental outcome. J perinatology 2014;34:125–9.

70. Niemarkt HJ, De Meij TG, van Ganzewinkel C, et al. Necrotizing enterocolitis, gut microbiota, and brain development: role of the brain-gut Axis. Neonatology 2019;115:423–31.

71. Shah TA, Meinzen-Derr J, Gratton T, et al. Hospital and neurodevelopmental outcomes of extremely low-birth-weight infants with necrotizing enterocolitis and spontaneous intestinal perforation. J Perinatol 2012;32:552–8.
72. Schulzke SM, Deshpande GC, Patole SK. Neurodevelopmental outcomes of very low-birth-weight infants with necrotizing enterocolitis: a systematic review of observational studies. Arch Pediatr Adolesc Med 2007;161:583–90.
73. Hintz SR, Kendrick DE, Stoll BJ, et al. Neurodevelopmental and growth outcomes of extremely low birth weight infants after necrotizing enterocolitis. Pediatrics 2005;115:696–703.
74. Chacko J, Ford WD, Haslam R. Growth and neurodevelopmental outcome in extremely-low-birth-weight infants after laparotomy. Pediatr Surg Int 1999;15:496–9.
75. Rees CM, Pierro A, Eaton S. Neurodevelopmental outcomes of neonates with medically and surgically treated necrotizing enterocolitis. Arch Dis Child Fetal Neonatal Ed 2007;92:193.
76. Wadhawan R, Oh W, Hintz SR, et al. Neurodevelopmental outcomes of extremely low birth weight infants with spontaneous intestinal perforation or surgical necrotizing enterocolitis. J Perinatol 2014;34:64–70.
77. Adesanya OA, O'Shea TM, Turner CS, et al. Intestinal perforation in very low birth weight infants: growth and neurodevelopment at 1 year of age. J Perinatol 2005;25:583–9.
78. Blakely ML, Tyson JE, Lally KP, et al. Laparotomy versus peritoneal drainage for necrotizing enterocolitis or isolated intestinal perforation in extremely low birth weight infants: outcomes through 18 months adjusted age. Pediatrics 2006;117:680.
79. Martin CR, Dammann O, Allred EN, et al. Neurodevelopment of extremely preterm infants who had necrotizing enterocolitis with or without late bacteremia. J Pediatr 2010;157:751–6.e1.

Neonatal Herpes Simplex Virus Disease

Updates and Continued Challenges

Nicole L. Samies, DO*, Scott H. James, MD,
David W. Kimberlin, MD

KEYWORDS

- Neonatal herpes • Antiviral agents • Herpes simplex virus
- Mother-to-child transmission • HSV-1 • HSV-2

KEY POINTS

- Early recognition and prompt initiation of intravenous acyclovir can aid in reducing the morbidity and mortality in infants with neonatal herpes simplex virus (HSV) disease.
- The introduction of polymerase chain reaction has improved diagnosis of neonatal HSV disease significantly, although viral culture remains the gold standard for detection of HSV in mucocutaneous lesions and in surface swabs, pending data comparing these 2 testing modalities.
- Rapid diagnostic tests at time of delivery may prove beneficial in detecting asymptomatic shedding of HSV in the maternal genital track to prevent transmission from mother to child.
- Efforts to find a prophylactic and therapeutic vaccine for both HSV type 1 and HSV type 2 are ongoing.
- Although new antiviral agents continue to be studied for the treatment of HSV infections, acyclovir remains the current drug of choice for the treatment of neonatal HSV disease.

INTRODUCTION

Over the past 40 years, significant advancements have been made in the diagnosis and management of neonatal herpes simplex virus (HSV) disease. Despite these advancements, neonatal HSV disease continues to be associated with high rates of morbidity and mortality. In the early 2000s, approximately 1500 infants out of an estimated 4 million births were diagnosed with neonatal HSV disease each year (approximately 3.75 per 10,000 births).[1] The incidence rate has continued to rise over the past

Department of Pediatrics, Division of Pediatric Infectious Diseases, University of Alabama at Birmingham, Children's Harbor Building 308, 1600 7th Avenue South, Birmingham, AL 35233-1711, USA
* Corresponding author.
E-mail address: nsamies@uabmc.edu

Clin Perinatol 48 (2021) 263–274
https://doi.org/10.1016/j.clp.2021.03.003
perinatology.theclinics.com

several years, with the last reported incidence rate in 2015 of 5.3 infants per 10,000 births.[2] This rarity should not preclude clinicians from evaluating any infant with suspicion of neonatal HSV disease. Early recognition and prompt initiation of acyclovir have been imperative to improving outcomes in infants.[3–7] Reduction of morbidity and mortality rates and prevention of mother-to-child transmission through vaccination or other preventative measures are continuing goals. This article highlights some of the significant advancements made over the past 40 years in the diagnosis and management of neonatal HSV disease and identifies areas where current research is seeking to continue to improve outcomes and to reduce the incidence of the disease. Specific challenges that hinder improvement also are addressed.

CLASSIFICATIONS OF NEONATAL HERPES SIMPLEX VIRUS DISEASE

Neonatal HSV disease is diagnosed primarily in infants between day 10 and day 19 of age but disease has been recognized in infants up to 42 days of age.[8,9] Patients can be classified into 3 groups: (1) skin, eye, and mouth (SEM); (2) central nervous system (CNS) disease; and (3) and disseminated disease (**Table 1**). Isolated SEM disease is the most common presentation, affecting approximately 45% of those with neonatal HSV,[10] and is defined as disease that remains localized to the skin or mucosal surfaces. Infants diagnosed with SEM disease usually present for care between day 10 and day 12 of life.[11,12] Infants with CNS disease may present with irritability, seizures, temperature instability, lethargy, poor feeding, and/or skin involvement and account for approximately 30% of all neonates affected. Infants with CNS disease typically develop symptoms between day 16 and day 19 of life.[10–12] The least common, but potentially most devastating in terms of mortality, manifestation of neonatal HSV disease is disseminated disease (25% of all infections).[10] Presentation of disseminated neonatal HSV disease may be confused with bacterial sepsis or a metabolic disorder because of an infant's ill appearance and multiorgan involvement, including hepatic, pulmonary, and/or adrenal. Infants with disseminated infections may have CNS and/or mucocutaneous involvement in addition to multisystem organ involvement. Infants with disseminated disease develop symptoms between day 10 and day 12 of life.[11,12]

TRANSMISSION

Transmission of HSV to an infant occurs primarily during the perinatal period (85%) by exposure to HSV (type 1 [HSV-1] or type 2 [HSV-2]) in the birth canal, but an infant also can be exposed postnatally (10%) by direct contact to the virus through either orolabial or other cutaneous lesions or, less commonly, via an in utero exposure (5%).[13] Congenitally infected infants typically have a very severe presentation, including skin findings indicative of previous in utero infection (eg, scarring and hypo/hyperpigmented lesions), active skin lesions, microcephaly, chorioretinitis, and/or cutis aplasia.[13,14]

The risk of perinatal HSV transmission has been linked to several factors, including the timing of infection present in the pregnant woman (first-episode primary, first-episode nonprimary, or recurrent infection, as determined by maternal antibody status and virus type present in the genital tract), the use of fetal scalp electrodes, mode of delivery (vaginal vs cesarean delivery), and duration of rupture of membranes.[9,10] An infant is most at risk of perinatal acquisition of HSV infection when there is maternal primary genital HSV infection because there is inadequate time for protective immunoglobulins against HSV to be passed transplacentally to the infant. A first-episode nonprimary genital infection poses a somewhat lesser risk to an infant because the mother has HSV IgG antibodies to 1 type of HSV that provide some cross-protection to her

Table 1
Disease classifications of neonatal herpes simplex virus disease

Disease Classification	Percentage of Those Diagnosed	Typical Age at Presentation (d)	Common Clinical Presentation	Diagnosis	Treatment
SEM	45	10–12	Vesicular lesions or ulcerations on eye or mucous membranes	Skin/mucosal culture/PCR +, CSF PCR −, blood PCR ±, ALT normal	Intravenous acyclovir (60 mg/kg/d divided 3 times/d) for 14 d Followed by oral acyclovir (300 mg/m^2/dose 3 times/d) to complete a 6-mo suppressive course
CNS	30	16–19	Irritability, seizures, temperature instability, lethargy, poor feeding	Skin/mucosal culture/PCR ±, CSF PCR +[a], blood PCR ±, ALT normal	Intravenous acyclovir (60 mg/kg/d divided 3 times/d) for at least 21 d, pending negative CSF PCR near the end of therapy Followed by oral acyclovir (300 mg/m^2/dose 3 times/d) to complete a 6-mo suppressive course
Disseminated	25	10–12	Respiratory failure, encephalitis, hepatic failure, hypoperfusion, Disseminated intravascular coagulation	Skin/mucosal culture/PCR ±, CSF PCR ±, blood PCR ±, ALT elevated[b]	Intravenous acyclovir (60 mg/kg/d divided 3 times/d) for at least 21 d pending negative CSF PCR (if CSF initially was positive) near the end of therapy Followed by oral acyclovir (300 mg/m^2/dose 3 times/d) to complete a 6-mo suppressive course

[a] Neonates with a negative CSF PCR but who otherwise appear to have CNS involvement (abnormal CSF indices, presented with or developed seizures, or has abnormal neuroimaging or EEG) should be treated as CNS disease.

[b] In the setting of a positive HSV PCR from skin/mucosal swab, blood, or CSF or HSV isolated from viral culture of skin or mucosal swab.

"+" refers to a positive test result.

"−" refers to a negative test result.

"±" refers to either a positive or negative test result.

newly acquired HSV type (eg, a pregnant mother previously had HSV-2 and newly acquires HSV-1 near delivery). Recurrent genital HSV infection, which is the most common form of HSV genital infection in pregnancy, refers to the reactivation of a previously acquired HSV type (as determined by existing maternal antibodies).[9,13] Determining the risk of mother-to-child transmission continues to be difficult because of the inability to detect asymptomatic shedding at time of delivery.

Historically, HSV-2 was associated with genital herpes and HSV-1 with orolabial infections, but over the past 2 decades HSV-1 has become the predominate cause of genital infections in Europe and the United States. The reasoning behind the increase in HSV-1 genital infections is secondary to changing sexual practices, with an increase in oral-genital contact and a lower incidence of HSV-1 orolabial infections during childhood.[15] Sacral ganglia reactivation of HSV-1 is less common than HSV-2. Therefore, HSV-1 may be associated with an increased risk of neonatal transmission, because, when present, HSV-1 genital lesions are more likely to represent a first-episode primary or a first-episode nonprimary infection in the pregnant woman, both of which are associated with a 10-fold to 30-fold increased risk of transmission to the neonate compared with a recurrent episode.[16]

DISCUSSION
Current Diagnostic Recommendations

The recommendations provided by the American Academy of Pediatrics Committee on Infectious Diseases for evaluating an infant with suspected neonatal HSV disease have continued to evolve. The introduction of new diagnostic tests, increasing knowledge of the pathogenicity and epidemiology of HSV, and disease presentation in neonates have resulted in revised recommendations for evaluation and management of neonates with known or suspected HSV infection. The current recommendations for diagnostic evaluation of infants with suspected HSV infection include (1) viral culture and polymerase chain reaction (PCR) from any mucocutaneous lesion concerning for HSV; (2) viral culture and PCR of swabs of conjunctiva, nasopharyngeal mucosa, oral mucosa, and anal mucosa (often collectively referred to as surface swabs); (3) cerebrospinal fluid (CSF) HSV PCR; (4) whole-blood HSV PCR; and (5) an alanine aminotransferase (ALT) level.[17] Infants with suspected HSV infection should empirically receive intravenous acyclovir, 20 mg/kg/dose every 8 hours, while awaiting the results of the recommended HSV studies. If a lumbar puncture is unable to be performed due to clinical instability in an infant undergoing HSV evaluation or a lumbar puncture was attempted but CSF was unable to be obtained, empiric acyclovir should not be withheld. In such cases, a lumbar puncture should be performed as early as possible to obtain CSF indices and evaluate the CSF for HSV DNA.

The introduction of PCR has revolutionized the process of diagnosing neonatal HSV disease, especially CNS disease. Prior to the availability of PCR, the diagnosis of CNS disease was dependent on viral culture and invasive measures, such as brain biopsy.[18,19] In the mid-1990s, studies evaluating the sensitivity and specificity of HSV PCR in CSF were performed and demonstrated the utility of the diagnostic test in detecting HSV DNA in the CSF of infants; prior to the availability of molecular testing, many neonates without obvious CNS symptoms likely were managed as if they had SEM disease.[20] A negative CSF PCR, however, does not eliminate CNS involvement, especially if the CSF indices, neuroimaging, or electroencephalogram (EEG) monitoring is abnormal, or if the patient has or develops seizures.[20]

PCR also has been used in the detection of HSV DNA in blood as an additional tool for diagnosis of neonatal HSV infection.[21] Detection of HSV DNA in the blood of neonates indicates infection but does not correlate with classification of disease; neonates may be viremic (and hence DNAemic) with isolated SEM or CNS disease. A positive HSV blood PCR result may be helpful to detect the presence of HSV DNA in neonates who may not have other diagnostic or clinical evidence of infection.[22–24]

The current recommendation for testing mucocutaneous lesions and surface swabs (specimens from mouth, nasopharynx, conjunctiva, and anus) is to perform both viral culture and molecular testing on these specimens because the sensitivity and specificity of PCR have not yet been established in infants. PCR has replaced viral culture in many institutions, however, due to the unavailability of viral culture facilities[25] as well as the more rapid turnaround time for molecular testing results. PCR test results typically are reported within 24 hours of sample collection whereas a viral culture may take between 2 days and 5 days to be reported.[9] Cultures also are more likely to be negative during the later stages (ulceration and crusting) of skin lesions whereas PCR testing is more likely to detect HSV DNA in more mature lesions where viral burden may be reduced.[26] Additional studies are needed to evaluate the sensitivity of PCR versus culture for skin and mucous membrane specimens in neonates.

Treatment

Over the past 40 years, treatment of neonatal herpes has improved significantly, with a corresponding reduction in morbidity and mortality. Prior to the use of antiviral agents for treatment of neonatal HSV disease, the mortality rate ranged from 50% to 85% in CNS and disseminated disease, respectively.[1] An older antiviral, vidarabine, proved effective in randomized controlled trials in the late 1970s.[3,4] In the 1980s, acyclovir, a nucleoside analog, was evaluated for the treatment of neonatal HSV disease and subsequently has become the mainstay of treatment.[6,27] Currently, high-dose acyclovir (60 mg/kg/d divided every 8 hours) reduces mortality to 4% in those with CNS disease and to 30% with disseminated disease.[27] Further reduction in mortality also can be achieved by initiating high-dose acyclovir within the first day of hospitalization rather than delaying to day 2 or day 3 while awaiting confirmatory test results.[7]

Duration of therapy is a minimum of 21 days of intravenous therapy in those with CNS and disseminated disease and 14 days for SEM disease.[28] Prior to discontinuing therapy at 21 days in neonates with an initial positive CSF HSV PCR, a repeat lumbar puncture is recommended to document clearance of viral DNA. If HSV DNA still is detected, the infant should receive an additional 7 days of weight-adjusted intravenous acyclovir and have a repeat lumbar puncture performed at the end of the fourth week of therapy to document clearance of HSV DNA. The extension of therapy for an additional 7 days followed by a repeat lumbar puncture should continue until clearance of viral DNA from the CSF is demonstrated.[29] Neonates who are receiving treatment with intravenous acyclovir should be hospitalized for the duration of their therapy to monitor for adverse effects of acyclovir including neutropenia and renal toxicity, which is reversible, as well as other clinical complications.[27] Following the completion of intravenous acyclovir, infants are transitioned to oral suppressive therapy with acyclovir for a 6-month course. This recommendation is based on the findings of a randomized, placebo-controlled study that infants who received oral suppressive acyclovir therapy had improved neurologic outcomes and fewer skin recurrences than infants who did not receive suppressive therapy.[30]

Other oral nucleoside analogs, valacyclovir and famciclovir, are available for use in HSV infections, specifically genital lesions, but have not been studied in neonatal HSV disease. Valacyclovir, the prodrug of acyclovir, is an oral agent that has improved bioavailability compared with oral acyclovir, but its pharmacokinetic profile in neonates is not yet known. The pharmacokinetics of valacyclovir have been evaluated down to 1 month of age, but variability in drug exposure in very young infants has limited dosing recommendations to infants 3 months and older.[31] Additional studies evaluating the pharmacokinetics of valacyclovir in neonates are needed prior to any recommendations being made on its use.

Two additional parenteral antiviral agents, cidofovir and foscarnet, are associated with significant toxicity and typically are reserved for the treatment of acyclovir-resistant HSV infections in immunocompromised patients.[32,33] Resistance of HSV to acyclovir to date is reported mainly in immunocompromised patients and not frequently in neonates[28]; therefore, these antiviral agents rarely are used in the neonatal population. Newer antiviral agents currently in development, brincidofovir and pritelivir, have been evaluated for the use in HSV disease. Brincidofovir, an orally bioavailable lipid acyclic nucleotide phosphonate, poses a possibility for use in HSV infections because its intracellular conversion to cidofovir diminishes the renal toxicity associated with the administration of cidofovir. Unlike cidofovir, however, brincidofovir was noted to cause significant gastrointestinal disturbances in stem cell transplant patients, and this has limited its further development.[33,34] Pritelivir is a helicase-primase inhibitor that offers a novel approach to preventing HSV replication and provides promise in treating HSV infections. One study evaluated its use in genital infections and noted a decrease in viral shedding and symptomatic lesions in those receiving higher doses of the novel antiviral agent.[35] Currently, no studies have evaluated its use in neonates, but it may pose a future option for use in pregnant women or seropositive partners in hopes of decreasing asymptomatic shedding of the virus and transmission to the neonate.

Combination therapies also have been considered for the treatment of severe HSV infections, with the addition of another antiviral agent to acyclovir in an effort to further reduce mortality.[28] This approach has not yet been addressed in neonates but is a possible future consideration that will require the accumulation of pharmacokinetic data.

How Can Neonatal Herpes Simplex Virus Disease Be Prevented?

In order to reduce mother-to-child transmission of HSV infection, the American College of Obstetricians and Gynecologists (ACOG) recommends cesaren delivery in all women noted to have active genital lesions or prodromal symptoms at time of labor, even if rupture of membranes already has occurred.[36] Cesarean delivery is not routinely recommended to reduce peripartum transmission in women with a history of recurrent genital herpes without active lesions at onset of labor, although, in order to account for the possible risk of prolonged viral shedding, it may be considered in women who have primary or nonprimary first-episode genital infection at any point during the third trimester.[36]

ACOG also recommends that suppressive antiviral therapy be started at 36 weeks' gestation in pregnant women who have a prior history of HSV genital lesions.[36] This therapy aids in reduction of active genital lesions at time of delivery in women with a prior history of genital herpes. Yet antenatal suppressive therapy does not completely prevent asymptomatic shedding at time of delivery and it also does not prevent transmission from HSV infections acquired late in pregnancy.[13,37] HSV infections have occurred in neonates born to women receiving antiviral suppressive therapy.[38]

Identification of pregnant women who are asymptomatically shedding HSV at the time of delivery would be beneficial in preventing mother-to-child transmission. Obtaining prenatal or perinatal genital cultures from pregnant women does not predict which women will be asymptomatically shedding at time of delivery.[37,39] The

Step 1: Obstetrician to collect a swab of maternal genital lesion and send for culture, HSV PCR, and HSV typing. Maternal serology to also be sent for HSV-1 and HSV-2 to determine type of maternal HSV infection.

    First-Episode Primary: genital lesion positive for HSV-1 or HSV-2 **AND** maternal antibody negative for both HSV-1 or HSV-2

    First-Episode NonPrimary: genital lesion positive for HSV-1 **AND** maternal antibody negative for HSV-1 but positive for HSV-2

                                              OR

          genital lesion positive for HSV-2 **AND** maternal antibody negative for HSV-2 but positive for HSV-1

    Recurrent: genital lesion positive for HSV-1 **AND** maternal antibody positive for HSV-1

                                              OR

    genital lesion positive for HSV-2 **AND** maternal antibody positive for HSV-2

Step 2: While awaiting maternal testing of genital lesion and serology, determine if mother had a prior history of genital lesions.

    A: If mother reports prior history of HSV: 1) obtain swabs for HSV cultures <u>AND</u> PCR from conjunctiva, nasopharynx, mouth, and anus on infant at 24 hours of life **PLUS** 2) HSV blood PCR. Do not automatically start IV acyclovir.

        1. If any above return positive, finish evaluation of infant with LP for CSF studies including HSV PCR and obtain serum ALT. Start IV acyclovir 20 mg/kg/dose every 8 hours and continue based on disease classification.
        2. If testing on infant remains negative, educate parents on neonatal HSV disease and arrange for close follow up.

    B: If mother reports **no** prior history of HSV: 1) obtain swabs for HSV cultures <u>AND</u> PCR from conjunctiva, nasopharynx, mouth, and anus on infant at 24 hours of life **PLUS** 2) HSV blood PCR **PLUS** 3) perform an LP for CSF to send for cell count, glucose, protein, and HSV PCR **PLUS** 4) obtain a serum ALT **PLUS** 5) start IV acyclovir 20 mg/kg/dose every 8 hours.

        1. If mother's genital lesion is determined to be a recurrent infection and all neonatal testing remains negative, stop IV acyclovir, educate family on neonatal HSV disease, and arrange for close follow up.
        2. If mother's genital lesion is determined to be a recurrent infection and the neonatal surface culture/PCR is positive, but CSF indices are normal, CSF and blood PCR are negative, ALT is normal, and infant remains asymptomatic, treat preemptively with IV acyclovir for a total of 10 days.
        3. If mother's genital lesion is determined to be a recurrent infection and neonate is symptomatic, surface culture/PCR is positive, CSF indices are abnormal, CSF and/or blood PCR are positive, and/or ALT is abnormal, continue IV acyclovir for 14–21 days, with the duration being based on disease classification.
        4. If mother's genital lesion is determined to be a first-episode primary/first-episode nonprimary and the neonatal surface culture/PCR is positive but the CSF indices are normal, CSF and blood PCR are negative, ALT is normal, and infant remains asymptomatic, treat preemptively with IV acyclovir for a total of 10 days.
        5. If mother's genital lesion is determined to be a first-episode primary/first-episode nonprimary and baby is symptomatic, surface culture/PCR is positive, CSF indices are abnormal, CSF and/or blood PCR are positive, and/or ALT is abnormal, continue IV acyclovir for 14–21 days, with the duration being based on disease classification.

Fig. 1. Steps to managing infants born to mothers with active genital lesions at delivery.

turnaround time from specimen collection to result for both culture and PCR testing precludes both from being practical informants of delivery modality. As a result, culture and PCR are not performed routinely at time of labor to assess for asymptomatic shedding. The introduction of a rapid, point-of-care molecular diagnostic test designed to screen for asymptomatic shedding of HSV at the onset of labor would be valuable in determining mode of delivery, benefit of intrapartum antiviral therapy, and in consideration of neonatal antiviral prophylaxis.[13,40] One multicenter clinical trial (ClinicalTrials Identifier: NCT01878383) is evaluating the use of a point-of-care PCR diagnostic in pregnant women at onset of labor; the results of this study currently are pending publication.

When evaluating the risk of transmission to an infant, relying on history to determine a maternal history of genital HSV infection is ineffective because a majority of women with infants who have neonatal HSV disease are unaware of having had a prior genital HSV infection.[37,41] The use of serology at time of delivery in women with active genital lesions may assist with classification as a first-episode primary, first-episode nonprimary, or recurrent infection. Serology performed at prenatal appointments could identify seronegative pregnant women who might benefit from counseling on strategies to prevent exposure during the third trimester, because this period of gestation poses the highest risk of mother-to-child transmission. Serology also could aid in counseling seropositive women to recognize the subtle symptoms of a reactivation,[41] and perhaps knowledge of seropositivity might decrease the use of fetal scalp electrodes.[10] The programmatic complexities of serologic assessments of pregnant women and their partners during pregnancy and the interpretation of reactive HSV-1 serology in a person who likely had HSV-1 disease as a child, however, are challenging.

The American Academy of Pediatrics published guidance in 2013 with recommendations for the evaluation and management of infants born to women with active genital lesions at the time of delivery (**Fig. 1**). This document bases the assessment of an infant's risk for developing HSV disease on classification of maternal genital infection as a primary, first-episode nonprimary, or recurrent episode and provides guidance for diagnostics and antiviral management.[9]

Vaccine Development

A vaccine is the most effective way to prevent mother-to-child transmission of HSV. A preventative vaccine that prevents acquisition of HSV-1 and HSV-2 in a seronegative woman and a therapeutic vaccine that decreases the likelihood of viral shedding in those who are seropositive each would have a substantial impact on the incidence of neonatal HSV infection and disease. One recent therapeutic vaccine demonstrated reduction in viral shedding and duration of symptomatic lesions, but these reductions were temporary.[42] Another recent therapeutic vaccine candidate being studied, HSV529, has had promising response in seronegative individuals, but continued efforts are being made to improve its immunogenicity.[43] Vaccine research remains an area of interest to both obstetricians and neonatologists, with several candidate vaccines under evaluation.

SUMMARY

Although understanding of neonatal HSV disease has grown exponentially over the past 40 years, with gains in diagnostics, treatment, and prevention, a rising incidence rate and continued poor outcomes in affected neonates are concerning. The need for further advances in point-of-care diagnostics and vaccination that could be applied to the prevention of mother-to-child transmission of HSV as well as efforts to optimize management to decrease the morbidity and mortality of infants with neonatal HSV disease continues to be a high priority.

CLINICS CARE POINTS

- Early detection is key to improving the morbidity and mortality of neonatal HSV disease.
- Culture remains the gold standard currently for evaluation of mucocutaneous lesions and surface swabs in neonates while the sensitivity of PCR in the detection of HSV DNA for these specimens continues to be evaluated.

- PCR has improved diagnosis of neonatal HSV CNS disease vastly. Neonatal HSV CNS infection may be diagnosed based on clinical presentation or other laboratory parameters, even if the CSF HSV PCR is negative.
- A blood PCR to detect HSV DNA is a helpful adjunct to detecting viremia in neonates without notable signs and symptoms of HSV infection.
- Mother-to-child transmission of HSV is highly dependent on timing and classification of maternal infection.
- Intravenous acyclovir is the mainstay of treatment of neonatal HSV disease.
- Despite multiple vaccine research trials, no vaccine has yet proved beneficial.

Best practices

What is the current practice for Neonatal Herpes Simplex Virus Disease?

Best Practice/Guideline/Care Path Objective(s) For Neonates Suspected of Having HSV Disease:
- Promptly evaluate any infant with suspected HSV disease with the following diagnostic tests: (1) viral culture and PCR on "surface swabs" and any mucocutaneous lesion if present, (2) CSF HSV PCR, (3) whole blood HSV PCR, and (4) serum ALT level.
- Initiate IV acyclovir 20 mg/kg/dose every 8 hours as soon as possible while awaiting results of diagnostic tests.
- In an infant suspected of having neonatal HSV disease, do not delay starting IV acyclovir therapy if unable to obtain CSF for HSV PCR testing. A lumbar puncture should be repeated or performed as soon as clinically able.
- Duration of IV acyclovir is dependent upon disease classification- 14 days for SEM disease and a minimum of 21 days for CNS and disseminated disease.
- A repeat lumbar puncture should be performed in all infants with an initial positive CSF HSV PCR near the end of 21 days of IV acyclovir to evaluate for clearance of viral DNA; continued PCR-positivity from CSF necessitates continuation of IV acyclovir for at least another 7 days, with another repeat lumbar puncture near the end of that extension of parenteral therapy (consultation with a pediatric infectious diseases specialist is advised in this situation).
- Upon completion of treatment course with IV acyclovir, all infants should be transitioned to suppressive therapy with oral acyclovir for 6 months to improve neurodevelopmental outcomes and reduce skin recurrences.

What changes in current practice are likely to improve outcomes?

- Have a heightened awareness of neonatal HSV in order to identify any infants who should be evaluated for neonatal HSV disease.
- Begin IV acyclovir without delay in such neonates.

Is there a Clinical Algorithm? If so, please include

See Fig. 1.

Bibliographic Source(s): [1,9,12,13,27,31,37,41]

DISCLOSURE

SHJ reports prior consulting fees from Bayer, outside the scope of this work.

REFERENCES

1. Kimberlin DW. Neonatal herpes simplex infection. Clin Microbiol Rev 2004; 17(1):1–13.

2. Mahant S, Hall M, Schondelmeyer AC, et al. Neonatal herpes simplex virus infection among medicaid-enrolled children: 2009-2015. Pediatrics 2019;143(4): e20183233.

3. Whitley RJ, Nahmias AJ, Soong SJ, et al. Vidarabine therapy of neonatal herpes simplex virus infection. Pediatrics 1980;66(4):495–501.

4. Whitley RJ, Yeager A, Kartus P, et al. Neonatal herpes simplex virus infection: follow-up evaluation of vidarabine therapy. Pediatrics 1983;72(6):778–85.

5. Whitley RJ, Corey L, Arvin A, et al. Changing presentation of herpes simplex virus infection in neonates. J Infect Dis 1988;158(1):109–16.

6. Whitley R, Arvin A, Prober C, et al. A controlled trial comparing vidarabine with acyclovir in neonatal herpes simplex virus infection. Infectious Diseases Collaborative Antiviral Study Group. N Engl J Med 1991;324(7):444–9.

7. Shah SS, Aronson PL, Mohamad Z, et al. Delayed acyclovir therapy and death among neonates with herpes simplex virus infection. Pediatrics 2011;128(6): 1153–60.

8. Curfman AL, Glissmeyer EW, Ahmad FA, et al. Initial presentation of neonatal herpes simplex virus infection. J Pediatr 2016;172:121–126 e1.

9. Kimberlin DW, Baley J, Committee on Infectious D, et al. Guidance on management of asymptomatic neonates born to women with active genital herpes lesions. Pediatrics 2013;131(2):383–6.

10. Corey L, Wald A. Maternal and neonatal herpes simplex virus infections. N Engl J Med 2009;361(14):1376–85.

11. Pinninti SG, Kimberlin DW. Management of neonatal herpes simplex virus infection and exposure. Arch Dis Child Fetal Neonatal Ed 2014;99(3):F240–4.

12. Kimberlin DW, Lin CY, Jacobs RF, et al. Natural history of neonatal herpes simplex virus infections in the acyclovir era. Pediatrics 2001;108(2):223–9.

13. James SH, Sheffield JS, Kimberlin DW. Mother-to-Child transmission of herpes simplex virus. J Pediatr Infect Dis Soc 2014;3(Suppl 1):S19–23.

14. Hutto C, Arvin A, Jacobs R, et al. Intrauterine herpes simplex virus infections. J Pediatr 1987;110(1):97–101.

15. Looker KJ, Magaret AS, May MT, et al. Global and Regional estimates of prevalent and incident herpes simplex virus type 1 infections in 2012. PLoS One 2015; 10(10):e0140765.

16. Gardella C, Brown Z. Prevention of neonatal herpes. BJOG 2011;118(2):187–92.

17. American Academy of Pediatrics. Herpes Simplex. In: Kimberlin DW, Brady MT, Jackson MA, et al. Red Book: 2018 Report of the Committee on Infectious Diseases. 31st edition. Itasca (IL): American Academy of Pediatrics; 2018: 437-49.

18. Malm G, Forsgren M. Neonatal herpes simplex virus infections: HSV DNA in cerebrospinal fluid and serum. Arch Dis Child Fetal Neonatal Ed 1999;81(1):F24–9.

19. Lakeman FD, Whitley RJ. Diagnosis of herpes simplex encephalitis: application of polymerase chain reaction to cerebrospinal fluid from brain-biopsied patients and correlation with disease. National Institute of Allergy and Infectious Diseases Collaborative Antiviral Study Group. J Infect Dis 1995;171(4):857–63.

20. Kimberlin DW, Lakeman FD, Arvin AM, et al. Application of the polymerase chain reaction to the diagnosis and management of neonatal herpes simplex virus disease. National Institute of Allergy and Infectious Diseases Collaborative Antiviral Study Group. J Infect Dis 1996;174(6):1162–7.

21. Diseases ACoI, Pickering LK, Baker CJ, Kimberlin DW, et al. Red book. 29th Edition 2012. p. 1098.

22. Samies N, Jariwala R, Boppana S, et al. Utility of surface and blood polymerase chain reaction assays in identifying infants with neonatal herpes simplex virus infection. Pediatr Infect Dis J 2019;38(11):1138–40.
23. Diamond C, Mohan K, Hobson A, et al. Viremia in neonatal herpes simplex virus infections. Pediatr Infect Dis J 1999;18(6):487–9.
24. Lyons TW, Cruz AT, Freedman SB, et al. Herpes simplex virus study group of the pediatric emergency medicine collaborative research C. Accuracy of herpes simplex virus polymerase chain reaction testing of the blood for central nervous system herpes simplex virus infections in infants. J Pediatr 2018;200:274–276 e1.
25. Dominguez SR, Pretty K, Hengartner R, et al. Comparison of herpes simplex virus PCR with culture for virus detection in multisource surface swab specimens from neonates. J Clin Microbiol 2018;56(10):e00632.
26. Scoular A, Gillespie G, Carman WF. Polymerase chain reaction for diagnosis of genital herpes in a genitourinary medicine clinic. Sex Transm Infect 2002; 78(1):21–5.
27. Kimberlin DW, Lin CY, Jacobs RF, et al. Safety and efficacy of high-dose intravenous acyclovir in the management of neonatal herpes simplex virus infections. Pediatrics 2001;108(2):230–8.
28. Whitley R, Baines J. Clinical management of herpes simplex virus infections: past, present, and future. F1000Res 2018;7.
29. Pinninti SG, Kimberlin DW. Neonatal herpes simplex virus infections. Pediatr Clin North Am 2013;60(2):351–65.
30. Kimberlin DW, Whitley RJ, Wan W, et al. Oral acyclovir suppression and neurodevelopment after neonatal herpes. N Engl J Med 2011;365(14):1284–92.
31. Kimberlin DW, Jacobs RF, Weller S, et al. Pharmacokinetics and safety of extemporaneously compounded valacyclovir oral suspension in pediatric patients from 1 month through 11 years of age. Clin Infect Dis 2010;50(2):221–8.
32. Strasfeld L, Chou S. Antiviral drug resistance: mechanisms and clinical implications. Infect Dis Clin North Am 2010;24(3):809–33.
33. De SK, Hart JC, Breuer J. Herpes simplex virus and varicella zoster virus: recent advances in therapy. Curr Opin Infect Dis 2015;28(6):589–95.
34. Marty FM, Winston DJ, Rowley SD, et al. CMX001 to prevent cytomegalovirus disease in hematopoietic-cell transplantation. N Engl J Med 2013;369(13):1227–36.
35. Wald A, Corey L, Timmler B, et al. Helicase-primase inhibitor pritelivir for HSV-2 infection. N Engl J Med 2014;370(3):201–10.
36. Management of genital herpes in pregnancy: ACOG practice bullotinaoog practice bulletin, Number 220. Obstet Gynecol 2020;135(5):e193–202.
37. Prober CG, Hensleigh PA, Boucher FD, et al. Use of routine viral cultures at delivery to identify neonates exposed to herpes simplex virus. N Engl J Med 1988; 318(14):887–91.
38. Pinninti SG, Angara R, Feja KN, et al. Neonatal herpes disease following maternal antenatal antiviral suppressive therapy: a multicenter case series. J Pediatr 2012; 161(1):134–8, e1-3.
39. Arvin AM, Hensleigh PA, Prober CG, et al. Failure of antepartum maternal cultures to predict the infant's risk of exposure to herpes simplex virus at delivery. N Engl J Med 1986;315(13):796–800.
40. Brown ZA, Wald A, Morrow RA, et al. Effect of serologic status and cesarean delivery on transmission rates of herpes simplex virus from mother to infant. JAMA 2003;289(2):203–9.

41. Brown ZA, Benedetti JK, Watts DH, et al. A comparison between detailed and simple histories in the diagnosis of genital herpes complicating pregnancy. Am J Obstet Gynecol 1995;172(4 Pt 1):1299–303.
42. Bernstein DI, Wald A, Warren T, et al. Therapeutic vaccine for genital herpes simplex virus-2 infection: findings from a randomized trial. J Infect Dis 2017;215(6): 856–64.
43. Dropulic LK, Oestreich MC, Pietz HL, et al. A randomized, double-blinded, placebo-controlled, phase 1 study of a replication-defective herpes simplex virus (HSV) type 2 vaccine, HSV529, in adults with or without HSV infection. J Infect Dis 2019;220(6):990–1000.

HIV in Neonates and Infants

Andres F. Camacho-Gonzalez, MD, MSc[a],*, Paul Palumbo, MD[b]

KEYWORDS

- HIV • Neonates • Prevention • Treatment

KEY POINTS

- Current perinatal HIV prevention strategies are effective, raising the possibility of eliminating mother-to-child transmission of HIV.
- Testing and early identification of infected pregnant women needs to be prioritized as the first pillar of the neonatal HIV prevention cascade
- Newer HIV therapies are becoming available and will increase the effectiveness of the treatment and prevention of neonatal HIV.

HISTORY, EPIDEMIOLOGY, AND ELIMINATION OF MOTHER-TO-CHILD TRANSMISSION

Historical Perspective

The initial recognition of AIDS in select populations in the early 1980s was soon recognized to be an issue for the broader, general population. Early cases suggesting maternal-to-infant transmission were met with disbelief, but case series from New Jersey, the Bronx, and Miami established vertical HIV transmission as a worrisome reality.[1–3] As the epidemic rapidly expanded in the 1980s, fueled in part by intravenous drug use, the number of newborns with HIV infection increased strikingly. In this setting, newly designed HIV diagnostics—serology, viral culture, and ultimately HIV polymerase chain reaction—were applied to the maternal–infant setting to identify affected individuals, even though prevention and treatment modalities were very limited or nonexistent.

A single antiviral agent—azidothymidine (AZT), zidovudine—derived from the anticancer viral research program at Burroughs Wellcome and, through collaborative testing with the National Cancer Institute, in vitro activity against HIV was demonstrated.[4] It was quickly taken up by investigative teams, prominently at the National Cancer Institute and by members of the AIDS Clinical Trials Group (ACTG), organized by the Division of AIDS at the National Institutes for Health, for the treatment of adults with HIV infection. Pediatric investigators within the ACTG jumpstarted phase I and II

[a] Division of Pediatric Infectious Diseases, Children's Healthcare of Atlanta, Emory University School of Medicine, 2015 Uppergate Drive, Suite 500, Atlanta, GA 30322, USA; [b] Section of Infectious Diseases and International Health, Geisel School of Medicine at Dartmouth, 1 Medical Center Drive, Lebanon, NH 03756, USA
* Corresponding author.
E-mail address: ACAMAC2@emory.edu

Clin Perinatol 48 (2021) 275–292
https://doi.org/10.1016/j.clp.2021.03.004
0095-5108/21/© 2021 Elsevier Inc. All rights reserved.
perinatology.theclinics.com

clinical trials targeting safety and dosing in children. As the only available antiviral in the mid and late 1980s, desperate clinician investigators boldly considered the possibility of using AZT for the prevention of maternal-to-child HIV transmission. The concept of administering a nucleic acid transcriptase–targeting compound to pregnant women and their fetuses was a concern. Ultimately, risk–benefit and ethical considerations led to the ACTG 076 trial (conducted in the United States and France), which administered, in a placebo-controlled fashion, oral AZT to pregnant women ($\geq$14 weeks gestation), intravenous AZT during labor, and oral AZT to their newborns for 6 weeks. Enrollment began in April 1991 and prematurely ended in December 1993 when an interim Data Safety Monitoring Board review detected a two-thirds protective effect in treatment versus placebo recipients.[5] The Centers for Disease Control and Prevention and the US Public Health Service quickly incorporated intrapartum AZT into standard of care. The 076 trial is arguably the most impactful HIV prevention trial during the first few decades of the HIV epidemic, responsible for preventing millions of transmissions globally.

The logistics of implementing 076 globally, especially in resource-limited settings, led to scaled down, short-course versions. Another milestone study, especially for regions where 076 implementation posed challenges, was the HIVNET 012 study conducted in Uganda from 1997 to 1999.[6] This comparative peripartum prevention trial randomized participants either to short course AZT (oral AZT to mother during labor and daily oral AZT to newborn for 7 days) versus single dose nevirapine (NVP) to mother while in labor and single dose NVP to her newborn within 72 hours of birth. Significant benefit was demonstrated for NVP over AZT through 16 weeks of life in this breastfeeding population (transmission risk of 25% vs 13%; relative efficacy rate of NVP compared with AZT = 47%). Interestingly, this beneficial effect was sustained through 18 months of life.[7]

Epidemiology

The understanding of mother-to-child transmission (MTCT) of HIV and the development and implementation of prevention programs have decreased the rates of transmission in both resource-available and resource-challenged countries in a way that the elimination of MTCT has become a possibility and a reality. Countries like Armenia, Belarus, Thailand, Cuba, and other Caribbean territories have effectively eliminated MTCT and have mapped the way for other countries to follow by combining strong public health approaches, political leadership, funding, and a coordinated effort.[8] In resource-available regions of the world, very low numbers of MTCT have been documented, with the Centers for Disease Control and Prevention reporting 39 HIV-infected children via MTCT identified in the United States in 2017.[9] Although remarkable progress has been accomplished regarding prevention of MTCT, it has been challenging to reach World Health Organization (WHO)–targeted goals, with approximately 150,000 new MTC infections recorded in 2019. Currently global antiretroviral therapy (ART) coverage in pregnant women is estimated to be 85%, a significant increase from 2010 levels, when only 45% of women were covered. A remaining challenge is that only 50% of HIV-exposed infants are tested by 2 months of age.[10] To continue the progress toward the elimination of MTCT, efforts are needed to enhance identification and ART coverage of infected mothers and their infants, as well as further advances in program implementation.

PREVENTION OF MOTHER-TO-CHILD TRANSMISSION OF HIV

Very early in the course of the disease, we learned that without intervention approximately 20% of formula-fed infants are infected, with one-third infected in utero and the remaining two-thirds infected during the peripartum period.[11,12] Postpartum transmission via breastfeeding increases transmission rates by another 20% to 25%, with increased risk during the initial lactation period, because a higher concentration of cell-associated virus exists in the colostrum, and with longer duration of breastfeeding.[13] Regardless of the transmission period, the major risk factor for neonatal infection is the level of maternal viral replication, and therefore every effort to achieve viral control is essential.[14]

Testing and Early Identification

The French perinatal study showed that there was a zero percent risk of MTCT of HIV when treatment and viral control was achieved before conception, with increased residual transmission risk, depending on which trimester of pregnancy antiretroviral treatment was initiated, regardless of achieving undetectable level of the virus at the time of delivery (**Table 1**).[14,15] Based on these findings, early testing (preconception or first trimester of pregnancy) becomes highly desirable, but unfortunately is not always achievable. The current guidelines recommend testing pregnant women at first health care encounter and also in the third trimester and during breastfeeding, based on studies that show increased risk of HIV acquisition per condom-less act during late pregnancy (adjusted risk ratio, 2.82; $P = .01$) and the postpartum period (adjusted risk ratio, 3.97; $P = .01$).[16–18] Concepts such as the perinatal HIV prevention cascade not only recognize the ideal scenario of preconception testing and viral control, but also highlight missed opportunities throughout pregnancy and delivery and the importance of multilevel interventions that can impact newborn transmission rates at each step of the cascade (**Fig. 1**).[19]

Antiretroviral Therapy Strategies

ART strategies for prevention of MTCT include both a "pre-exposure prophylaxis" (mother on ART) and "postexposure prophylaxis" (infant on ART) approach. Our understanding of ART pharmacokinetics and pharmacodynamics during both pregnancy and the early neonatal period (especially if preterm) is limited because only few ARTs have been studied during this period. In general, the recommendation for pregnant women is to continue the same treatment, but if the infection is newly identified during pregnancy then certain ARTs are preferred over others.[16] For neonates, the choice of ART depends on the transmission risk as established by maternal viral load close to delivery as well as gestational age (**Table 2**). For those neonates considered to be high risk (born to mothers with no antepartum or intrapartum ART or in whom viral control near delivery is not achieved, mothers who received only intrapartum ART,

Table 1 Transmission rate based on initiation of ART		
Maternal ART Timing	Percentage Positive (Confidence Interval)	Odds Ratio
Preconception	0.2 (0.06–0.4)	1
First trimester	0.4 (0.09–1.2)	2.9
Second trimester	0.9 (0.5–1.3)	6
Third trimester	2.2 (1.4–3.3)	7.8

Data from Connor EM, Sperling RS, Gelber R, et al. Reduction of maternal-infant transmission of human immunodeficiency virus type 1 with zidovudine treatment. Pediatric AIDS Clinical Trials Group Protocol 076 Study Group. N Engl J Med. 1994;331(18):1173 to 1180.

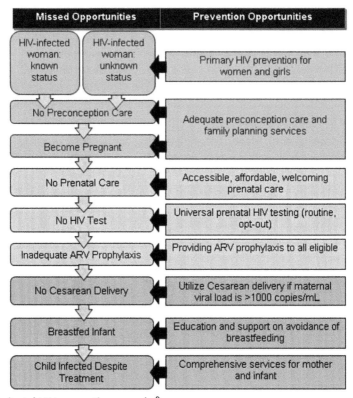

Fig. 1. Perinatal HIV prevention cascade.[9]

mothers with acute HIV infection during pregnancy, or infants who are breastfed), presumptive HIV therapy with triple ART should be started to complete 6 weeks of therapy (see **Table 2**). For neonates considered to be low risk (born to mothers who received ART during pregnancy with a viral load near delivery of <50 copies/mL and no concerns about ART adherence) ART prophylaxis with 4 weeks of zidovudine should be provided (see **Table 2**).

Breastfeeding

Despite our understanding that HIV can be transmitted through breastfeeding, safer alternatives may not be available or may not be possible in culturally sensitive areas, and the risk of death from malnutrition, diarrhea, or pneumonia may exceed the risks of potential HIV transmission. Multiple studies have shown significant decreases in transmission when ART therapy is administered to the breastfeeding mother, the infant, or both. The postpartum PROMISE study showed transmission rates of less than 1% with either maternal triple ART while breastfeeding or daily infant NVP, after 18 months of exclusive breastfeeding.[20] Similarly, a study in rural Tanzania showed no HIV transmission among infants whose mothers received triple ART while breastfeeding.[21] The success of breastfeeding strategies in resource-constrained countries has questioned the need to avoid breastfeeding by HIV-infected women in high-income countries. US guidelines continue to advocate for exclusive formula feeding as a zero percent risk strategy, highlighting concerns that cell-associated virus may still pose some transmission risk.[16,22]

Table 2
Antiretroviral prophylaxis regimens and dosing recommendations based on maternal risk and gestational age

Medication	Duration	Gestational Age	Dosing[a]
Low Risk			
AZT[b]	4 wk	≥ 35 wk	4 mg/kg/dose
		≥30–<35 wk	Birth–age 2 wk: 2 mg/kg/dose
			2 weeks–4 weeks: 3 mg/kg/dose
		<30 wk	Birth–age 4 wk: 2 mg/kg/dose
High risk (combination therapy of AZT + 3TC + NVP or raltegravir)			
AZT	6 wk	≥35 wk	4 mg/kg/dose
		≥30–<35 wk	Birth–age 2 wk: 2 mg/kg/dose
			2 weeks–6 weeks: 3 mg/kg/dose
		<30 wk	Birth–age 4 wk: 2 mg/kg/dose
			4 weeks–6 weeks: 3 mg/kg/dose
3TC[b]	6 wk	≥32 wk	Birth–age 4 wk: 2 mg/kg/dose
			>4 wk: 4 mg/kg/dose
NVP	6 wk	≥37 wk	Birth–age 6 wk: 6 mg/kg/dose
		≥34–<37 wk	Birth–age 1 wk: 4 mg/kg/dose
			Age 1–6 wk: 6 mg/kg/dose
Raltegravir[c]	6 wk	Birth–1 wk	Once daily dosing
			2–<3 kg 4 mg
			3–<4 kg 5 mg
			4–5 7 mg
		1-4 weeks (approx 3 mg/kg/dose)	Twice daily dosing
			2–<3 kg 8 mg
			3–<4 kg 10 mg
			4–5 kg 15 mg
		4-6 weeks (approx 6 mg/kg/dose)	Twice daily dosing
			3–4 kg 25 mg
			4–<6 kg 30 mg
			6–<8 kg 40 mg

[a] All dosing is orally and twice a day
[b] AZT = zidovudine; 3TC = lamivudine; NVP= Nevirapine.
[c] At ≥37 wk gestation and ≥2 kg.

Future Potential Prevention Mother-to-Child Transmission Strategies

Passive immunotherapy

The development of new approaches that would complement the current MTCT efforts include passive immunotherapy with human anti–HIV-1 broadly neutralizing monoclonal antibodies (bNAbs). The advantages of such technology include longer lasting protection and immediate protection to the infant born to women with viremia at the time of delivery or acute seroconversion during breastfeeding.[23] The IMPAACT study P1112 was a phase I study evaluating safety and tolerability of VRCO1 (bNAb specific for the HIV-1 CD4 binding site)[24,25] in HIV-exposed infants. Breastfed and nonbreastfed infants were enrolled, with the former receiving monthly subcutaneous injections until the cessation of breastfeeding. Doses of 40 mg/kg achieved serum concentrations above the threshold for neutralization of more than 90% of tested viruses. No systemic reactions were seen in formula-fed infants who received a single dose, although a small number of breastfed infants developed grade 1 systemic reactions that included fever, irritability, and sleepiness. Local reactions were common, but self-limited.[26] The armamentarium of bNAbs has been expanding, targeting not only CD4 binding sites, but also the V3glycan patch, V1/V2, and the membrane proximal extracellular region.[27–32] The breadth and potency of these newer bNAbs allow dose reduction and decreases the likelihood of neutralization escape. Studies of VRCO7-523LS and VRC01LS are being conducted currently in HIV-exposed infants.[33]

Long-acting antiretroviral therapy

Challenges with ART adherence as well as the difficulty and resources required to maintain daily dosing strategies, has led to innovations in drug development and delivery. Long-acting ARTs (LA-ARTs) are now available for HIV treatment, but their role in MTCT is not yet clear. Similar to other ART strategies, scenarios can be predicted where women become pregnant while on LA-ARTs for their own HIV control and/or the neonate is given a single or multiple doses of LA-ARTs depending on the duration of exposure (eg, breastfeeding). Understanding the impact of LA-ARTs on a developing fetus as well as the pharmacokinetics and pharmacodynamics of LA-ARTs in pregnant women, neonates, and in human milk will be essential for integrating these new technologies in MTCT strategies. A myriad of products are in development highlighting the importance of studying these compounds in pregnant women and infants.[34–37] The IMPAACT 2026 study will evaluate the pharmacokinetics and pharmacodynamics parameters of these LA-ART in both neonates and pregnant women.[38]

NEONATAL HIV TREATMENT
Early Initiation Versus Late Initiation Antiretroviral Therapy

The neonatal intervention field has moved from no options in the 1980s to multiple, although limited, options currently. An important component of neonatal intervention has been the timing of initiation. There is now robust evidence for the broad benefits of treatment intervention as soon as possible after diagnosis (early initiation). The pivotal CHER study conducted in South Africa first brought attention to the health and survival benefits of initiating treatment before 6 months of age.[39] Subsequent large cohorts have confirmed and built on this base.[40,41] Improved neurodevelopmental outcomes are a key benefit that have emerged from the early initiation investigations,[42] with better outcomes associated with timing of initiation—the earlier the better.[43,44]

Complimentary virologic benefits have also been demonstrated together with the clinical effects: early initiation of treatment is associated with improved control of viral load; lower levels of circulating, cell-associated DNA[45], slower viral evolution[46]; and decreased viral reservoir.[47,48]

The famous "Mississippi Baby" illustrates the influence that 1 clinical case can exert on the field. Born to a mother who was diagnosed with HIV infection at the time of delivery, her physician (Dr Hannah Gay) recognized the high-risk nature of the event and prescribed triple therapy with AZT, 3TC, and NVP at 30 hours of age.[49] Initial virologic diagnostic testing of the newborn was positive and she experienced a benign clinical course with rapid control of viral replication. The first 18 months of life were remarkable for her normal CD4 count, nondetectable viral load, and eventual reversion to HIV antibody negativity. She was lost to medical care for 5 months, experiencing an unplanned treatment interruption. Upon return to care, her medical team was surprised to observe a healthy infant with nondetectable plasma viral RNA and a normal CD4 count. Additional diagnostics revealed very little, if any, evidence of residual virus. This case raises the possibility of HIV cure in the setting of aggressive treatment with ARVs initiated as close as possible to the time of infection. The daunting challenge of very small (nondetectable) amounts of residual latent virus evident after 22 months of observation, when the child relapsed with virologic rebound and was replaced on ARV treatment.[50] Multiple trials to further test very early neonatal ARV initiation in the context of cure, or the now more fashionable term viral remission, ensued and are currently ongoing.

Antiretroviral Therapy for Infected Neonates

In the absence of ART, more than one-half of perinatally HIV-infected neonates will die by 2 years of age. Therefore, the current guidelines recommend ART administration to all infants and children suspected or known to be infected with HIV.[51] However, the paucity of drug choices and dosing information in neonates, as well as potential long-term toxicity of ART, pose challenges to the prescriber and may lead to suboptimal treatment of HIV-infected neonates. Available ARTs for neonates lack the innovation and potency of adult treatments with formulations that are not palatable or easy to administer. Only 5 of the 6 options approved by the US Food and Drug Administration are available for use in full-term neonates (zidovudine, lamivudine, emtricitabine, NVP, and raltegravir) and of those, only zidovudine has been studied sufficiently in preterm neonates.[52] This reality contrasts with the increasing evidence that early ART treatment limits HIV reservoirs, favors immune recovery, and improves the survival, growth, and development of infected infants.[39,45,53–55]

Current guidelines recommend treatment initiation with triple ART consisting of 2-nucleoside reverse transcriptase inhibitors (NRTIs) and either an integrase strand transfer inhibitor or a non-NRTI or a protease inhibitor within days of diagnosis (**Table 3**).[51] For term infants, zidovudine, lamivudine, and either NVP or raltegravir are the ARTs of choice. For premature infants, there are data to support dosing recommendations for zidovudine and lamivudine, as well as experimental dosing for NVP (see **Table 3**). Raltegravir can replace NVP in term infants 37 weeks of gestation or older and weighing 2 kg or more. Lopinavir/ritonavir should only be used in term neonates at age 14 days or older, or when premature infants reach a postmenstrual age of 42 weeks or older and a postnatal age of at least 2 weeks. Although there are limited studies comparing available ART in neonates, the IMPAACT P1060 study favored lopinavir/ritonavir over NVP based on better mortality and virologic failure rates and toxicity outcomes.[56] There are no studies comparing raltegravir with either lopinavir/ritonavir or NVP.

ALTERNATIVES TO FIRST LINE ANTIRETROVIRAL REGIMEN AND THERAPIES UNDER INVESTIGATION
Nucleoside Reverse Transcriptase Inhibitors

Abacavir, an NRTI licensed for use in infants older than 3 months of age, is recommended by the WHO as a first-line alternative in HIV-infected children 4 weeks of age and older and weighing 3 kg or more. Recent data from South African and European cohorts supports the WHO recommendations, and provides additional safety data for children weighing less than 3 kg using same dosing as infants older than 3 months

Table 3
Antiretroviral treatment regimens for neonates and infants

| | Combination Therapy of AZT + 3TC + NVP or Raltegravir | |
Medication	Gestational Age	Dosing[a]
AZT[b]	≥35 wk	Birth to age 4 wk: 4 mg/kg/dose
		Age > 4 wk: 12 mg/kg/dose
	≥30–<35 wk	Birth–age 2 wk: 2 mg/kg/dose
		2 weeks–8 weeks: 3 mg/kg/dose
		Age >8 wk: 12 mg/kg/dose
	<30 wk	Birth–age 4 wk: 2 mg/kg/dose
		4 weeks–10 weeks: 3 mg/kg/dose
		Age> 10 wk: 12 mg/kg/dose
3TC[b]	≥32 wk	Birth–age 4 wk: 2 mg/kg/dose
		>4 wk: 4 mg/kg/dose
NVP	≥37 wk	Birth–age 4 wk: 6 mg/kg/dose
		Age >4 wk: 200 mg/m²/dose
	≥34–<37 wk	Birth–age 1 wk: 4 mg/kg/dose
		Age 1–4 wk: 6 mg/kg/dose
		Age > 4 wk: 200 mg/m²/dose
Raltegravir[c]	Birth–1 wk	*Once daily dosing*
		2–<3 kg 4 mg
		3–<4 kg 5 mg
		4–5 7 mg
	1-4 weeks	*Twice daily dosing*
		2–<3 kg 8 mg
		3–<4 kg 10 mg
		4–5 kg 15 mg
	> 4 weeks	*Twice daily dosing*
		3–4 kg 25 mg
		4–< 6 kg 30 mg
		6–<8 kg 40 mg

[a] All dosing is orally and twice a day.
[b] AZT = zidovudine; 3TC = lamivudine; NVP, nevirapine.
[c] At ≥37 wk gestation and ≥2 kg.

of age (8 mg/kg twice daily), with minimal side effects (gastroenteritis and respiratory infection) and no hypersensitivity reactions reported.[57–59]

Integrase Inhibitors

The US Food and Drug Administration has also recently approved dolutegravir (DTG), a second-generation integrase strand transfer inhibitor, for children at least 4 week old and weighing 3 kg or more. The dose for children between 3 kg and less than 6 kg is 5 mg/d (dispersible tablets of 5 mg to be dissolve in 5 mL of water). Data from the IMPAACT 1093 study showed that 62% of pediatric patients taking DTG tablets or DTG dispersible tablets had an undetectable viral load at week 24, increasing to 69% at week 48.[60] Similarly, studies using physiologically based pharmacokinetic modeling to identify an age-appropriate dose of DTG for neonates between 0 and 28 days of age show that a dose of 5 mg every 48 hours for the first 3 weeks followed by daily dosing during the fourth week may achieve plasma exposure needed for treatment.[61] The progress of DTG drug development in newborns and young infants may soon allow the achievement of WHO's vision to feature DTG as a first-line option for all age groups. Similarly physiologically based pharmacokinetic modeling on biktegravir, another second-generation integrase strand transfer inhibitor, showed that starting neonates on a 5 mg once a day dose, increasing to 7.5 to 10.0 mg once daily after day 11 resulted in exposure comparable with adults.[62]

Broadly Neutralizing Antibodies

BNAbs have the potential of neutralizing the virus through the Fab domain, clear infected cells through the Fc domain and form antigen–antibody complexes that increases antigen presentation.[63–66] All of these characteristics highlight the potential that bNAbs have in both treatment and prevention strategies. Animal studies in both mice and nonhuman primates show that a combination of bNAbs can control viral replication and delay time to viral rebound.[67,68] Similarly, studies done in adults show promising results by increasing time to viral rebound after treatment interruption, as well as decreasing the size of the latent viral reservoir. Safety trials in neonates for prevention purposes have been reassuring and currently ongoing trials are evaluating combinations of bNAbs and ART for clearance of infected cells as well as for maintenance of viral suppression.[26,69,70]

Vaccines

HIV immunization in neonates and young infants is appealing. There are target applications of interest for both the mother and the infant: maternal immunization before or during pregnancy to minimize transmission risk and newborn immunization to prevent peripartum and breast milk infection. The challenges are daunting, not the least of which is the longstanding lack of an efficacious preventive vaccine. There is also understandable hesitancy to involve neonates, and pregnant women early in the vaccine development process, before safety and immunogenicity is established in general adult populations. Many perinatologists and neonatologists have encouraged relatively early involvement of these at-risk populations and have convened think tanks to probe the ethics and science.[71,72]

Early vaccine candidates have undergone phase I study in neonates and young infants, including viral vector prime/protein boost approaches, viral vector alone using canarypox/ALVAC vectors, and protein subunit vaccines. These early studies have demonstrated safety in small cohorts as well as modest immunogenicity, both in the United States and internationally.[73–76] Harnessing the potential of the neonatal and young infant immune response remain a high priority for both HIV prevention and treatment purposes.[23]

COMPLICATIONS IN HIV-EXPOSED AND -INFECTED CHILDREN

Complications in infants born to HIV-infected mothers, whether infected or not, can be multifactorial and not necessarily all directly linked with HIV and its treatment. Poverty, lack of health care, drug addiction, co-infections, and social vulnerability affect the overall health and development of these children. Additionally, there are specific health-related issues that can be directly attributed to HIV and its treatment.

Antiretroviral Therapy Toxicities

Mitochondrial toxicity

Potential mitochondrial toxicity from NRTIs result from the inhibition of polymerase-γ, blocking the synthesis of mitochondrial DNA. The mechanisms of inhibition can be secondary to either chain termination by incorporation of the nucleoside analogue during mitochondrial DNA synthesis, direct inhibition of polymerase-γ without incorporation, inhibition of DNA polymerase-γ exonuclease activity, or alteration of the fidelity of mitochondrial DNA synthesis by polymerase-γ.[77–79] Clinical manifestations vary depending on the degree of mitochondrial damage and include lactic acidosis, hepatic steatosis, pancreatitis, muscular weakness and rhabdomyolysis, peripheral neuropathies, lipodystrophy, nephrotoxicity, central nervous system dysfunction, osteopenia, and myopathies.[78] Perinatal NRTI exposure has been implicated in several studies with asymptomatic hyperlactatemia ranging from 13.1% to 50.0%.[80–83] Symptomatic disease was seen in 12 of 2644 children in a French cohort, presenting mainly with motor and cognitive delays and seizures.[84] Other symptoms may include weight loss, fatigue, abdominal pain, tachycardia, tachypnea, and liver failure.[85] Patients with symptomatic hyperlactatemia should discontinue ART and implement supportive measures to reverse metabolic acidosis, which may include fluid and electrolyte corrections, ventilator support, and dialysis if needed. Once acidosis resolves, ART may be resumed with an NRTI-sparing regimen, but a different NRTI backbone with a lower risk of mitochondrial toxicity may be considered.[86]

Growth and Development

In the pre-ART era stunting and growth delays were more common in both HIV-exposed but uninfected infants and HIV-infected infants when compared with HIV-unexposed/uninfected infants.[87] During the ART era the association of growth delay and HIV-exposed but uninfected infants is less clear; however, recent studies continue to suggest that HIV-exposed but uninfected infants tend to have a higher risk of growth delays.[88] Similarly, HIV-infected children have progressive decreases in both height and weight velocity when compared with uninfected children. Although the etiology is usually multifactorial, HIV infection itself seems to be an independent factor.[89] A longitudinal prospective study in England showed HIV-unexposed/uninfected infants were 22% heavier and 5.6% taller than HIV-infected children after 10 years of follow-up.[90] Similar trends were seen in underdeveloped countries.[91,92] The use of ART has been associated with recovery of the patient's nutritional status with better outcomes obtained with earlier initiation of therapy.[93]

In terms of development, it has been observed that HIV-infected infants have poorer developmental staging scores when compared with uninfected infants.[94,95] However, this association has not been as clear with HIV-exposed but uninfected infants. Recently a subanalysis of the PROMISE study compared neurodevelopmental outcomes of ante- and postpartum ART exposure of HIV-exposed but uninfected infants and HIV-unexposed/uninfected infants children up to 60 months of age and found no difference between the 2 groups.[96] Similarly, other studies in developed countries have found reassuring results,[97,98] although others have reported a greater incidence of language delay, worse fine motor development, poorer school performance, and lower IQs among HIV-exposed but uninfected infants.[99,100] Microcephaly is a likely surrogate of poor neurologic outcomes in both HIV-exposed but uninfected infants and HIV-infected infants.[101] It is not clear if the increased risk is related to viral exposure, ART exposure, or a combination of both. An observational study in Latin America reported higher rates of microcephaly in HIV-exposed but uninfected infants than in the general population, but this finding was not associated with maternal ART use during pregnancy.[102] A study in the United States compared the presence of microcephaly as well as other anthropometric measurements in HIV-exposed but uninfected infants to HIV-unexposed children younger than 2 years of age and observed no difference.[103] More recently, the SMARTT study found that HIV-exposed but uninfected infants exposed to efavirenz were more likely to have microcephaly than those who received non–efavirenz-containing regimens, with a higher risk if efavirenz was combined with zidovudine and lamivudine. More important, the presence of microcephaly was associated with neurodevelopmental deficits at 1 and 5 years of age.[104] Fortunately, the use of efavirenz in pregnant women has significantly decreased with the increased use of DTG.

Increased Risk of Bacterial Infections

An increased risk of bacterial infections has been documented among HEU (HIV-Exposed uninfected) when compared with HIV-unexposed/uninfected infants, especially to encapsulated bacteria. This association seems to be related to decreased passage of maternal antibody, especially in mothers with significant immunosuppression, more than to an intrinsic defect of the infant's immune system, highlighting the increased need to expand vaccination programs among exposed and infected infants and children.[105,106]

THE FUTURE AND NEED

Recent advances in HIV management make a world where infected children have the hope of simpler and more tolerable HIV treatments, where new therapies may allow safe treatment interruptions decreasing medication toxicity, and where prevention strategies could lead to the elimination of pediatric HIV. From a prevention standpoint, the expansion of sexual and reproductive health services and HIV screening programs, in addition to persistent efforts to expand antiretroviral coverage and the retention of both the infected mother and the newborn infant in care, are essential as the starting point of the prevention cascade.[107] The implementation of pre-exposure prophylaxis services for pregnant and breastfeeding women are important as more data support its use during these periods.[108–111] Increased political will, funding, and strong and coordinated public health responses will increase the likelihood of achieving these goals, but and independent country-level analysis may be required to better outline strengths, weaknesses, and areas needing reinforcement.[112]

From a pharmacologic perspective, further development of newer maternal and pediatric antiretroviral formulations that are safer, easier to administer, with less adverse effects will also be important. The WHO-led Pediatric Antiretroviral Drug Optimization group met in 2018 and recommended an antiretroviral priority list for the next 3 to 5 years that included dispersible combination tablets with DTG and either lamivudine/abacavir or tenofovir/emtricitabine, lower dose tablets of darunavir/ritonavir and DTG, and a combination formulations of tenofovir/emtricitabine or lamivudine. It also recommended the development of novel delivery technologies and expansion of pediatric research on bNAbs, LA-ART, and testing and approval of newer medications such as doravirine and islatavir.[113]

A combined effort that includes strategies to prevent maternal disease, early identification of infected women, and expansion of prophylactic measures and treatment strategies will lead to significant decreases in and the elimination of MTCT, as well as safer treatment for HIV-infected infants and children.

DISCLOSURES

A.F. Camacho-Gonzalez receives research support from Gilead Sciences, Janssen Pharmaceuticals and Merck & Co Pharmaceuticals. P. Palumbo Serves on the Data Safety Monitoring Boards for Gilead and Janssen.

REFERENCES

1. Oleske J, Minnefor A, Cooper R Jr, et al. Immune deficiency syndrome in children. JAMA 1983;249(17):2345–9.
2. Rubinstein A, Sicklick M, Gupta A, et al. Acquired immunodeficiency with reversed T4/T8 ratios in infants born to promiscuous and drug-addicted mothers. JAMA 1983;249(17):2350–6.
3. Scott GB, Buck BE, Leterman JG, et al. Acquired immunodeficiency syndrome in infants. N Engl J Med 1984;310(2):76–81.
4. Mitsuya H, Weinhold KJ, Furman PA, et al. 3'-Azido-3'-deoxythymidine (BW A509U): an antiviral agent that inhibits the infectivity and cytopathic effect of human T-lymphotropic virus type III/lymphadenopathy-associated virus in vitro. Proc Natl Acad Sci U S A 1985;82(20):7096–100.
5. Connor EM, Sperling RS, Gelber R, et al. Reduction of maternal-infant transmission of human immunodeficiency virus type 1 with zidovudine treatment. Pediatric AIDS Clinical Trials Group Protocol 076 Study Group. N Engl J Med 1994; 331(18):1173–80.
6. Guay LA, Musoke P, Fleming T, et al. Intrapartum and neonatal single-dose nevirapine compared with zidovudine for prevention of mother-to-child transmission of HIV-1 in Kampala, Uganda: HIVNET 012 randomised trial. Lancet 1999;354(9181):795–802.
7. Jackson JB, Musoke P, Fleming T, et al. Intrapartum and neonatal single-dose nevirapine compared with zidovudine for prevention of mother-to-child transmission of HIV-1 in Kampala, Uganda: 18-month follow-up of the HIVNET 012 randomised trial. Lancet 2003;362(9387):859–68.
8. Organization WH. WHO validation for the elimination of mother-to-child transmission of HIV and/or syphilis. 2021. Available at: https://www.who.int/reproductivehealth/congenital-syphilis/WHO-validation-EMTCT/en/. Accessed February 19, 2021.
9. Prevention CfDCA. HIV surveillance report, 2018; vol. 31. Available at: https://www.cdc.gov/hiv/library/reports/hiv-surveillance/vol-31/index.html. Accessed December 2, 2020.
10. Organization WH. HIV/AIDS key facts 2020. Available at: https://www.who.int/news-room/fact-sheets/detail/hiv-aids. Accessed December 2, 2020.
11. Blanche S, Rouzioux C, Moscato ML, et al. A prospective study of infants born to women seropositive for human immunodeficiency virus type 1. HIV Infection in Newborns French Collaborative Study Group. N Engl J Med 1989;320(25): 1643–8.
12. Luzuriaga K, Mofenson LM. Challenges in the elimination of pediatric HIV-1 infection. N Engl J Med 2016;374(8):761–70.
13. Van de Perre P, Rubbo PA, Viljoen J, et al. HIV-1 reservoirs in breast milk and challenges to elimination of breast-feeding transmission of HIV-1. Sci Transl Med 2012;4(143):143sr143.
14. Mock PA, Shaffer N, Bhadrakom C, et al. Maternal viral load and timing of mother-to-child HIV transmission, Bangkok, Thailand. Bangkok collaborative perinatal HIV transmission study group. AIDS 1999;13(3):407–14.
15. Mandelbrot L, Tubiana R, Le Chenadec J, et al. No perinatal HIV-1 transmission from women with effective antiretroviral therapy starting before conception. Clin Infect Dis 2015;61(11):1715–25.
16. Transmission PoToPWwHIaPoP. Recommendations for the use of antiretroviral drugs in pregnant women with HIV infection and interventions to reduce

perinatal HIV transmission in the United States. 2020. Available at: https://clinicalinfo.hiv.gov/en/guidelines/perinatal/whats-new-guidelines.   Accessed November 19, 2020.

17. Organization WH. Consolidated guidelines on the use of antiretroviral drugs for treating and preventing HIV infection: recommendations for a public health approach 2016. Available at: http://apps.who.int/iris/bitstream/10665/208825/1/9789241549684_eng.pdf. Accessed November 19, 2020.

18. Thomson KA, Hughes J, Baeten JM, et al. Increased risk of HIV acquisition among women throughout pregnancy and during the postpartum period: a prospective per-coital-act analysis among women with HIV-infected partners. J Infect Dis 2018;218(1):16–25.

19. Nesheim S, Harris LF, Lampe M. Elimination of perinatal HIV infection in the USA and other high-income countries: achievements and challenges. Curr Opin HIV AIDS 2013;8(5):447–56.

20. Flynn PM, Taha TE, Cababasay M, et al. Prevention of HIV-1 transmission through breastfeeding: efficacy and safety of maternal antiretroviral therapy versus infant nevirapine prophylaxis for duration of breastfeeding in HIV-1-Infected women with high CD4 cell count (IMPAACT PROMISE): a randomized, open-label, clinical trial. J Acquir Immune Defic Syndr 2018;77(4):383–92.

21. Luoga E, Vanobberghen F, Bircher R, et al. Brief report: no HIV transmission from virally suppressed mothers during breastfeeding in rural Tanzania. J Acquir Immune Defic Syndr 2018;79(1):e17–20.

22. Waitt C, Low N, Van de Perre P, et al. Does U=U for breastfeeding mothers and infants? Breastfeeding by mothers on effective treatment for HIV infection in high-income settings. Lancet HIV 2018;5(9):e531–6.

23. Voronin Y, Jani I, Graham BS, et al. Recent progress in immune-based interventions to prevent HIV-1 transmission to children. J Int AIDS Soc 2017;20(4).

24. Wu X, Yang ZY, Li Y, et al. Rational design of envelope identifies broadly neutralizing human monoclonal antibodies to HIV-1. Science 2010;329(5993):856–61.

25. Zhou T, Georgiev I, Wu X, et al. Structural basis for broad and potent neutralization of HIV-1 by antibody VRC01. Science 2010;329(5993):811–7.

26. Cunningham CK, McFarland EJ, Morrison RL, et al. Safety, tolerability, and pharmacokinetics of the broadly neutralizing human immunodeficiency virus (HIV)-1 monoclonal antibody VRC01 in HIV-exposed newborn infants. J Infect Dis 2020;222(4):628–36.

27. Rudicell RS, Kwon YD, Ko SY, et al. Enhanced potency of a broadly neutralizing HIV-1 antibody in vitro improves protection against lentiviral infection in vivo. J Virol 2014;88(21):12669–82.

28. Huang J, Kang BH, Ishida E, et al. Identification of a CD4-binding-site antibody to HIV that evolved near-Pan neutralization breadth. Immunity 2016;45(5):1108–21.

29. Scheid JF, Mouquet H, Ueberheide B, et al. Sequence and structural convergence of broad and potent HIV antibodies that mimic CD4 binding. Science 2011;333(6049):1633–7.

30. Doria-Rose NA, Bhiman JN, Roark RS, et al. New member of the V1V2-directed CAP256-VRC26 lineage that shows increased breadth and exceptional potency. J Virol 2016;90(1):76–91.

31. Sok D, van Gils MJ, Pauthner M, et al. Recombinant HIV envelope trimer selects for quaternary-dependent antibodies targeting the trimer apex. Proc Natl Acad Sci U S A 2014;111(49):17624–9.

32. Huang J, Ofek G, Laub L, et al. Broad and potent neutralization of HIV-1 by a gp41-specific human antibody. Nature 2012;491(7424):406–12.

33. Clinicaltrials.gov. Evaluating the safety and pharmacokinetics of VRC01, VRC01LS, and VRC07-523LS, potent anti-HIV neutralizing monoclonal antibodies, in HIV-1-Exposed infants. Available at: https://clinicaltrials.gov/ct2/show/NCT02256631. Accessed November 6, 2020.

34. Cortez JM Jr, Quintero R, Moss JA, et al. Pharmacokinetics of injectable, long-acting nevirapine for HIV prophylaxis in breastfeeding infants. Antimicrob Agents Chemother 2015;59(1):59–66.

35. Sillman B, Bade AN, Dash PK, et al. Creation of a long-acting nanoformulated dolutegravir. Nat Commun 2018;9(1):443.

36. McMillan J, Szlachetka A, Slack L, et al. Pharmacokinetics of a long-acting nanoformulated dolutegravir prodrug in rhesus macaques. Antimicrob Agents Chemother 2018;62(1):e01316.

37. Rizzardini G, Overton ET, Orkin C, et al. Long-acting injectable cabotegravir + rilpivirine for HIV maintenance therapy: week 48 pooled analysis of phase 3 ATLAS and FLAIR trials. J Acquir Immune Defic Syndr 2020;85(4):498–506.

38. IMPAACT Network 2026 Study: pharmacokinetic properties of antiretroviral and anti-Tuberculosis drugs during pregnancy and postpartum. Available at: https://impaactnetwork.org/studies/IMPAACT2026.asp.

39. Violari A, Cotton MF, Gibb DM, et al. Early antiretroviral therapy and mortality among HIV-infected infants. N Engl J Med 2008;359(21):2233–44.

40. Shiau S, Strehlau R, Technau KG, et al. Early age at start of antiretroviral therapy associated with better virologic control after initial suppression in HIV-infected infants. AIDS 2017;31(3):355–64.

41. Schomaker M, Leroy V, Wolfs T, et al. Optimal timing of antiretroviral treatment initiation in HIV-positive children and adolescents: a multiregional analysis from Southern Africa, West Africa and Europe. Int J Epidemiol 2017;46(2):453–65.

42. Laughton B, Cornell M, Grove D, et al. Early antiretroviral therapy improves neurodevelopmental outcomes in infants. AIDS 2012;26(13):1685–90.

43. Laughton B, Naidoo S, Dobbels E, et al. Neurodevelopment at 11 months after starting antiretroviral therapy within 3 weeks of life. South Afr J HIV Med 2019;20(1):1008.

44. Benki-Nugent S, Wamalwa D, Langat A, et al. Comparison of developmental milestone attainment in early treated HIV-infected infants versus HIV-unexposed infants: a prospective cohort study. BMC Pediatr 2017;17(1):24.

45. Kuhn L, Paximadis M, Da Costa Dias B, et al. Age at antiretroviral therapy initiation and cell-associated HIV-1 DNA levels in HIV-1-infected children. PLoS One 2018;13(4):e0195514.

46. Persaud D, Ray SC, Kajdas J, et al. Slow human immunodeficiency virus type 1 evolution in viral reservoirs in infants treated with effective antiretroviral therapy. AIDS Res Hum Retroviruses 2007;23(3):381–90.

47. Persaud D, Patel K, Karalius B, et al. Influence of age at virologic control on peripheral blood human immunodeficiency virus reservoir size and serostatus in perinatally infected adolescents. JAMA Pediatr 2014;168(12):1138–46.

48. Uprety P, Patel K, Karalius B, et al. Human immunodeficiency virus type 1 DNA decay dynamics with early, long-term virologic control of perinatal infection. Clin Infect Dis 2017;64(11):1471–8.

49. Bocci V. Administration of interferon at night may increase its therapeutic index. Cancer Drug Deliv 1985;2(4):313–8.

50. Luzuriaga K, Gay H, Ziemniak C, et al. Viremic relapse after HIV-1 remission in a perinatally infected child. N Engl J Med 2015;372(8):786–8.

51. HIV PoATaMMoCLw. Guidelines for the use of antiretroviral agents in pediatric HIV infection. 2020. Available at: http://aidsinfo.nih.gov/contentfiles/lvguidelines/pediatricguidelines.pdf. Accessed November 20, 2020.

52. Capparelli EV, Mirochnick M, Dankner WM, et al. Pharmacokinetics and tolerance of zidovudine in preterm infants. J Pediatr 2003;142(1):47–52.

53. Barlow-Mosha L, Musiime V, Davies MA, et al. Universal antiretroviral therapy for HIV-infected children: a review of the benefits and risks to consider during implementation. J Int AIDS Soc 2017;20(1):21552.

54. Azzoni L, Barbour R, Papasavvas E, et al. Early ART results in Greater immune reconstitution benefits in HIV-infected infants: working with data missingness in a longitudinal dataset. PLoS One 2015;10(12):e0145320.

55. Garcia-Broncano P, Maddali S, Einkauf KB, et al. Early antiretroviral therapy in neonates with HIV-1 infection restricts viral reservoir size and induces a distinct innate immune profile. Sci Transl Med 2019;11(520).

56. Violari A, Lindsey JC, Hughes MD, et al. Nevirapine versus ritonavir-boosted lopinavir for HIV-infected children. N Engl J Med 2012;366(25):2380–9.

57. De Waal RRH, Technau K, Eley B, et al. Abacavir safety and efficacy in young infants in South African observational cohorts, CROI 2020. 2020. Available at: https://2jg4quetidw2blbbq2ixwziw-wpengine.netdna-ssl.com/wp-content/uploads/sites/2/posters/2020/1430_7_DeWaal_00845.pdf. Accessed November 13, 2020.

58. Cressey TBA, Cababasay M, Wang J, et al, for the IMPAACT P1106 Team. Abacavir safety and pharmacokinetics in normal and low Birth weight infants with HIV. CROI 2020. 2020. Available at: https://2jg4quetidw2blbbq2ixwziw-wpengine.netdna-ssl.com/wp-content/. Accessed November 13, 2020.

59. Crichton SCI, Turkova A, Ene L, et al, for the European Pregnancy and Paediatric HIV Cohort Collaboration (EPPICC). Abacavir dosing, effectiveness and safety in young infants living with HIV in Europe, CROI 2020 2020. Available at: https://2jg4quetidw2blbbq2ixwziw-wpengine.netdna-ssl.com/wp-content/uploads/sites/2/posters/2020/1430_6_Crichton_00844.pdf. Accessed November 13, 2020.

60. Ruel TFM, Alvero C, Acosta E, et al, the P1093 Team. Twenty-four week Safety, tolerability and efficacy of dolutegravir dispersible tablets in children 4 weeks to <6 years old with HIV-1: results from IMPAACT P1093. AIDS 2020 2020. Available at: https://impaactnetwork.org/DocFiles/AIDS2020/PEB0293_DTG_DT_24wkOutcomesFINAL_6.26.20.pdf. Accessed November 14, 2020.

61. Bunglawala F, Rajoli RKR, Mirochnick M, et al. Prediction of dolutegravir pharmacokinetics and dose optimization in neonates via physiologically based pharmacokinetic (PBPK) modelling. J Antimicrob Chemother 2020;75(3):640–7.

62. Bunglawala FRR, Kinvig H, Cottura N, et al. Siccardi M identification of age-appropriate dosing strategies of bictegravir in neonates. CROI 2020 2020. Available at: https://2jg4quetidw2blbbq2ixwziw-wpengine.netdna-ssl.com/wp-content/uploads/sites/2/posters/2020/1430_1_Bunglawala_00839.pdf. Accessed November 14, 2020.

63. Chun TW, Murray D, Justement JS, et al. Broadly neutralizing antibodies suppress HIV in the persistent viral reservoir. Proc Natl Acad Sci U S A 2014;111(36):13151–6.

64. Bruel T, Guivel-Benhassine F, Amraoui S, et al. Elimination of HIV-1-infected cells by broadly neutralizing antibodies. Nat Commun 2016;7:10844.

65. Lu CL, Murakowski DK, Bournazos S, et al. Enhanced clearance of HIV-1-infected cells by broadly neutralizing antibodies against HIV-1 in vivo. Science 2016;352(6288):1001–4.

66. Schoofs T, Klein F, Braunschweig M, et al. HIV-1 therapy with monoclonal antibody 3BNC117 elicits host immune responses against HIV-1. Science 2016; 352(6288):997–1001.

67. Klein F, Halper-Stromberg A, Horwitz JA, et al. HIV therapy by a combination of broadly neutralizing antibodies in humanized mice. Nature 2012;492(7427): 118–22.

68. Mendoza P, Gruell H, Nogueira L, et al. Combination therapy with anti-HIV-1 antibodies maintains viral suppression. Nature 2018;561(7724):479–84.

69. ClinicalTrials.gov. Phase I/II multisite, randomized, controlled study of monoclonal antibody VRC01 with combination antiretroviral therapy to promote clearance of HIV-1-Infected cells in infants. Available at: https://clinicaltrials.gov/ct2/show/NCT03208231. Accessed November 17, 2020.

70. ClinicalTrials.gov. Dual bNAb treatment in children. Available at: https://clinicaltrials.gov/ct2/show/NCT03707977. Accessed November 17, 2020.

71. Hoff R, McNamara J, Fowler M, et al. HIV vaccine development and clinical trials. Acta Paediatr Suppl 1994;400:73–7.

72. Goswami R, Berendam SJ, Li SH, et al. Harnessing early life immunity to develop a pediatric HIV vaccine that can protect through adolescence. PLoS Pathog 2020;16(11):e1008983.

73. McFarland EJ, Borkowsky W, Fenton T, et al. Human immunodeficiency virus type 1 (HIV-1) gp120-specific antibodies in neonates receiving an HIV-1 recombinant gp120 vaccine. J Infect Dis 2001;184(10):1331–5.

74. Kintu K, Andrew P, Musoke P, et al. Feasibility and safety of ALVAC-HIV vCP1521 vaccine in HIV-exposed infants in Uganda: results from the first HIV vaccine trial in infants in Africa. J Acquir Immune Defic Syndr 2013;63(1):1–8.

75. McFarland EJ, Johnson DC, Muresan P, et al. HIV-1 vaccine induced immune responses in newborns of HIV-1 infected mothers. AIDS 2006;20(11):1481–9.

76. Johnson DC, McFarland EJ, Muresan P, et al. Safety and immunogenicity of an HIV-1 recombinant canarypox vaccine in newborns and infants of HIV-1-infected women. J Infect Dis 2005;192(12):2129–33.

77. White AJ. Mitochondrial toxicity and HIV therapy. Sex Transm Infect 2001;77(3): 158–73.

78. Kakuda TN. Pharmacology of nucleoside and nucleotide reverse transcriptase inhibitor-induced mitochondrial toxicity. Clin Ther 2000;22(6):685–708.

79. Brinkman K, ter Hofstede HJ, Burger DM, et al. Adverse effects of reverse transcriptase inhibitors: mitochondrial toxicity as common pathway. AIDS 1998; 12(14):1735–44.

80. Noguera A, Fortuny C, Munoz-Almagro C, et al. Hyperlactatemia in human immunodeficiency virus-uninfected infants who are exposed to antiretrovirals. Pediatrics 2004;114(5):e598–603.

81. Ekouevi DK, Toure R, Becquet R, et al. Serum lactate levels in infants exposed peripartum to antiretroviral agents to prevent mother-to-child transmission of HIV: Agence Nationale de Recherches Sur le SIDA et les Hepatites Virales 1209 study, Abidjan, Ivory Coast. Pediatrics 2006;118(4):e1071–7.

82. Desai N, Mathur M, Weedon J. Lactate levels in children with HIV/AIDS on highly active antiretroviral therapy. AIDS 2003;17(10):1565–8.

83. Noguera A, Fortuny C, Sanchez E, et al. Hyperlactatemia in human immunode-ficiency virus-infected children receiving antiretroviral treatment. Pediatr Infect Dis J 2003;22(9):778–82.

84. Barret B, Tardieu M, Rustin P, et al. Persistent mitochondrial dysfunction in HIV-1-exposed but uninfected infants: clinical screening in a large prospective cohort. AIDS 2003;17(12):1769–85.

85. Falco V, Rodriguez D, Ribera E, et al. Severe nucleoside-associated lactic acidosis in human immunodeficiency virus-infected patients: report of 12 cases and review of the literature. Clin Infect Dis 2002;34(6):838–46.

86. Lonergan JT, Barber RE, Mathews WC. Safety and efficacy of switching to alter-native nucleoside analogues following symptomatic hyperlactatemia and lactic acidosis. AIDS 2003;17(17):2495–9.

87. Omoni AO, Ntozini R, Evans C, et al. Child growth according to maternal and child HIV status in Zimbabwe. Pediatr Infect Dis J 2017;36(9):869–76.

88. le Roux SM, Abrams EJ, Donald KA, et al. Growth trajectories of breastfed HIV-exposed uninfected and HIV-unexposed children under conditions of universal maternal antiretroviral therapy: a prospective study. Lancet Child Adolesc Health 2019;3(4):234–44.

89. Miller TL. Nutritional aspects of HIV-infected children receiving highly active an-tiretroviral therapy. AIDS 2003;17(Suppl 1):S130–40.

90. Newell ML, Borja MC, Peckham C, et al. Height, weight, and growth in children born to mothers with HIV-1 infection in Europe. Pediatrics 2003;111(1):e52–60.

91. Buonora S, Nogueira S, Pone MV, et al. Growth parameters in HIV-vertically-infected adolescents on antiretroviral therapy in Rio de Janeiro, Brazil. Ann Trop Paediatr 2008;28(1):59–64.

92. Villamor E, Fataki MR, Bosch RJ, et al. Human immunodeficiency virus infection, diarrheal disease and sociodemographic predictors of child growth. Acta Pae-diatr 2004;93(3):372–9.

93. McGrath CJ, Diener L, Richardson BA, et al. Growth reconstitution following an-tiretroviral therapy and nutritional supplementation: systematic review and meta-analysis. AIDS 2015;29(15):2009–23.

94. Le Doare K, Bland R, Newell ML. Neurodevelopment in children born to HIV-infected mothers by infection and treatment status. Pediatrics 2012;130(5): e1326–44.

95. Hoare J, Ransford GL, Phillips N, et al. Systematic review of neuroimaging studies in vertically transmitted HIV positive children and adolescents. Metab Brain Dis 2014;29(2):221–9.

96. Boivin MJ, Maliwichi-Senganimalunje L, Ogwang LW, et al. Neurodevelopmental effects of ante-partum and post-partum antiretroviral exposure in HIV-exposed and uninfected children versus HIV-unexposed and uninfected children in Uganda and Malawi: a prospective cohort study. Lancet HIV 2019;6(8): e518–30.

97. Alimenti A, Forbes JC, Oberlander TF, et al. A prospective controlled study of neurodevelopment in HIV-uninfected children exposed to combination antiretro-viral drugs in pregnancy. Pediatrics 2006;118(4):e1139–45.

98. Sirois PA, Huo Y, Williams PL, et al. Safety of perinatal exposure to antiretroviral medications: developmental outcomes in infants. Pediatr Infect Dis J 2013; 32(6):648–55.

99. Kerr SJ, Puthanakit T, Vibol U, et al. Neurodevelopmental outcomes in HIV-exposed-uninfected children versus those not exposed to HIV. AIDS Care 2014;26(11):1327–35.

100. Rice ML, Zeldow B, Siberry GK, et al. Evaluation of risk for late language emergence after in utero antiretroviral drug exposure in HIV-exposed uninfected infants. Pediatr Infect Dis J 2013;32(10):e406–13.

101. Evans C, Chasekwa B, Ntozini R, et al. Head circumferences of children born to HIV-infected and HIV-uninfected mothers in Zimbabwe during the preantiretroviral therapy era. AIDS 2016;30(15):2323–8.

102. Spaulding AB, Yu Q, Civitello L, et al. Neurologic outcomes in HIV-Exposed/Uninfected infants exposed to antiretroviral drugs during pregnancy in Latin America and the Caribbean. AIDS Res Hum Retroviruses 2016;32(4):349–56.

103. Neri D, Somarriba GA, Schaefer NN, et al. Growth and body composition of uninfected children exposed to human immunodeficiency virus: comparison with a contemporary cohort and United States National Standards. J Pediatr 2013; 163(1):249–54, e241-242.

104. Williams PL, Yildirim C, Chadwick EG, et al. Association of maternal antiretroviral use with microcephaly in children who are HIV-exposed but uninfected (SMARTT): a prospective cohort study. Lancet HIV 2020;7(1):e49–58.

105. Brennan AT, Bonawitz R, Gill CJ, et al. A meta-analysis assessing all-cause mortality in HIV-exposed uninfected compared with HIV-unexposed uninfected infants and children. AIDS 2016;30(15):2351–60.

106. Jones CE, Naidoo S, De Beer C, et al. Maternal HIV infection and antibody responses against vaccine-preventable diseases in uninfected infants. JAMA 2011;305(6):576–84.

107. Fatti G, Shaikh N, Jackson D, et al. Low HIV incidence in pregnant and postpartum women receiving a community-based combination HIV prevention intervention in a high HIV incidence setting in South Africa. PLoS One 2017;12(7): e0181691.

108. Pollock L, Levison J. Role of preexposure prophylaxis in the reproductive health of women at risk for human immunodeficiency virus infection. Obstet Gynecol 2018;132(3):687–91.

109. Heffron R, Pintye J, Matthews LT, et al. PrEP as peri-conception HIV prevention for women and men. Curr HIV/AIDS Rep 2016;13(3):131–9.

110. Kinuthia J, Pintye J, Abuna F, et al. Pre-exposure prophylaxis uptake and early continuation among pregnant and post-partum women within maternal and child health clinics in Kenya: results from an implementation programme. Lancet HIV 2020;7(1):e38–48.

111. Seidman DL, Weber S, Cohan D. Offering pre-exposure prophylaxis for HIV prevention to pregnant and postpartum women: a clinical approach. J Int AIDS Soc 2017;20(Suppl 1):21295.

112. UNICEF UW. Key considerations for programming and prioritization Going the 'Last Mile' to EMTCT: a road map for ending the HIV epidemic in children 2020. Available at: http://www.childrenandaids.org/sites/default/files/2020-02/Last-Mile-To-EMTCT_WhitePaper_UNICEF2020.pdf. Accessed November 19, 2020.

113. Penazzato M, Townsend CL, Rakhmanina N, et al. Prioritising the most needed paediatric antiretroviral formulations: the PADO4 list. Lancet HIV 2019;6(9): e623–31.

Syphilis in Neonates and Infants

Alexandra K. Medoro, MD[a,b], Pablo J. Sánchez, MD[a,b],*

KEYWORDS

- Syphilis • Congenital syphilis • Maternal syphilis • Syphilis screening • Infant
- Reverse sequence syphilis screening

INTRODUCTION

In 1905 in Germany, Fritz Schaudinn, a zoologist, and Erich Hoffmann, a dermatologist, discovered the causal agent of syphilis, the bacterium *Spirochaeta pallida*, later known as *Treponema pallidum* subsp. *pallidum,* from a vulvar lesion in a woman with secondary syphilis.[1] Soon thereafter in 1906, bacteriologist August Paul von Wassermann along with 2 dermatologists, Albert Neisser and Carl Bruck, developed the first serologic test for syphilis,[2] although it has been supplanted by newer but still imperfect assays. The organism is markedly fastidious, surviving only briefly outside of the human host, and only recently has it been able to be cultured in artificial media.[3] The complete genome of the organism has been sequenced, bringing renewed hope for better understanding of pathogenesis and improved diagnostic assays using a polymerase chain reaction methodology.[4–7]

Syphilis infection in neonates and infants is almost always a consequence of fetal infection after maternal spirochetemia. Despite decades of experience with syphilis in adults and infants, it remains a significant health problem worldwide.[8] Congenital syphilis is a major cause of fetal and neonatal mortality globally.[9,10] In addition, syphilis, a genital ulcerative disease, has been shown to facilitate the transmission and acquisition of infection with HIV.

EPIDEMIOLOGY

In 2000, the rate of primary and secondary syphilis reported to the Centers for Disease Control and Prevention (CDC) was the lowest since 1941,[11] the year before penicillin

Potential Conflicts of Interest: The authors have no conflicts of interest relevant to this article
[a] Department of Pediatrics, Division of Neonatology, Nationwide Children's Hospital, The Ohio State University College of Medicine, Center for Perinatal Research, Abigail Wexner Research Institute at Nationwide Children's Hospital, 700 Children's Drive, RB3, WB5245, Columbus, OH 43205-2664, USA; [b] Department of Pediatrics, Division of Pediatric Infectious Diseases, Nationwide Children's Hospital, The Ohio State University College of Medicine, Center for Perinatal Research, Abigail Wexner Research Institute at Nationwide Children's Hospital, 700 Children's Drive, RB3, WB5245, Columbus, OH 43205-2664, USA
* Corresponding author. Department of Pediatrics, Division of Neonatology, Nationwide Children's Hospital, The Ohio State University College of Medicine, Center for Perinatal Research, Abigail Wexner Research Institute at Nationwide Children's Hospital, 700 Children's Drive, RB3, WB5245, Columbus, OH 43205-2664.
E-mail address: pablo.sanchez@nationwidechildrens.org

Clin Perinatol 48 (2021) 293–309
https://doi.org/10.1016/j.clp.2021.03.005

was first used for the treatment of streptococcal sepsis after a miscarriage. Since then, syphilis among adults has increased steadily, mostly among men who have sex with men.[12,13] However, since 2013, the number of cases among women of childbearing ages has increased substantially, resulting in a concurrent increase in congenital syphilis.[14,15]

Cases of congenital syphilis are reported to state health departments and subsequently to CDC using a surveillance case definition (https://wwwn.cdc.gov/nndss/conditions/congenital-syphilis/case-definition/2018/).[16] The original case definition used the Kaufman criteria, which required abnormalities in the clinical, laboratory, or radiographic evaluation that was consistent with a diagnosis of syphilis in infants and children.[17] It was revised in 1988 with minor clarifications in 1996 to provide a more accurate assessment of the substantial public health impact of maternal syphilis on infants.[18,19] The case definition now includes stillbirths as well as all infants and children born to mothers with untreated or inadequately treated syphilis, regardless of signs of syphilis in the infant or child.

The rate of reported congenital syphilis cases has increased each year since 2012 (**Fig. 1**). In 2018, there were 1306 cases of congenital syphilis reported to the CDC, including 78 syphilitic stillbirths and 16 infant deaths, for a national rate of 33 cases per 100,000 live births (https://www.cdc.gov/nchhstp/newsroom/2019/2018-STD-surveillance-report.html). This rate represented a 40% increase relative to 2017 (24 cases per 100,000 live births) and a 185% increase relative to 2014 (11 cases per 100,000 live births). As has been observed historically, this increase in the congenital syphilis rate paralleled increases in primary and secondary syphilis among all women and reproductive-aged women from 2014 to 2018 (173% and 165% increases, respectively). This recent increase in syphilis among women has been associated with methamphetamine, injection drug, and heroin use.[20,21]

In 2018, the increase in congenital syphilis cases in the United States occurred primarily in the West (49 cases per 100,000 live births) and South (45 cases per 100,000 live births), followed by the Midwest (12 cases per 100,000 live births) and the Northeast (9 cases per 100,000 live births). Rates were highest among Blacks (87 cases per 100,000 live births) and American Indians/Alaskan Natives (79 cases per 100,000 live births), followed by Hispanics (45 cases per 100,000 live births), Whites (14 cases per 100,000 live births), and Asians/Pacific Islanders (9 cases per 100,000 live births).[14]

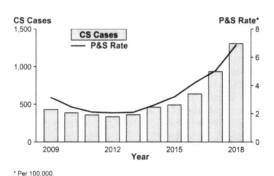

* Per 100,000.

Fig. 1. Reported cases of congenital syphilis to the CDC by year of birth and rates of reported cases of primary and secondary syphilis among females aged 15 to 44 years in the United States from 2009 to 2018. CS, congenital syphilis; P&S, primary and secondary syphilis. (Content source: Division of STD Prevention, National Center for HIV/AIDS, Viral Hepatitis, STD, and TB Prevention, Centers for Disease Control and Prevention.)

TRANSMISSION

Vertical transmission of *T pallidum* primarily occurs transplacentally during maternal spirochetemia. Transplacental transmission is supported by the isolation of *T pallidum* from amniotic fluid and umbilical cord blood by rabbit infectivity testing.[22–24] Furthermore, clinical disease such as hepatomegaly has been seen in utero by ultrasound examination and at birth,[25] and specific IgM antibody to *T pallidum* has been detected in fetal serum obtained by cordocentesis and in neonatal serum obtained at birth.[26–28]

It also is possible that the newborn can be infected during delivery from contact with maternal genital lesions such as condyloma lata that are teeming with spirochetes (**Fig. 2**). Although rare, postnatal transmission could occur from contact with open and weeping nongenital lesions on a caregiver. Transmission through human milk also is rare if it occurs at all, and breastfeeding is not contraindicated, unless the untreated mother has a chancre of the breast.

Fetal infection can occur at any time in gestation, and spirochetes have been detected in aborted fetal tissue at 9 and 10 weeks of gestation[29] and in amniotic fluid as early as 14 weeks of pregnancy by rabbit infectivity testing.[23] The previous belief that the Langhans' cell layer of the early placenta prevented fetal infection before the 18th week of pregnancy has been dispelled. Nevertheless, the risk of fetal infection increases as the pregnancy advances. Importantly, the rate of transmission is related to the stage of maternal syphilis, with congenital syphilis occurring in approximately 25%, 60%, 40%, and 7% of fetuses and infants born to mothers with untreated primary, secondary, early latent (syphilis less than a year's duration), and late latent infection (syphilis greater than a year's duration), respectively.[30–32]

CLINICAL MANIFESTATIONS

In addition to the clinical features of acquired syphilis (see **Fig. 2**), maternal syphilis is associated with adverse pregnancy outcomes such as preterm labor, spontaneous

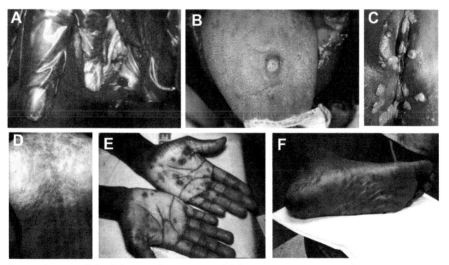

Fig. 2. Chancre of the (*A*) vaginal opening and (*B*) tongue representing the primary stage of syphilis. (*C*) Condyloma lata of perineum and rash involving the (*D*) back, (*E*) palms, and (*F*) soles of secondary syphilis. (Division of STD Prevention, National Center for HIV/AIDS, Viral Hepatitis, STD, and TB Prevention, Centers for Disease Control and Prevention).

abortion, stillbirth, and perinatal mortality.[33] Placental abnormalities of congenital syphilis include large size and pallor, and histopathologic examination reveals necrotizing funisitis ("barber's pole" appearance), villous enlargement, and acute villitis.[34] Placental and umbilical cord histopathology should be performed on every suspected case because it may aid in the diagnosis of congenital syphilis.

Clinical signs of infection in the fetus may present as hepatomegaly, anemia, and nonimmune hydrops resulting in preterm birth or perinatal death. Similar to other congenital infections, however, the majority of infants born to mothers with untreated syphilis at delivery lack clinical, laboratory, or radiographic signs of infection. If untreated in the neonatal period, these infants may develop signs of disease later in infancy, childhood, adolescence, or even adulthood.[35,36]

The clinical, laboratory, and radiographic abnormalities associated with congenital syphilis are a consequence of active infection with *T pallidum* and the resultant inflammatory response induced in various body organs. Congenital syphilis has been somewhat arbitrarily classified into 2 characteristic syndromes of clinical disease, namely, early and late congenital syphilis. Early congenital syphilis refers to those infants and children who present in the first 2 years of age, whereas late congenital syphilis includes older children and adults.

The clinical manifestations that characterize early congenital syphilis are shown in **Box 1**, with hepatomegaly occurring frequently owing to hepatitis or extramedullary hematopoiesis.[37] Other systemic manifestations may include intrauterine growth restriction or small for gestational age, adenopathy, pneumonia ("pneumonia alba"), anemia, or splenomegaly. Thrombocytopenia may be the only manifestation. Fever may be a presenting sign among older infants.[35,38]

Cutaneous manifestations also are frequent and vary from a generalized maculopapular copper-colored rash that may involve the palms and soles to a bullous eruption with subsequent desquamation referred to as pemphigus syphiliticus (**Fig. 3**).[39] A less frequent manifestation is condylomata lata, which present as white, flat or minimally raised, moist plaques on the perioral, oral, perineal, perirectal, or intertriginous areas. Some infants also present with nasal discharge commonly referred to as the "snuffles," which is initially watery but may become purulent or blood tinged (**Fig. 4**). Both the rash and rhinitis of congenital syphilis are highly infectious because they contain high concentrations of spirochetes.

Ocular findings are rare, but may include cataracts, chorioretinitis, uveitis, or glaucoma. Clinical signs of central nervous system involvement also are rare, but hypopituitarism with diabetes insipidus has been reported.[40,41] The vast majority of infants in whom *T pallidum* was detected in cerebrospinal fluid (CSF) by rabbit infectivity testing had no clinical signs of neurosyphilis such as irritability, seizures, or cranial nerve palsies.[42]

Radiographic abnormalities consisting of osteochondritis or periostitis are frequent, occurring in as many as 70% of infants approximately at 5 and 16 weeks, respectively, after fetal infection (**Fig. 5**).[43] The delayed visualization of periostitis helps to explain why osteochondritis involving the metaphases is a more frequent manifestation. In addition, skeletal survey of stillborn infants demonstrating characteristic osseous lesions may aid in the diagnosis of fetal infection. Radiographic findings are usually symmetric with preferential involvement of the lower versus the upper extremities. The bone lesions of congenital syphilis may be painful and result in refusal to move the affected extremity.[38] This so-called pseudoparalysis of Parrot results from a subepiphyseal fracture and epiphyseal dislocation. Another classic radiographic abnormality known as the Wimberger sign refers to the demineralization and osseous destruction of the proximal medial tibial metaphysis.[44] The bony lesions of congenital syphilis resolve within months with no long-term consequences among treated infants.

Box 1
Clinical, laboratory, and radiographic findings in congenital syphilis

1) Early congenital syphilis (<2 years of age)
   a) Clinical and physical examination findings: normal[b]; stillborn; preterm; nonimmune hydrops fetalis; intrauterine growth restriction; small for gestational age; fever; hepatomegaly[a] with or without jaundice; splenomegaly[a]; rash[a]; rhinitis (snuffles); mucous patch; condylomata lata; adenopathy (epitrochlear nodes); pseudoparalysis of Parrot; chorioretinitis; cataract; irritability; cranial nerve palsies; seizures; pancreatitis; myocarditis; gastrointestinal malabsorption
   b) Laboratory findings: anemia, thrombocytopenia[a]; hypoglycemia; liver transaminitis[c] and direct hyperbilirubinemia; cerebrospinal fluid pleocytosis, elevated protein content, reactive VDRL test; proteinuria (nephrotic syndrome); hypopituitarism (diabetes insipidus)
   c) Radiographic findings: periostitis; osteochondritis[a]; pneumonia alba

2) Late congenital syphilis (>2 years of age)
   a) Hutchinson's teeth[d]; Mulberry molars; interstitial keratitis[d]; optic nerve atrophy; healed chorioretinitis; rhagades; gummas; cranial nerve VIII nerve deafness[d]
   b) Intellectual disability; hydrocephalus; seizures, juvenile general paresis, cranial nerve palsies
   c) Frontal bossing, saddle nose deformity, protuberant mandible, short maxilla, high palatal arch, perforation of the hard palate, saber shin, sternoclavicular joint thickening (Higouménakis sign), Clutton's joints

Abbreviation: VDRL, Venereal Disease Research Laboratory.

[a] Prominent feature.
[b] The majority of infected newborns and infants seem to be clinically normal with a normal physical examination and no signs of central nervous system involvement.
[c] Liver transaminases may worsen after initiation of penicillin therapy and may represent a localized Jaresch–Herxheimer reaction.
[d] Comprise Hutchinson's triad, which is specific for congenital syphilis.

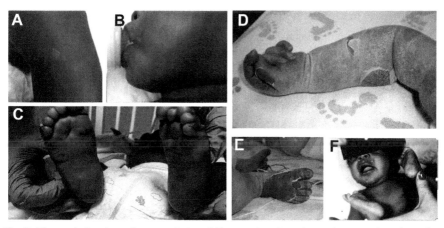

Fig. 3. The varied rashes of congenital syphilis, ranging from hypopigmented oval patches of the leg and face (*A*, *B*), hyperpigmented macules on soles of feet (*C*), desquamation of skin characteristic of "pemphigus syphiliticus" (*D*, *E*), and papular lesions periorally in infants with congenital syphilis (*F*). (*From [A–C]* Lanata MM, Bressler CJ, McKnight LV, Sanchez PJ, Tscholl JJ, Kasick RT. A Case of Fever, Rash, and a Painful Limb in an Infant. Clin Pediatr (Phila). 2019;58(6):711-714; with permission; [*D, E*] Wang EA, Chambers CJ, Silverstein M. A rare presentation of congenital syphilis: Pemphigus syphiliticus in a newborn infant with extensive desquamation of the extremities. Pediatr Dermatol. 2018;35(2):e110-e113; with permission; and [*F*] Centers for Disease Control and Prevention, courtesy of Susan Lindsley.)

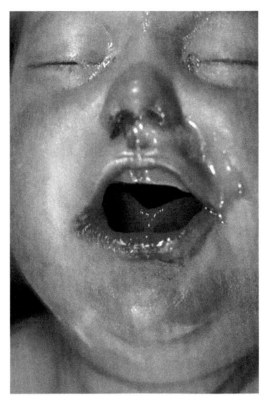

Fig. 4. Rhinitis or "snuffles" in an infant with congenital syphilis. (Division of STD Prevention, National Center for HIV/AIDS, Viral Hepatitis, STD, and TB Prevention, Centers for Disease Control and Prevention).

The manifestations and stigmata of late congenital syphilis usually appear near puberty or adolescence and result from persistent inflammation or scarring from the initial fetal infection that was untreated, inadequately treated, or treated beyond early infancy.[36] The classic Hutchinson's triad consists of interstitial keratitis, eighth cranial nerve deafness from osteochondritis of the otic capsule, and Hutchinson's teeth. The latter are small, widely spaced, notched, barrel-shaped permanent upper and occasionally lower central incisors (**Fig. 6**). Another late dental manifestation is mulberry molars in which the first lower molars have many small cusps instead of the usual four (see **Fig. 6**). In addition, frontal bone periostitis can result in frontal bossing, tibial periostitis may lead to tibial bowing or saber shins, and clavicular periostitis may result in sternoclavicular thickening (Higoumenakis sign). Syphilitic rhinitis in early infancy may involve the underlying cartilage and bone leading to a "saddle nose" deformity. Perforation of the palate and nasal septum also may occur, along with cracks or fissures around the mouth or nose (rhagades). Interstitial keratitis is often bilateral with the cornea having a ground glass appearance with vascularization of the adjacent sclera, resulting in blindness (see **Fig. 6**).[45] Central nervous system sequalae include intellectual disability, paresis, personality changes, seizure disorder, hydrocephalus, and optic atrophy.

DIAGNOSIS, EVALUATION, AND TREATMENT

The diagnosis of congenital syphilis remains problematic as detection of *T pallidum* in body fluids or from lesions rarely is able to be performed successfully. Unlike in older

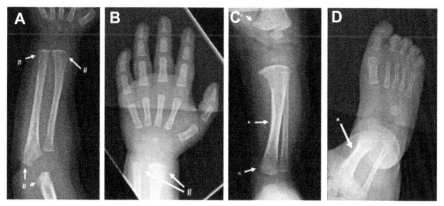

Fig. 5. Multiple bony lesions characteristic of early congenital syphilis involving the right upper extremity (*A, B*), left lower extremity (*C*), and right lower extremity (*D*). Metaphyseal lytic lesions (#) and periosteal reactions (*) were noted throughout the skeletal survey. A lytic (ˆ) lesion was interpreted as a metaphyseal fracture. (*From* Lanata MM, Bressler CJ, McKnight LV, Sanchez PJ, Tscholl JJ, Kasick RT. A Case of Fever, Rash, and a Painful Limb in an Infant. Clin Pediatr (Phila). 2019;58(6):711-714, with permission.)

children and adults, the reliance on serologic antibody assays is complicated by the transplacental passage of maternal IgG antibodies. Maternal nontreponemal and treponemal IgG antibodies can be transferred through the placenta to the fetus, complicating the interpretation of reactive serologic tests for syphilis in neonates and children less than 18 months of age. Therefore, treatment decisions frequently must be made on the basis of (1) diagnosis of syphilis in the mother, (2) adequacy of maternal treatment for syphilis, (3) presence of clinical, laboratory, or radiographic signs of syphilis in the infant, and (4) comparison of maternal (at delivery) and neonatal

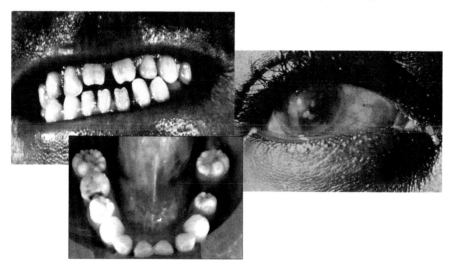

Fig. 6. Manifestations of late congenital syphilis include Hutchinson's teeth in which the teeth are widely spaced and surfaces of the incisors are notched, mulberry molars where the molars have multiple cusps instead of the usual four, and interstitial corneal keratitis, a chronic progressive keratitis of the corneal stroma, often resulting in blindness. (*From* the Centers for Disease Control and Prevention (Courtesy of Robert Sumpter).)

nontreponemal serologic titers using the same test, preferably conducted by the same laboratory.[46]

Serologic tests for syphilis are classified as nontreponemal and treponemal assays.[47,48] The nontreponemal tests include the rapid plasma reagin (RPR) test and the Venereal Disease Research Laboratory (VDRL) test. The RPR test is more sensitive than the VDRL test and therefore preferred for screening of pregnant women. These tests contain an antigen consisting of lecithin, cholesterol, and cardiolipin (diphosphatidylglycerol) that detects an IgG antibody against cardiolipin present in sera of individuals with syphilis. These tests are quantitative and therefore useful to assess adequacy of treatment (ie, a ≥4-fold decrease in titer) and reinfection (a ≥4-fold increase in titer). Additional benefits of nontreponemal tests include low cost and rapid results, but the test is not automated and needs to be performed on each individual patient's serum. Nontreponemal tests may be nonreactive in early primary syphilis, late latent syphilis, and late congenital syphilis.[49] In addition, the serum of some individuals with syphilis may exhibit a prozone phenomenon whereby the nontreponemal test result is falsely negative owing to high antibody titers, which interfere with the formation of the antigen–antibody complex necessary to visualize a positive flocculation test.[50] The prozone phenomenon can occur in primary and secondary syphilis when the nontreponemal antibody titers are disproportionately high, but can be overcome by dilution of the serum specimen that results in a positive flocculation reaction.[51,52] False-positive nontreponemal tests also can occur with connective tissue diseases, most commonly systemic lupus erythematosus, as well as with viral infections such as infectious mononucleosis, varicella, hepatitis, and measles. It also can be seen with lymphoma, tuberculosis, malaria, endocarditis, injection drug use, and during pregnancy. In newborns, performance of the RPR test on umbilical cord blood that is contaminated with Wharton's jelly may yield a false-positive reaction.

Treponemal tests such as the *T pallidum* particle agglutination (TP-PA) test and the fluorescent treponemal antibody absorbed (FTA-ABS) test become reactive before the nontreponemal tests in individuals with syphilis.[47] These tests are generally nonquantitative and, because they remain reactive indefinitely after the initial syphilis infection, they are not useful for distinguishing active versus past infection or assessing adequacy of treatment. In addition, because the treponemal assays detect mostly IgG antibodies, they are not useful in the evaluation of infants born to mothers with syphilis because they cannot distinguish maternal from infant antibody response. The 1 circumstance where the performance of a treponemal test on an infant would be helpful is when the mother is unavailable for testing. A reactive treponemal test in the infant would indicate likely exposure to maternal syphilis. Treponemal tests also are positive in individuals with other spirochetal infections such as yaws, pinta, leptospirosis, ratbite fever, relapsing fever, and Lyme disease.

Traditionally, the diagnosis of acquired syphilis involved the performance of a nontreponemal test, such as the RPR, and if reactive, followed by a confirmatory treponemal test, preferably the TP-PA test. Recently, automated and efficient treponemal tests using a high-throughput platform consisting of enzyme immunoassay, chemiluminescence immunoassay, and multiplex flow immunoassay have been developed that can test many patient sera simultaneously.[53] Many hospital laboratories have transitioned to a "reverse sequence" syphilis screening algorithm where a treponemal immunoassay is performed first and, if positive, a quantitative RPR test is done; if the RPR is also reactive, the diagnosis of syphilis is confirmed (**Fig. 7**). If the RPR is nonreactive, then the results are considered discordant and a confirmatory TP-PA is performed.[54] If the TP-PA is reactive, then syphilis (active or past) is diagnosed, but if nonreactive, then the initial positive treponemal immunoassay is most likely a false-positive result.[46,54] As many as 65% of mothers with discordant syphilis screening results have false-positive treponemal IgG immunoassay results and thus the need for reflexive testing with a TP-PA is imperative to diagnose syphilis and guide newborn management (**Fig. 8**).[55,56]

The treatment of pregnant women for syphilis is the same as the penicillin regimen appropriate for the stage of infection recommended for all adults.[47] The treatment for primary, secondary, and early latent syphilis is a single dose of intramuscular penicillin G 2.4 million units, whereas for late latent infection and syphilis of unknown duration, the treatment regimen is 3 weekly intramuscular injections of benzathine penicillin G 2.4 million units.[57] Pregnant women who miss any doses must repeat the full course of therapy for late latent syphilis or syphilis of unknown duration. Pregnant women who are allergic to penicillin should be desensitized and treated with penicillin.[47,58] Treatment may precipitate the Jarisch–Herxheimer reaction, an acute inflammatory response likely owing to the rapid killing of spirochetes.[59] Symptoms may include fever, contractions, or decreased fetal movement, resulting in fetal distress and premature labor.[60]

Infants born to mothers with syphilis should have a nontreponemal test performed and a careful examination for signs and symptoms of congenital syphilis. The nontreponemal test should be performed on infant serum rather than umbilical cord blood to avoid contamination with maternal blood or Wharton's jelly that could yield a falsely positive reaction. An infant serum quantitative nontreponemal titer that is 4-fold higher than the maternal serologic titer confirms congenital infection.[27] However, the absence of such a finding does not exclude a diagnosis of congenital syphilis, because the majority of infected infants have RPR titers that are the same or less than the maternal titer. Currently, no commercially available treponemal IgM assay is recommended for use infants and children owing to suboptimal sensitivity and specificity.

The determination of central nervous invasion with *T pallidum* is also problematic. In neonates, serum IgG antibodies cross the blood–brain barrier and could explain a reactive CSF VDRL test, irrespective of blood contamination resulting from a traumatic lumbar puncture.[61] Rabbit infectivity testing of CSF of infants born to mothers with untreated syphilis has yielded sensitivities and specificities of a reactive CSF VDRL test, pleocytosis, and elevated protein content of 53% and 90%, 38% and 88%, and 56% and 78%, respectively.[42] Overall, approximately 50% of infants with clinical, laboratory, or radiographic abnormalities consistent with congenital syphilis have spirochetes detected in CSF by rabbit infectivity testing. In contrast, central nervous system infection is infrequent among infants with normal results on clinical, laboratory, and radiographic evaluations.

An approach to the management of infants born to mothers with reactive serologic tests for syphilis is shown in **Fig. 8**. All mothers with syphilis should be tested for HIV infection, although HIV exposure or infection does not change the recommended neonatal evaluation and treatment for syphilis. Neonates with proven or highly probable congenital syphilis are those who have an abnormal physical examination that is consistent with syphilis, a serum quantitative nontreponemal titer that is 4-fold or greater than the mother's titer, or a positive darkfield test or if available, positive *T pallidum* DNA polymerase chain reaction of lesions or body fluid.[47] These infants should have a complete blood cell count and platelet count, examination of the CSF for VDRL, cell count, and protein, and other tests (eg, long bone radiographs, chest radiograph, liver function tests, ophthalmologic examination, neuroimaging, and hearing testing) as indicated clinically. They should receive 10 days of intravenous aqueous penicillin G or intramuscular procaine penicillin G (see **Fig. 8**). If more than 1 day of therapy is missed, the entire course should be restarted. When possible, a full 10-day course of penicillin is preferred, even if ampicillin was initially provided for possible sepsis.

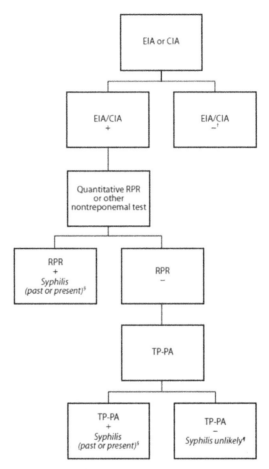

Fig. 7. Recommended algorithm for reverse sequence syphilis screening (treponemal test screening followed by nontreponemal test confirmation). The CDC recommends that a specimen with reactive enzyme immunoassay/chemiluminescence immunoassay results be tested reflexively with a quantitative nontreponemal test (eg, RPR or VDRL). If test results are discordant, the specimen should be tested reflexively using the TP-PA test as a confirmatory treponemal test. EIA/CIA = enzyme immunoassay/chemiluminescence immunoassay; RPR = rapid plasma reagin; TP-PA = *Treponema pallidum* particle agglutination.† If incubating or primary syphilis is suspected, treat with benzathine penicillin G 2.4 million units intramuscularly in a single dose.§ Evaluate clinically, determine whether treated for syphilis in the past, assess risk for infection, and administer therapy according to CDC's 2015 STD Treatment Guidelines.[47]¶ If at risk for syphilis, repeat RPR in several weeks. From Centers for Disease C, Prevention. Discordant results from reverse sequence syphilis screening–five laboratories, United States, 2006-2010. MMWR Morbidity and mortality weekly report. 2011;60(5):133-137.

Infants with possible congenital syphilis are those who have a normal physical examination, a serum quantitative nontreponemal titer equal to or less than 4-fold the maternal titer, and 1 of the following: (1) the mother was not treated, inadequately treated, or has no documentation of having received treatment, (2) the mother was treated with a nonpenicillin G regimen,[62] or (3) the mother received recommended treatment appropriate for the stage of syphilis, but the first penicillin dose was less

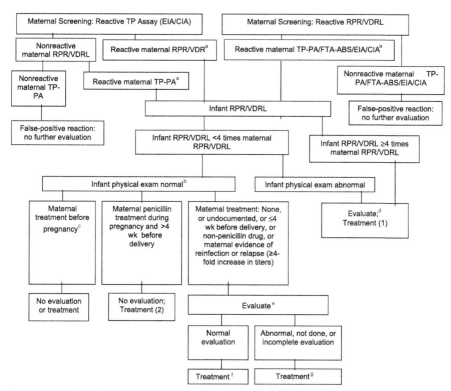

Fig. 8. Algorithm for evaluation and treatment of infants born to mothers with reactive serologic tests for syphilis. CBC, complete blood cell count; EIA/CIA, enzyme immunoassay/chemiluminescence immunoassay; FTA-ABS, fluorescent treponemal antibody absorbed; IM, intramuscular. [a] Test for HIV-antibody. Infants of HIV-infected mothers do not require different evaluation or treatment. [b] If the infant's RPR/VDRL is nonreactive AND the mother has had no treatment, undocumented treatment, treatment during pregnancy, or evidence of reinfection or relapse ($\geq$ 4-fold increase in titers), THEN treat infant with a single IM injection of benzathine penicillin (50,000 U/kg). No additional evaluation is needed. [c] Women who maintain a VDRL titer $\leq$1:2 (RPR $\leq$1:4) beyond 1 year following successful treatment are considered serofast. [d] Evaluation consists of CBC, platelet count; CSF examination for cell count, protein, and quantitative VDRL. Other tests as clinically indicated: long-bone x-rays, neuroimaging, auditory brainstem response, eye exam, chest x-ray, liver function tests. [e] CBC, platelet count; CSF examination for cell count, protein, and quantitative VDRL; long-bone x-rays. Treatment: [f] Aqueous penicillin G 50,000 U/kg IV q 12 hr ($\leq$1 wk of age), q 8 hr (>1 wk), or procaine penicillin G 50,000 U/kg IM single daily dose, x 10 days. [g] Benzathine penicillin G 50,000 U/kg IM x 1 dose. TP-PA, Treponema pallidum (italics)-particle agglutination; RPR, Rapid Plasma Reagin; VDRL, Venereal Disease Research Laboratory. *From* Cooper JM, Sánchez PJ. Congenital Syphilis. Seminars in Perinatology. 2018;42:181; with permission.

than 4 weeks before delivery.[47] The evaluation of these neonates should include complete blood cell count, platelet count, CSF examination (VDRL, cell count, and protein), and long bone radiographs. If the evaluation is completely normal, then the infant may receive a single intramuscular injection of benzathine penicillin G (see **Fig. 8**). Failure of benzathine penicillin G to treat congenital syphilis has only been reported in infants who have not had a complete evaluation.[63] If the evaluation is abnormal, incomplete, or unable to be performed, then 10 days of intravenous aqueous penicillin G or intramuscular procaine penicillin G is recommended. If the neonate's nontreponemal test is nonreactive and the physical examination is normal, treatment with a single intramuscular dose of benzathine penicillin G for possible incubating syphilis can be provided without an evaluation.[64,65]

Neonates in whom congenital syphilis is less likely are those who have a normal physical examination and a serum quantitative nontreponemal titer equal to or less than 4-fold the maternal titer, and the mother was treated appropriately during pregnancy with the first dose of penicillin administered more than 4 weeks before delivery, and she had no evidence of reinfection or relapse.[47] These infants do not require an evaluation, but many experts recommend a single dose of intramuscular penicillin G for the possibility of fetal treatment failure, which may occur in 2% to 14% of pregnancies (see **Fig. 8**).[30,66] Alternatively, close serologic follow-up of the infant is mandatory to confirm adequate fetal treatment.

Congenital syphilis is unlikely when maternal treatment for syphilis was adequate before pregnancy and the nontreponemal serologic titer remained low and stable (ie, serofast) before and during pregnancy and at delivery.[47] These infants do not require evaluation or treatment (see **Fig. 8**).

In infants older than 1 month of age born to mothers with untreated or inadequately treated syphilis, the evaluation should consist of complete blood cell count, platelet count, and CSF analysis for VDRL, cell count, and protein, with other tests such as long bone radiographs as clinically indicated.[47] The recommended treatment consists of aqueous penicillin G (200,000–300,000 U/kg/d intravenously, administered as 50,000 U/kg every 4–6 hours) for 10 days. If the infant has no clinical manifestations of congenital syphilis and the evaluation (including the CSF examination) is normal, treatment with up to 3 weekly doses of benzathine penicillin G, 50,000 U/kg IM can be considered. A single intramuscular dose of benzathine penicillin G (50,000 U/kg) can be considered after the 10-day course of intravenous aqueous penicillin to provide more comparable duration of treatment as in those who have no clinical manifestations and normal CSF.

In circumstances where penicillin is unavailable, a 10-day course of ceftriaxone may be considered with close clinical and serologic follow-up, including CSF evaluation.[47] However, ceftriaxone should not be used in neonates who are receiving calcium-containing products, such as total parenteral nutrition, owing to the formation of lethal precipitates in the lungs and kidneys.[67] In addition, ceftriaxone should be used cautiously, if at all, in neonates with jaundice given the in vitro risk of bilirubin displacement from albumin-binding sites.[68] For these reasons, ampicillin has been advocated as an alternative agent, even though the efficacy data are insufficient to recommend any alternative to penicillin. The use of agents other than penicillin requires close serologic follow-up to assess adequacy of therapy. Infants with a penicillin allergy should undergo desensitization with subsequent treatment with penicillin.

After treatment with penicillin, some infants and children will experience a Jarisch–Herxheimer reaction manifested by fever, hemodynamic instability, accentuation of cutaneous lesions, worsening of hepatic transaminases,[37,69] and even cardiovascular collapse.[70] Neither preemptive nor definitive treatment beyond supportive care is available.

PROGNOSIS AND FOLLOW-UP

The neurodevelopmental outcome of infants with congenital syphilis represents an important and vexing knowledge gap. Anecdotally, infants who receive prompt treatment in early infancy have an excellent prognosis with few if any long-term sequelae.

These infants should have careful follow-up examinations with nontreponemal serologic testing every 2 to 3 months until nonreactive or the titer has decreased by 4-fold.

Nontreponemal tests should become nonreactive or decrease by 4-fold within 6 to 12 months after appropriate treatment. Infants who were not infected often have nonreactive RPR test results by 6 months of age. If serum nontreponemal titers increase 4-fold at any time, the infant should be reevaluated and (re)treated with 10 days of intravenous penicillin G. It remains unclear what the best option is for previously treated children who maintain low stable titers beyond 18 to 24 months of age. The serologic response after therapy may be slower for infants and children who received appropriate treatment beyond the neonatal period. The finding of a reactive treponemal test beyond 18 to 24 months of age confirms a diagnosis of congenital syphilis because the maternal antibodies are no longer present. If the child was not treated previously, then treatment is indicated as for late congenital syphilis with 10 days of intravenous penicillin G.

As many as 30% of children who had confirmed congenital syphilis by detection of spirochetes in blood or CSF by rabbit infectivity testing and received appropriate penicillin treatment have nonreactive treponemal tests at 18 months of age or older. The previous recommendation of repeating a lumbar puncture at 6 months after therapy if the initial CSF evaluation was abnormal is no longer recommended, as long as the infant remains well and has an adequate serologic response to treatment. However, if a lumbar puncture is performed and is abnormal, retreatment is indicated if the abnormalities cannot be attributed to a cause other than syphilis.

PREVENTION

The prevention of congenital syphilis requires the identification and timely treatment of all infected pregnant women and their partners, which can only be achieved with universal prenatal care.[14,21,71,72] All pregnant women should be screened for syphilis at the first prenatal care visit with subsequent testing at 28 weeks' gestation and again at delivery in those with ongoing risk behaviors or residence in high prevalence communities.[73] Furthermore, their sexual partner(s) need to be identified and treated to prevent maternal reinfection. All women with a stillbirth at greater than 20 weeks of gestational age should be tested for syphilis. No newborn should be discharged from the birth hospital without the mother's serologic syphilis status known at least once during the pregnancy. Finally, all cases of syphilis must be reported to the local public health department for contact tracing and identification of core populations and environments.

DISCLOSURE

Supported in part by grants (1R29 AI 34932-01 to Dr. Sánchez from the National Institute of Allergy and Infectious Diseases and by a contract (C1000 689) with the Centers for Disease Control and Prevention.

REFERENCES

1. Thorburn AL. Fritz Richard Schaudinn, 1871-1906: protozoologist of syphilis. Br J Vener Dis 1971;47(6):459–61.
2. Von Wassermann ANA, Bruck C. Specific diagnostic blood test for syphilis. Dtsch Med Wochenschr 1906;32.
3. Edmondson DG, Hu B, Norris SJ. Long-term in vitro culture of the syphilis spirochete Treponema pallidum subsp. Pallidum. Mbio 2018;9(3).

4. Fraser CM, Norris SJ, Weinstock GM, et al. Complete genome sequence of Treponema pallidum, the syphilis spirochete. Science 1998;281(5375):375–88.

5. Radolf JD, Deka RK, Anand A, et al. Treponema pallidum, the syphilis spirochete: making a living as a stealth pathogen. Nat Rev Microbiol 2016;14(12):744–59.

6. Wang C, Cheng Y, Liu B, et al. Sensitive detection of Treponema pallidum DNA from the whole blood of patients with syphilis by the nested PCR assay. Emerg Microbes Infect 2018;7(1):83.

7. Wang C, Hu Z, Zheng X, et al. A new specimen for syphilis diagnosis: evidence by high loads of Treponema pallidum DNA in saliva. Clin Infect Dis 2020.

8. Diseases GBD, Injuries C. Global burden of 369 diseases and injuries in 204 countries and territories, 1990-2019: a systematic analysis for the Global Burden of Disease Study 2019. Lancet 2020;396(10258):1204–22.

9. Newman L, Kamb M, Hawkes S, et al. Global estimates of syphilis in pregnancy and associated adverse outcomes: analysis of multinational antenatal surveillance data. PLoS Med 2013;10(2):e1001396.

10. Su JR, Brooks LC, Davis DW, et al. Congenital syphilis: trends in mortality and morbidity in the United States, 1999 through 2013. Am J Obstet Gynecol 2016; 214(3):381, e381-389.

11. Centers for Disease C, Prevention. Primary and secondary syphilis–United States, 2000-2001. MMWR Morb Mortal Wkly Rep 2002;51(43):971–3.

12. de Voux A, Kidd S, Grey JA, et al. State-specific rates of primary and secondary syphilis among men who have sex with men - United States, 2015. MMWR Morb Mortal Wkly Rep 2017;66(13):349–54.

13. Peterman TA, Su J, Bernstein KT, et al. Syphilis in the United States: on the rise? Expert Rev Anti Infect Ther 2015;13(2):161–8.

14. Kimball A, Torrone E, Miele K, et al. Missed Opportunities for prevention of congenital syphilis - United States, 2018. MMWR Morb Mortal Wkly Rep 2020; 69(22):661–5.

15. Cooper JM, Porter M, Bazan JA, et al. Re-emergence of congenital syphilis in Ohio. Pediatr Infect Dis J 2018;37(12):1286–9.

16. Centers for Disease C. Congenital syphilis–New York city, 1986-1988. MMWR Morb Mortal Wkly Rep 1989;38(48):825–9.

17. Dunn RA, Webster LA, Nakashima AK, et al. Surveillance for geographic and secular trends in congenital syphilis–United States, 1983-1991. MMWR CDC Surveill Summ 1993;42(6):59–71.

18. Zenker P. New case definition for congenital syphilis reporting. Sex Transm Dis 1991;18(1):44–5.

19. Introcaso CE, Gruber D, Bradley H, et al. Challenges in congenital syphilis surveillance: how are congenital syphilis investigations classified? Sex Transm Dis 2013;40(9):695–9.

20. Kidd SE, Grey JA, Torrone EA, et al. Increased methamphetamine, injection drug, and heroin use among women and heterosexual men with primary and secondary syphilis - United States, 2013-2017. MMWR Morb Mortal Wkly Rep 2019; 68(6):144–8.

21. Smullin C, Wagman J, Mehta S, et al. A narrative review of the epidemiology of congenital syphilis in the United States from 1980 to 2019. Sex Transm Dis 2021;48(2):71–8.

22. Wendel GD Jr, Sanchez PJ, Peters MT, et al. Identification of Treponema pallidum in amniotic fluid and fetal blood from pregnancies complicated by congenital syphilis. Obstet Gynecol 1991;78(5 Pt 2):890–5.

23. Nathan L, Twickler DM, Peters MT, et al. Fetal syphilis: correlation of sonographic findings and rabbit infectivity testing of amniotic fluid. J Ultrasound Med 1993; 12(2):97–101.

24. Nathan L, Bohman VR, Sanchez PJ, et al. In Utero infection with Treponema pallidum in early pregnancy. Prenat Diagn 1997;17(2):119–23.

25. Hollier LM, Harstad TW, Sanchez PJ, et al. Fetal syphilis: clinical and laboratory characteristics. Obstet Gynecol 2001;97(6):947–53.

26. Sanchez PJ, McCracken GH Jr, Wendel GD, et al. Molecular analysis of the fetal IgM response to Treponema pallidum antigens: implications for improved serodiagnosis of congenital syphilis. J Infect Dis 1989;159(3):508–17.

27. Sanchez PJ, Wendel GD Jr, Grimprel E, et al. Evaluation of molecular methodologies and rabbit infectivity testing for the diagnosis of congenital syphilis and neonatal central nervous system invasion by Treponema pallidum. J Infect Dis 1993;167(1):148–57.

28. Dobson SR, Taber LH, Baughn RE. Recognition of Treponema pallidum antigens by IgM and IgG antibodies in congenitally infected newborns and their mothers. J Infect Dis 1988;157(5):903–10.

29. Harter C, Benirschke K. Fetal syphilis in the first trimester. Am J Obstet Gynecol 1976;124(7):705–11.

30. Sheffield JS, Sanchez PJ, Morris G, et al. Congenital syphilis after maternal treatment for syphilis during pregnancy. Am J Obstet Gynecol 2002;186(3):569–73.

31. Ingraham NR Jr. The value of penicillin alone in the prevention and treatment of congenital syphilis. Acta Derm Venereol Suppl 1950;31(Suppl. 24):60–87.

32. Fiumara NJ, Fleming WL, Downing JG, et al. The incidence of prenatal syphilis at the Boston City Hospital. N Engl J Med 1952;247(2):48–52.

33. Gomez GB, Kamb ML, Newman LM, et al. Untreated maternal syphilis and adverse outcomes of pregnancy: a systematic review and meta-analysis. Bull World Health Organ 2013;91(3):217–26.

34. Sheffield JS, Sanchez PJ, Wendel GD Jr, et al. Placental histopathology of congenital syphilis. Obstet Gynecol 2002;100(1):126–33.

35. Dorfman DH, Glaser JH. Congenital syphilis presenting in infants after the newborn period. N Engl J Med 1990;323(19):1299–302.

36. Fiumara NJ, Lessell S. The stigmata of late congenital syphilis: an analysis of 100 patients. Sex Transm Dis 1983;10(3):126–9.

37. Long WA, Ulshen MH, Lawson EE. Clinical manifestations of congenital syphilitic hepatitis: implications for pathogenesis. J Pediatr Gastroenterol Nutr 1984;3(4): 551–5.

38. Lanata MM, Dressler CJ, McKnight LV, et al. A case of fever, rash, and a painful Limb in an infant. Clin Pediatr (Phila) 2019;58(6):711–4.

39. Wang EA, Chambers CJ, Silverstein M. A rare presentation of congenital syphilis: pemphigus syphiliticus in a newborn infant with extensive desquamation of the extremities. Pediatr Dermatol 2018;35(2):e110–3.

40. Benzick AE, Wirthwein DP, Weinberg A, et al. Pituitary gland gumma in congenital syphilis after failed maternal treatment: a case report. Pediatrics 1999;104(1):e4.

41. Nolt D, Saad R, Kouatli A, et al. Survival with hypopituitarism from congenital syphilis. Pediatrics 2002;109(4):e63.

42. Michelow IC, Wendel GD Jr, Norgard MV, et al. Central nervous system infection in congenital syphilis. N Engl J Med 2002;346(23):1792–8.

43. Dunn RA, Zenker PN. Why radiographs are useful in evaluation of neonates suspected of having congenital syphilis. Radiology 1992;182(3):639–40 [discussion 641].

44. Stephens JR, Arenth J. Wimberger sign in congenital syphilis. J Pediatr 2015; 167(6):1451.
45. Probst LE, Wilkinson J, Nichols BD. Diagnosis of congenital syphilis in adults presenting with interstitial keratitis. Can J Ophthalmol 1994;29(2):77–80.
46. Cooper JM, Sanchez PJ. Congenital syphilis. Semin Perinatol 2018;42(3):176–84.
47. Workowski KA, Bolan GA, Centers for Disease C, Prevention. Sexually transmitted diseases treatment guidelines, 2015. MMWR Recomm Rep 2015; 64(RR-03):1–137.
48. Tuddenham S, Katz SS, Ghanem KG. Syphilis laboratory guidelines: performance characteristics of nontreponemal antibody tests. Clin Infect Dis 2020; 71(Supplement_1):S21–42.
49. Sanchez PJ, Wendel GD, Norgard MV. Congenital syphilis associated with negative results of maternal serologic tests at delivery. Am J Dis Child 1991;145(9): 967–9.
50. Spydell LE. Congenital syphilis and the prozone phenomenon: a case study. Adv Neonatal Care 2018;18(6):446–50.
51. Liu LL, Lin LR, Tong ML, et al. Incidence and risk factors for the prozone phenomenon in serologic testing for syphilis in a large cohort. Clin Infect Dis 2014;59(3): 384–9.
52. Levine Z, Sherer DM, Jacobs A, et al. Nonimmune hydrops fetalis due to congenital syphilis associated with negative intrapartum maternal serology screening. Am J Perinatol 1998;15(4):233–6.
53. Centers for Disease C, Prevention. Syphilis testing algorithms using treponemal tests for initial screening–four laboratories, New York City, 2005-2006. MMWR Morb Mortal Wkly Rep 2008;57(32):872–5.
54. Centers for Disease C, Prevention. Discordant results from reverse sequence syphilis screening–five laboratories, United States, 2006-2010. MMWR Morb Mortal Wkly Rep 2011;60(5):133–7.
55. Williams JEP, Bazan JA, Turner AN, et al. Reverse sequence syphilis screening and discordant results in pregnancy. J Pediatr 2020;219:263–6.e261.
56. Mmeje O, Chow JM, Davidson L, et al. Discordant syphilis immunoassays in pregnancy: perinatal outcomes and implications for clinical management. Clin Infect Dis 2015;61(7):1049–53.
57. Wendel GD Jr, Sheffield JS, Hollier LM, et al. Treatment of syphilis in pregnancy and prevention of congenital syphilis. Clin Infect Dis 2002;35(Suppl 2):S200–9.
58. Wendel GD Jr, Stark BJ, Jamison RB, et al. Penicillin allergy and desensitization in serious infections during pregnancy. N Engl J Med 1985;312(19):1229–32.
59. Rac MW, Greer LG, Wendel GD Jr. Jarisch-Herxheimer reaction triggered by group B streptococcus intrapartum antibiotic prophylaxis. Obstet Gynecol 2010;116(Suppl 2):552–6.
60. Klein VR, Cox SM, Mitchell MD, et al. The Jarisch-Herxheimer reaction complicating syphilotherapy in pregnancy. Obstet Gynecol 1990;75(3 Pt 1):375–80.
61. Thorley JD, Kaplan JM, Holmes RK, et al. Passive transfer of antibodies of maternal origin from blood to cerebrospinal fluid in infants. Lancet 1975; 1(7908):651–3.
62. Zhou P, Qian Y, Xu J, et al. Occurrence of congenital syphilis after maternal treatment with azithromycin during pregnancy. Sex Transm Dis 2007;34(7):472–4.
63. Beck-Sague C, Alexander ER. Failure of benzathine penicillin G treatment in early congenital syphilis. Pediatr Infect Dis J 1987;6(11):1061–4.
64. Wozniak PS, Cantey JB, Zeray F, et al. Congenital syphilis in neonates with nonreactive nontreponemal test results. J Perinatol 2017;37(10):1112–6.

65. Peterman TA, Newman DR, Davis D, et al. Do women with persistently negative nontreponemal test results transmit syphilis during pregnancy? Sex Transm Dis 2013;40(4):311–5.
66. Alexander JM, Sheffield JS, Sanchez PJ, et al. Efficacy of treatment for syphilis in pregnancy. Obstet Gynecol 1999;93(1):5–8.
67. Donnelly PC, Sutich RM, Easton R, et al. Ceftriaxone-associated biliary and Cardiopulmonary adverse events in neonates: a systematic review of the literature. Paediatr Drugs 2017;19(1):21–34.
68. Fink S, Karp W, Robertson A. Ceftriaxone effect on bilirubin-albumin binding. Pediatrics 1987;80(6):873–5.
69. Anand NK, Chellani HK, Wadhwa A, et al. Congenital syphilitic hepatitis. Indian Pediatr 1991;28(2):157–9.
70. Wang C, He S, Yang H, et al. Unique manifestations and risk factors of Jarisch-Herxheimer reaction during treatment of child congenital syphilis. Sex Transm Infect 2018;94(8):562–4.
71. Stafford IA, Sanchez PJ, Stoll BJ. Ending congenital syphilis. JAMA 2019; 322(21):2073–4.
72. Cooper JM, Michelow IC, Wozniak PS, et al. In time: the persistence of congenital syphilis in Brazil - more progress needed! Revi Paul Pediatr 2016;34(3):251–3.
73. Lin JS, Eder ML, Bean SI. Screening for syphilis infection in pregnant women: updated evidence report and systematic review for the US preventive services task force. JAMA 2018;320(9):918–25.

Ebola, Dengue, Chikungunya, and Zika Infections in Neonates and Infants

Annabelle de St. Maurice, MD, MPH[a],[*],[1], Elizabeth Ervin, MPH[b],[1], Alison Chu, MD[c]

KEYWORDS

- Ebola • Zika virus • Chikungunya • Dengue • Congenital infection • Pregnancy

KEY POINTS

- Emerging infectious diseases, such as Ebola, chikungunya, Zika, and dengue, may have significant impacts on maternal and fetal health.
- Although treatment of these infections during pregnancy consists mostly of supportive care, the recent development of novel therapeutics for Ebola virus disease in promising.
- Women largely have been excluded from clinical vaccine trials for Ebola, dengue, chikungunya, and Zika; therefore, data on immunogenicity and safety of these vaccines in pregnant women are limited.

BACKGROUND

Pregnant women may be more susceptible to severe infections than nonpregnant women, particularly for certain infections, such as influenza and malaria.[1] The severity of infection in pregnant women likely is due to hormones (eg, estradiol) affecting cellular and adaptive humoral immunity.[1]

Emerging infectious diseases, such as Ebola, dengue, chikungunya virus (CHIKV), and Zika virus, pose specific challenges for obstetricians and neonatologists (**Fig. 1**). Few of these viral diseases have treatments that have been well studied in pregnant women or neonates. Some emerging infections can be severe in pregnant women and can result in infant mortality and lead to congenital malformations.

---

[a] Division of Pediatric Infectious Diseases, Department of Pediatrics, Los Angeles, 924 Westwood Boulevard, Suite 900, CA 90095, USA; [b] Post-baccalaureate Premedical Program, University of Michigan, Office of Graduate and Postdoctoral Studies, 2960 Taubman Health Science Library, 1135 Catherine Street, Ann Arbor, MI 48109, USA; [c] Division of Neonatology and Developmental Biology, Department of Pediatrics, 10833 Le Conte Avenue, MDCC B2-411, Los Angeles, CA 90095, USA
[1] Share first authorship.
* Corresponding author.
E-mail address: adestmaurice@mednet.ucla.edu

Clin Perinatol 48 (2021) 311–329
https://doi.org/10.1016/j.clp.2021.03.006

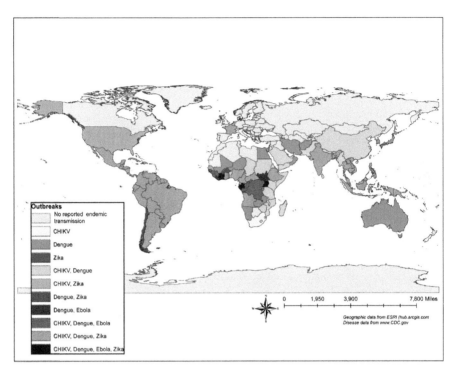

Fig. 1. Map of countries with endemic transmission of Zika, dengue, chikungunya (CHIKV), and Ebola. Each color represents endemic transmission of 1 or more viruses. Yellow: areas with CHIKV only; light blue: areas with dengue only; light red: areas with Zika only; light green: CHIKV and dengue; orange: CHIKV and Zika; purple: dengue and Zika; dark blue: dengue and Ebola; dark green: CHIKV, dengue, and Ebola; tan: CHIKV, dengue, and Zika; and dark red: CHIKV, dengue, Ebola, and Zika.

This review describes the epidemiology and presentation of Ebola, dengue, chikungunya, and Zika virus in pregnant women and infants and reviews the development of therapeutics and vaccines (**Table 1**).

EBOLA VIRUS DISEASE
Epidemiology

Ebola virus is an enveloped, negative strand RNA virus in the *Filoviridae* family.[2] Ebola virus first was identified following an outbreak near the Ebola river in the Democratic Republic of the Congo (DRC) and southern Sudan in 1976.[3] Since 1976, there have been several Ebola outbreaks, the largest of which occurred in West Africa from 2014 to 2016.[4] The second largest Ebola outbreak occurred from 2018 to 2020 in the North and South Kivu regions of the DRC.[5] The outbreak was declared over in June 2020.

Ebola outbreaks typically occur through a spillover event from a zoonotic reservoir to the human population.[4,6] Subsequent human-to-human transmission of Ebola virus occurs through direct human-to-human contact, through contact with infected tissues or bodily fluids, or less commonly via indirect contact with contaminated surfaces or objects.[6]

Disease Presentation

The incubation period for Ebola is 2 days to 21 days (mean 4–10 days).[4] Ebola virus disease (EVD) symptoms include fever, chills, fatigue, and myalgia.[4] EVD then progresses to widespread systemic symptoms, including gastrointestinal, respiratory, vascular, and neurologic symptoms, culminating in a hemorrhagic phase characterized by petechiae, ecchymoses, and internal and external bleeding. Laboratory studies demonstrate leukopenia, lymphopenia, and neutrophilia as well as thrombocytopenia, elevated serum liver enzymes, and prothrombin and partial thromboplastin times consistent with diffuse intravascular coagulopathy. The case fatality rate of EVD is between 40% and 50%, although it does vary by study.[6] Mortality may vary across populations due to differences in access to health care, genetics, overall health of the affected population, and testing availability.

Treatment

Supportive care is the mainstay of treatment of EVD; however, clinical trials during the recent EVD outbreak in the DRC have identified novel treatments, including monoclonal antibodies.[7] The 2 most promising therapies were mAb114 (Cook Pharmaca LLC, Bloomington, IN, USA) and REGN-EBS (Regeneron Pharmaceuticals, New York, USA) which reduced mortality substantially and had the most benefit when given early in the disease course. REGN-EB3 is the only Food and Drug Administration (FDA)-approved medication for the treatment of EVD in the United States.[8] Because safety and efficacy data for these therapies in pregnant women are sparse, the risks and benefits need to be weighed when considering their use in pregnant women.[9] The World Health Organization (WHO) recommends that these therapies be used in pregnant women only in the context of clinical research or under the Monitored Emergency Use of Unregistered Investigational Interventions protocols.[9]

Ebola Virus Disease and Pregnancy

The interaction between Ebola virus infection and pregnancy is poorly understood. Prior to 2014, pregnant women with EVD with poor outcomes were described in outbreaks in Sudan and Zaire (now DRC).[3,10–12] Cases of pregnant women from the 1976 Sudan outbreak and the Zaire outbreak demonstrated high case fatality, high rates of fetal demise and neonatal death, and no evidence of neonatal survival.[3,12] In a case series of pregnant women with EVD in the Kikwit area of the DRC in 1995, mortality was very high (95.5%).[11] Evidence accrued during the 2014 Ebola epidemic suggests that pregnant women with EVD have a high mortality rate and that there are very high rates of adverse pregnancy outcomes, including fetal demise and neonatal death.[13] The interaction between EVD infection and pregnancy, however, is not well understood.[13] Reports from the 2014 outbreak in West Africa demonstrated high mortality rates among pregnant women as well, although perhaps not as high as those reported in Kikwit; however, few cases of EVD in pregnancy were reported overall.[14,15] Data from a small study demonstrated that of 77 pregnant women admitted to an Ebola treatment unit managed by Médecins Sans Frontières, only 36 survived (47%).[14]

Given the limited data that exist on Ebola infection in pregnancy, it is difficult to conclude whether timing of EVD infection in pregnancy affects maternal or neonatal outcomes. WHO guidelines recommend supportive care for pregnant women with EVD, including the conditional use of investigational interventions.[9] Induction of labor or invasive procedures are not recommended for fetal indications in women with EVD.[9] Breastfeeding is not recommended in women with acute EVD, and separation of the mother from the infant is recommended to prevent additional exposures.[9] Ebola virus RNA has been identified in the breastmilk of women with both acute and convalescent EVD and possible evidence of mother-to-child transmission through breastmilk exists.[16] For women who have recovered from EVD, breastfeeding may be an option.[9] Testing of the breastmilk by reverse transcription–polymerase chain reaction (RT-PCR) to assess for persistent viral shedding is recommended prior to initiation of breastfeeding.[9]

Risk of Congenital Transmission and Prognosis for Infected Infants

There are reports of Ebola virus detection in vaginal swabs, amniotic fluid, fetal cord blood, and placental tissue.[17–23] There are few reports, however, of histopathologic examinations of infected fetal tissue.[22] RT-PCR, ELISAs, transmission electron microscopy, and histopathologic examination of maternal and fetal specimens collected from 2 pairs of women and their infants in Gulu, Uganda, and in Isiro, DRC,[22] demonstrated evidence of Ebola virus antigen in the placenta by immunohistochemical staining; however, there was no evidence of positive antigen staining in the fetal tissue. The syncytiotrophoblast and extravillous trophoblast also had evidence of Ebola virus by immunohistochemical staining. This suggests that Ebola virus may cross the placental-epithelial barrier, resulting in fetal infection in utero.

The pathogenesis of Ebola infection in neonates is not well understood,[22] with sparse information about the teratogenic effects of Ebola infection. The longest recorded neonatal survival in the setting of maternal infection with acute EVD was 19 days prior to the 2014 Ebola pandemic.[3,24] Some reports describe fetuses delivered to women with EVD as being deformed,[19] whereas other reports describe neonates born to EVD-infected mothers as appearing morphologically normal at birth.[23] Moreover, some liveborn neonates developed symptoms only after several days.[21,22] It is unclear if these neonates were infected while in utero or became infected in the peripartum or postpartum time period (eg, transvaginally or through breastfeeding).

There is only 1 report of neonatal survival in an infant born to a previously healthy 25-year-old woman with symptom onset 8 days prior to delivery and diagnostic evidence of acute EVD infection.[25] The mother was treated with favipiravir on day 5 of her illness and died on the eighth day of her illness (hospital day 5) after a spontaneous vaginal delivery, due to severe vaginal bleeding. Her infant was treated with monoclonal antibodies (ZMapp), a buffy coat transfusion from an Ebola survivor, and the antiviral drug GS-5734 (remdesivir). Aside from seizure-like activity, the infant had no other symptoms and was discharged with normal development and growth at 12 months of age.[25]

Vaccination of Pregnant Mothers

The WHO prequalified the first vaccine for Ebola, rVSV-ZEBOV-GP (Ervebo, Merck, New Jersey, USA), in November 2019.[9] The FDA also approved the vaccine in the United States in December 2019.[26] This live, attenuated recombinant vesicular stomatitis vaccine has been found to be protective when used as part of a ring-vaccination strategy of exposed individuals.[27] Although initial studies excluded pregnant women, some women became pregnant while enrolled in the trial and 1 vaccine trial demonstrated that the risk of fetal loss among vaccinated women was not substantially different from unvaccinated women.[28] Based on an analysis of safety data from clinical trials and cohort studies and weighing the risks and benefits of vaccination, the WHO recommended that pregnant and lactating women should be offered vaccination using rVSV-ZEBOV-GP during an active Zaire EVD outbreak, as part of a research study, or for compassionate use.[9]

ZIKA VIRUS
Epidemiology

Zika virus is an enveloped positive-sense RNA virus in the Flaviviridae family.[29] First identified in 1947 in the Zika Forest in Uganda, Zika virus circulating among nonhuman primates and mosquitoes resulted in occasional transmission to humans in rural settings. In 2007, outbreaks occurred in Micronesia and French Polynesia with evidence of transmission in urban settings.[30] By 2015, Zika was endemic in Brazil, where the association of congenital microcephaly and maternal Zika virus infection first was described.[31,32] Microcephaly resulting from congenital transmission has been subsequently described in additional settings.[30,31,33,34]

Zika virus transmission to humans occurs through the bite of infected mosquitoes; however, human-to-human transmission may occur through mucosal exposure to infected blood or body fluids.[30] Examples of human-to-human transmissions include blood transfusion, transplantation of bone marrow or solid organs, and sexual activity.[30]

Disease Presentation

The incubation period of Zika ranges from 3 days to 14 days.[29] Zika virus infection most often is asymptomatic, but symptomatic disease is characterized by a mild febrile illness associated with rash, arthralgia, myalgia, and conjunctivitis.[29] Severe complications, including Guillain-Barré syndrome, meningoencephalitis, transient myocarditis, and thrombocytopenia, may occur rarely. Mortality is estimated to be less than 0.01%, and deaths occur among immunocompromised individuals and those with comorbidities.[29] The manifestations of Zika virus infections in pregnant and nonpregnant women are similar.[31]

Zika Treatment

There are no specific treatments for self-limited Zika virus infections; the mainstay of therapy is supportive care.[30] Those with severe complications, such as Guillain-Barré syndrome, may require hospitalization and further therapy. Because of the potential person-to-vector-to-person risk of transmission, infected individuals should avoid mosquito bites while they are symptomatic, to avoid further transmission to others.

Zika Virus and Congenital Malformations

Congenital Zika virus infection has been associated with a spectrum of anomalies,[29] notably severe microcephaly, characterized by premature closure of the fontanels and overlapping sutures.[29] Children with congenital Zika syndrome may have neurologic abnormalities, including decreased myelination, cerebellar hypoplasia, abnormalities of neuronal migration, and enlarged ventricles.[29] As a result, children may have seizures, neurodevelopmental delay, hearing loss, and visual impairment. Ocular abnormalities, including pigmented retinal mottling and chorioretinal atrophy, are most common, with ocular calcifications, microphthalmia, lens subluxation, and iris colobomas occurring less frequently.[8] Musculoskeletal abnormalities include arthrogryposis, hip dislocation, and talipes equinovarus or club foot.

The risk of congenital Zika syndrome is greatest when infection occurs in the first trimester[25,33]; however, infection in the second or third trimester may result in notable anomalies.[31,35] The odds ratio (OR) for having a child with microcephaly is reported to be as high as 21.9 for women with Zika virus infection during pregnancy compared with women with no Zika virus infection.[32] A recent meta-analysis found that the prevalence of microcephaly in pregnant women with symptomatic Zika virus was 63%

compared with 46% in asymptomatic pregnant women with Zika virus infection.[36] Zika virus has been identified in the amniotic fluid of pregnant women,[37] in placental tissue[38] and in multiple organs in infants with congenital Zika syndrome.[34]

Vaccine Development for Pregnant Women

Following the 2017 Zika virus outbreak, multiple public and private organizations began research initiatives to develop a safe and effective vaccine based on a variety of formulations.[39] Because the number of Zika virus infections has decreased substantially, phase III trials to assess efficacy have been more difficult to conduct with decreased Zika virus prevalence. A recent placebo-controlled phase I trial of a purified inactivated Zika virus vaccine candidate demonstrated safety and immunogenicity in a small number of people.[40] Currently, there are no US FDA-licensed vaccines to prevent Zika virus infections. Further vaccine studies should be conducted in pregnant women to understand the efficacy of these vaccines in preventing congenital malformations.

CHIKUNGUNYA
Epidemiology

CHIKV is a mosquito-borne virus first isolated in the *Aedes aegypti* mosquito,[41] in 1952, in present-day Tanzania.[42] Isolated cases or sporadic outbreaks have been reported mostly in Africa,[43,44] until 2004, when an outbreak that may have started in Kenya spread to India and across tropical Asia, affecting millions of people in large epidemics over the next several years.[42,43] In 2013, the first autochthonous outbreak of CHIKV in the Americas was confirmed in the Caribbean island of Saint Martin. CHIKV has continued to spread in the region[41,45] and, to date, more than 100 countries globally report local transmission.[41,46] Several additional *Aedes* mosquito species, notably *A albopictus*, have been found to be competent vectors for CHIKV.[42,43,47]

Disease Presentation

The mean incubation period is approximately 3 days.[42] A majority of people infected with CHIKV develop symptoms; however, CHIKV rarely is fatal.[42,43] Acute chikungunya fever typically presents with rapid-onset of fever followed by asthenia, arthralgia, myalgia, headache, and maculopapular rash. Joint pain is common, seen in 90% of patients, and usually is symmetric across arms and legs.[43,47] Rash also is common, seen in 20% to 80% of acute cases.

Treatment

Current treatment is supportive therapy only, with no specific antiviral option. Anti-inflammatory drugs can be used to alleviate symptoms and control joint swelling.[41,43]

Risk of Congenital Transmission and Prognosis For Infected Infants

CHIKV infection typically is not associated with increased risk of complications in pregnant women, and its major morbidity instead is related to adverse neonatal outcomes related to neonatal infection after intrapartum transmission.[44] A study of 1400 pregnant women affected during the 2006 epidemic in La Réunion showed that rates of stillbirth, congenital anomalies, premature birth, and low birthweight were not significantly higher in CHIKV-infected women compared with those who were uninfected.[48] Although congenital infection before 22 weeks of gestation has been associated with fetal loss, congenital malformations have not been reported.[49,50] Maternal CHIKV infection after 22 weeks of gestation does not appear to be associated with worse fetal outcomes. Of 739 women with CHIKV infection diagnosed during pregnancy, 700 were symptomatic in the antepartum period and none of their neonates developed CHIKV infection.[51] A large systematic review of 13 studies demonstrated that the pooled risk of symptomatic neonatal disease was 50% for intrapartum infections versus 0% for antepartum/peripartum maternal infections.[52] Smaller individual studies support these rates of neonatal disease, with perinatal transmission reported in up to 50% of viremic mothers (within 48 hours before or after delivery).[48,51,53,54] Although the overall pooled risk of mother-to-child transmission was 15.5%,[52] these studies taken together suggest that prenatal and postnatal exposure of the fetus or neonate to CHIKV does not result in increased risk of neonatal infection whereas intrapartum transmission does result in neonatal infection with both short-term and long-term sequelae.

The typical clinical course for neonatal CHIKV infection after intrapartum transmission is an infant who is asymptomatic at birth, who develops fever, poor feeding, joint swelling, rash, and hematologic and hepatic laboratory abnormalities (including transaminitis, hypoalbuminemia, hyperbilirubinemia, and prolonged partial thromboplastin time) 3 days to 5 days after birth.[51] More severely infected neonates develop respiratory distress, sepsis, meningoencephalitis, cardiac abnormalities, necrotizing enterocolitis, and/or myocarditis.[55,56] In a large cohort study of more than 7500 pregnant women, 100% of affected newborns were symptomatic, with more than half presenting with encephalopathy.[51]

In neonates, intrapartum exposure has led to severe disease with encephalopathy and long-term neurologic sequelae.[42–44] Among perinatally CHIKV-infected neonates who developed encephalitis, magnetic resonance imaging revealed severe white matter injury that progresses in 3 stages: cytotoxic brain edema (ischemia), vasogenic edema (reperfusion), and mass reduction (demyelination).[51,57] Long-term outcomes are guarded; newborns infected via intrapartum transmission during the CHIKV epidemic in La Réunion scored poorly in developmental testing at 2 years of age in motor, language, and social domains, with approximately 12% of infected newborns categorized as having severe developmental delay, including microcephaly and cerebral palsy.[57] In contrast, fetuses or neonates exposed to CHIKV in the prenatal or postnatal period (outside of the intrapartum period) do not demonstrate worse neurodevelopmental outcomes at 2 years of age.[58] It is suggested that severe CHIKV disease can be linked to unique viral genotypes, and on the other hand, divergent and geographically distinct CHIKV genotypes can induce similar disease syndromes. This is an important clinicopathologic consideration, because it provides context for studies of neonatal outcomes from geographically and temporally specific outbreaks.[59]

Vaccine

There is no licensed vaccine for use in humans, although efforts to develop a vaccine have been ongoing for decades. A few candidates have progressed to phase I and phase II trials and still are in development.[60]

DENGUE
Epidemiology

Dengue is the fastest-spreading disease caused by an arthropod-borne virus (arbovirus),[61,62] with 40% to over 50% of the world's population[64] reported to be at risk in more than 100 countries, now considered dengue endemic. Globally, 100 million of 400 million people are estimated to have symptomatic infection,[61] resulting in between 10,000 to 22,000 deaths annually.[63–65]

Four dengue virus (DENV) serotypes cause disease in humans. Recovery from infection of 1 serotype is thought to provide long-lasting or even lifelong immunity to that serotype; however, there is little or transient cross-immunity to other serotypes.[61,66,67] An individual, therefore, can be infected 4 times[61,63] and subsequent infections have been linked to increased risk of severe disease.[61,65]

The major vectors for transmission of DENV to humans are the *A aegypti* and *A albopictus* mosquitoes. DENV is transmitted to humans through the bite of an infected female mosquito, and humans with DENV viremia also can infect mosquitos. Once infectious, the mosquito can transmit virus for the rest of its life, leading to further human transmission.[61]

Disease Presentation

Identification of dengue can be challenging because most infections are believed to have little to no symptoms or to have mild, self-limiting illness.[67] Symptomatic patients commonly present with sudden onset of fever and other symptoms, including headache, vomiting, myalgia, arthralgia, malaise, asthenia, and generalized rash.[61,66,68–70] Severe forms of DENV infections progress to dengue hemorrhagic fever or dengue shock syndrome.[61,67,68] Features of severe dengue include persistent vomiting, increasing abdominal pain or tenderness, and hemorrhagic signs, including petechiae and mucosal bleeding.[61,70] An increase in hematocrit along with a decrease in platelet count also is seen in severe dengue.[61] There may be increased risk for poor pregnancy outcome in women with clinical symptoms of dengue fever.[67]

Treatment

Treatment of symptomatic DENV infections is supportive care.

Vaccine

The FDA announced the approval of Dengvaxia (Sanofi Pasteur, Lyon, France), a vaccine for dengue prevention[71] in people ages 9 years to 16 years who have laboratory-confirmed previous dengue infection and who live in endemic areas of the United States, including Puerto Rico, the US Virgin Islands, American Samoa, and Guam, in May of 2019. Dengvaxia, or CYD-TDV, is a live, attenuated, recombinant tetravalent vaccine. It has been recommended for limited use by the WHO in 2016 and with revised guidance in 2018. WHO recommendations state that vaccination should be based on country-specific data in the population at greatest risk but can include people between ages 9 years and 45 years. The vaccine has been shown to be safe and efficacious in persons with previous dengue infection, which should be laboratory confirmed prior to vaccination. Vaccination in persons without prior infection may lead to increased risk of severe dengue disease if natural dengue infection occurs after vaccination.

Although approval for use of CYD-TDV does not include neonates or infants, women of reproductive age are included in the WHO recommendations. From a limited data set accrued from 19 CYD-TDV clinical trials, a small number of women were reported to have received inadvertent vaccination with of CYD-TDV. In assessing pregnancy outcomes, there was no evidence of higher than baseline adverse pregnancy outcomes in women inadvertently vaccinated in early pregnancy compared with control groups.[72]

Risk of Congenital Transmission and Prognosis for Infected Infants

Dengue can be vertically transmitted (transplacental) or transmitted during the perinatal period. Many studies have reported maternal-to-fetal transmission of DENV.[73–78]

Table 1
Summary of infection and treatment in pregnant women, congenital syndromes and vaccine development for Ebola, Chikungunya, Dengue and Zika infections

Disease	Infection in Pregnant Women	Treatment in Pregnant Women	Congenital Syndromes	Vaccine Development
Ebola	Based on limited evidence, pregnant women infected with Ebola demonstrate high case fatality, high rates of abortions, and no (to extremely low) evidence of neonatal survival.	Supportive care, including conditional use of investigational interventions, is advised in pregnant women infected with EVD. Induction of labor or invasive procedures are not indicated for fetal indications.	Only 1 report of neonatal survival after acute maternal EVD infection late in pregnancy. The baby was treated with monoclonal antibodies (ZMapp) and the antiviral GS-5734. There was normal growth and development reported at 12 mo of age. Reports of fetuses or newborns who died shortly after birth have varied from normal appearing to having gross deformities. Other reports describe symptoms developing several days after birth.	rVSV-ZEBOV GP is a live, attenuated recombinant vesicular stomatitis vaccine that is effective when used as part of a ring-vaccination strategy. This vaccine should be offered to pregnant and lactating women during active EVD outbreaks as part of a research study or for compassionate use.
Chikungunya	Evidence suggests the highest risk to neonates occurs during maternal-fetal blood exchange in delivery (Burt, Weave).[42,43] Data suggest that although antepartum congenital infection has been detected in miscarried fetuses, there is the lack of epidemiologic evidence overall to suggest a causal association between infection and miscarriage (Mehta).[44]	Treatment is supportive.	Overall, rates of stillbirth, congenital anomalies, premature birth and low birthweight are similar in neonates born to infected mothers compared with uninfected mothers. Congenital infections prior to 20 wk gestational age, however, have been associated with fetal loss, whereas congenital infection after 22 wk is not associated	Many in development, some phase I and phase II clinical trials

(continued on next page)

Table 1
(continued)

Disease	Infection in Pregnant Women	Treatment in Pregnant Women	Congenital Syndromes	Vaccine Development
			with worse fetal outcomes. Perinatal transmission has been reported, however, in up to 50% of viremic mother, 100% of affected newborns were reported as symptomatic; 50% of symptomatic infants present with encephalopathy. The typical course of perinatally acquired congenital infection is the development of symptoms, including fever, poor feeding, joint swelling, rash, and hematologic and hepatic laboratory abnormalities 3–5 d after birth. More severe infections are characterized by respiratory distress, sepsis, meningoencephalitis, cardiac abnormalities, necrotizing enterocolitis, and/or myocarditis. Long-term outcomes of infected neonates, especially those with meningoencephalitis, may include developmental delays, microcephaly and cerebral palsy.	
Dengue	Although symptoms can vary widely, infected patients commonly present with sudden-	Treatment is supportive.	Dengue can be vertically transmitted or perinatally transmitted. Overall maternal-	Dengvaxia, or CYD-TDV, is a live, attenuated recombinant tetravalent vaccine, and limited

	onset of fever and systemic symptoms, including headache, vomiting, myalgia, arthralgia, malaise, asthenia, and rash. Severe infections can progress to dengue hemorrhagic fever or dengue shock syndrome	fetal transmission rate has been estimated to be ~ 20%, though this may be close to 50% when considering perinatal transmission. Maternal infection has not been consistently shown to be significantly associated with worse fetal outcomes, including premature birth, SGA status, or fetal loss. Mothers with severe infection, however, may have higher risk of preterm birth or low-birthweight neonates. Congenital malformations have been reported in association with maternal DENV infection. Neonates with primary infection experience symptoms, such as fever, rash, hepatitis and thrombocytopenia. Severe neonatal disease is rare and can include sepsis and encephalitis. Long-term outcomes are good.	data on its inadvertent use in pregnant women suggest no evidence of higher-than-normal adverse pregnancy outcomes.
Zika	Presenting similarly to nonpregnant infected individuals, pregnant women may have a mild febrile illness or by asymptomatic.	Congenital Zika syndrome risk is greatest if maternal infection occurs in the first trimester. Infections in any trimester, however, can lead to significant congenital anomalies. Severe microcephaly, characterized by premature closure of the fontanelles and overlapping sutures, may occur. Other	Phase III trials have been difficult to conduct, given the natural occurrence of the disease is less prevalent. A recent placebo-controlled phase I trial of a purified inactivated zika virus vaccine candidate, however, demonstrated safety and immunogenicity in a small number of patients.

(continued on next page)

Table 1
(continued)

Disease	Infection in Pregnant Women	Treatment in Pregnant Women	Congenital Syndromes	Vaccine Development
			neurologic abnormalities include decreased myelination, cerebellar hypoplasia, abnormalities of neuronal migration, calcifications, and enlarged ventricles. These structural abnormalities are associated with seizures, neurodevelopmental delays, and hearing and vision impairment. Ophthalmologic abnormalities also are common, such as microphthalmia, pigmented retinal mottling, chorioretinal atrophy, lens subluxation, and iris colobomas. Musculoskeletal abnormalities include arthrogryposis, hip dislocation, and talipes equinovarus.	

In case reports, DENV has been detected in placental samples from aborted fetuses, and specific IgM, nonstructural (NS1) antigen, and DENV RNA have been detected in newborn sera.[79–81] In 1 review of 19 case reports and 9 case series, the overall vertical transmission rate was 34 of 168 infants (20%). Similarly, in a prospective cohort study of 54 women, the overall risk of vertical transmission was estimated to be between 18.5% and 22.7%. When considering only maternal infections detected within approximately 2 weeks prior to and 2 days after delivery, the risk of vertical transmission increased to approximately 56.2%.[79]

Low levels of viremia may lead to false-negative diagnostic results in the first 2 days after birth.[82] Neonates with a primary infection may experience a longer phase of fever and duration of viremia due to a limited immunologic response. For these reasons, asymptomatic high-risk infants at birth should be monitored closely, even with a negative diagnostic test at birth. Repeat screening using the NS1 antigen in newborns born to mothers with dengue should be considered, because NS1 antigen may be detected up to 7 days after birth, with a peak on the fifth postnatal day.[82] Serology can take up to 2 weeks from infection to have detectable antibody.

The fetal/neonatal outcomes of perinatally acquired Dengue are not well characterized. Studies of dengue infection in pregnancy and neonatal outcomes have been conducted in small cohorts, with the exception of a few studies in Brazil, French Guiana, Sudan, and Mexico. One study of 82 maternal-infant dyads in 2013 from 9 centers in Mexico found no deaths nor vertical transmission prior to hospital discharge in full-term neonates with normal birthweight.[83] Similarly, a matched cohort study of 292 pregnant women in French Guiana, 73 of whom had symptomatic dengue, suggested that exposure to DENV was not significantly associated with prematurity, small-for-gestational-age (SGA) status, or in utero demise, although there was a trend toward significance ($P = .09$) for fetal loss.[84] A systematic review and meta-analysis of original studies reporting fetal outcomes suggest that among 6071 pregnant women, the most commonly reported adverse outcomes were preterm birth (OR 1.71; 95% CI, 1.06–2.76) and low birthweight. Low birthweight, defined as either SGA (birthweight below the tenth percentile) or a birthweight less than 2500 g, was not associated with maternal DENV infection. There also was a minor association with pregnancy loss at less than 22 weeks' gestation and maternal DENV infection (OR 3.51; 95% CI, 1.15–10.77).[67] Significant heterogeneity among included studies, however, may limit the interpretation of these findings.

The risk of premature birth and fetal loss has been associated with severity of maternal disease.[85] A large population-based cohort of Brazilian women and their infants from 2006 to 2012 found an increased risk of adverse birth outcomes (preterm birth and low birthweight <2500 g) in women with severe dengue infection during pregnancy.[86]

Congenital malformations have not been associated definitively with DENV infection. One large population-based study in Brazil suggested an association of maternal dengue infection with congenital malformations of the brain; however, this study was limited by suboptimal reporting and accounting of confounding variables, such as co-infection, maternal age, and drug exposures.[87] A large retrospective cohort study of more than 3800 pregnant patients in Brazil with symptomatic DENV infection did not report an increased risk of congenital malformations in infants born to dengue-infected women compared with infants born to dengue-uninfected pregnant women.[88]

Up to 85% of neonates with perinatally acquired DENV infection in a cohort in Brazil were symptomatic.[89] Fever, rash, hepatitis, and thrombocytopenia were more common than severe neonatal disease, which was rare (eg, sepsis and encephalitis).

Overall, the clinical course of neonatal dengue typically is mild and characterized by nonspecific fever and hematologic abnormalities, with a good prognosis.[90] To date, there have not been documented long-term sequelae in the neonate infected with DENV.

SUMMARY

Emerging infectious diseases, such as Ebola, chikungunya, Zika, and dengue, may have a significant impact on maternal and fetal health. Although treatment of these infections during pregnancy consists mostly of supportive care, the recent development of novel therapeutics for EVD in promising. Women largely have been excluded from clinical vaccine trials for Ebola, dengue, chikungunya, and Zika; therefore, data on immunogenicity and safety are limited. Further research on therapeutic and preventative measures should be conducted in pregnant women for these and other emerging diseases.

CLINICS CARE POINTS

- Emerging infectious diseases caused by Ebola, chikungunya, Zika, and dengue viruses impact pregnant women and their neonates.
- Pregnant women infected with Ebola have high mortality and there is low neonatal survival.
- Maternal chikungunya infection carries high rates of perinatal transmission and affected neonates have variable disease severity.
- Dengue can be transmitted to neonates via vertical or perinatal transmission.
- Zika virus causes mild disease in pregnant women, but can cause severe congenital infections.

Best practices

What is the current practice?

- Ebola, Dengue, chikungunya, and Zika virus infections should be suspected in symptomatic mothers with a history of travel to areas where these viruses are endemic
- Providers should obtain a thorough maternal history of travel and infectious symptoms during pregnancy, particularly in symptomatic neonates (Table 1)
- Testing for Ebola, Dengue, chikungunya, and Zika should be considered in symptomatic infants whose mother's have risk factors for infection
- Promising vaccines are in development for these emerging infectious diseases

DISCLOSURE

The authors have nothing to disclose.

REFERENCES

1. Kourtis AP, Read JS, Jamieson DJ. Pregnancy and infection. N Engl J Med 2014; 370(23):2211–8.
2. Feldmann H, Sanchez A, Geisbert TW. Filoviridae: marburg and ebola viruses. In: Knipe DM, Howley PM, editors. Fields Virology, vol. 1. Philadelphia, PA: Lippincott Williams & Wilkins; 2013. p. 1995–9.

3. WHO. Ebola haemorrhagic fever, in Zaire, 1976. Bulletin of the World Health Organization. 1978;56:271-293.

4. Feldmann H, Geisbert TW. Ebola haemorrhagic fever. Lancet 2011;377(9768): 849-62.

5. WHO. Ebola Virus Disease Democratic Republic of the Congo. External Situation Report 98. June 23 2020 2020.

6. Jacob ST, Crozier I, Fischer WA 2nd, et al. Ebola virus disease. Nat Rev Dis Primers 2020;6(1):13.

7. Iversen PL, Kane CD, Zeng X, et al. Recent successes in therapeutics for Ebola virus disease: no time for complacency. Lancet Infect Dis 2020;20(9):e231-7.

8. FaDA. FDA Approves first treatment for Ebola virus. Available at: https://www.fda. gov/news-events/press-announcements/fda-approves-first-treatment-ebola-virus.

9. WHO. Guidelines for the management of pregnant and breastfeeding women in the context of Ebola Virus Disease 2020. Available at: https://apps.who.int/iris/bitstream/handle/10665/330851/9789240001381-eng.pdf?ua=1. Accessed November 11, 2020.

10. Francesconi P, Yoti Z, Declich S, et al. Ebola hemorrhagic fever transmission and risk factors of contacts, Uganda. Emerg Infect Dis 2003;9(11):1430-7.

11. Mupapa K, Mukundu W, Bwaka MA, et al. Ebola hemorrhagic fever and pregnancy. J Infect Dis 1999;179(Suppl 1):S11-2.

12. WHO. Ebola haemorrhagic fever in Sudan, 1976. Bulletin of the World Health Organization. 1978;56:247-270.

13. Jamieson DJ, Uyeki TM, Callaghan WM, et al. What obstetrician-gynecologists should know about ebola: a perspective from the centers for disease control and prevention. Obstet Gynecol 2014;124(5):1005-10.

14. Caluwaerts S, Lagrou D, Weber PL, et al. Blood, birthing and body fluids: delivering and staying alive in an Ebola Treatment Centre (West Africa epidemic, 1/4/2014-1/1/2016 2016. Available at: https://f1000research.com/slides/1000081.

15. Chertow DS, Kleine C, Edwards JK, et al. Ebola virus disease in West Africa–clinical manifestations and management. N Engl J Med 2014;371(22):2054-7.

16. Foeller ME, Carvalho Ribeiro do Valle C, Foeller TM, et al. Pregnancy and breastfeeding in the context of Ebola: a systematic review. Lancet Infect Dis 2020;20(7): e149-58.

17. Akerlund E, Prescott J, Tampellini L. Shedding of ebola virus in an asymptomatic pregnant woman. N Engl J Med 2015;372(25):2467-9.

18. Baggi FM, Taybi A, Kurth A, et al. Management of pregnant women infected with Ebola virus in a treatment centre in Guinea, June 2014. Euro Surveill 2014;19(49): 20983.

19. Bower H, Grass JE, Veltus E, et al. Delivery of an ebola virus-positive stillborn infant in a rural community health center, Sierra Leone, 2015. Am J Trop Med Hyg 2016;94(2):417-9.

20. Caluwaerts S, Fautsch T, Lagrou D, et al. Dilemmas in managing pregnant women with ebola: 2 case reports. Clin Infect Dis 2016;62(7):903 5.

21. Kratz T, Roddy P, Tshomba Oloma A, et al. Ebola virus disease outbreak in Isiro, democratic Republic of the Congo, 2012: signs and symptoms, management and outcomes. PLoS One 2015;10(6):e0129333.

22. Muehlenbachs A, de la Rosa Vazquez O, Bausch DG, et al. Ebola virus disease in pregnancy: clinical, histopathologic, and immunohistochemical findings. J Infect Dis 2016;215(1):64-9.

23. Oduyebo T, Pineda D, Lamin M, et al. A pregnant patient with ebola virus disease. Obstet Gynecol 2015;126(6):1273–5.
24. Nelson JM, Griese SE, Goodman AB, et al. Live neonates born to mothers with Ebola virus disease: a review of the literature. J Perinatol 2016;36(6):411–4.
25. Dörnemann J, Burzio C, Ronsse A, et al. First newborn Baby to receive Experimental therapies survives ebola virus disease. J Infect Dis 2017;215(2):171–4.
26. First FDA-approved vaccine for the prevention of Ebola virus disease, marking a critical milestone in public health preparedness and response [press release]. December 19, 2019 2020.
27. Henao-Restrepo AM, Longini IM, Egger M, et al. Efficacy and effectiveness of an rVSV-vectored vaccine expressing Ebola surface glycoprotein: interim results from the Guinea ring vaccination cluster-randomised trial. The Lancet 2015; 386(9996):857–66.
28. Legardy-Williams JK, Carter RJ, Goldstein ST, et al. Pregnancy outcomes among women receiving rVSVDelta-ZEBOV-GP ebola vaccine during the Sierra Leone trial to Introduce a vaccine against ebola. Emerg Infect Dis 2020;26(3):541–8.
29. Musso D, Ko AI, Baud D. Zika virus infection — after the Pandemic. N Engl J Med 2019;381(15):1444–57.
30. Musso D, Gubler DJ. Zika virus. Clin Microbiol Rev 2016;29(3):487.
31. Brasil P, Pereira JP, Moreira ME, et al. Zika virus infection in pregnant women in Rio de Janeiro. N Engl J Med 2016;375(24):2321–34.
32. Krow-Lucal ER, Biggerstaff BJ, Staples JE. Estimated incubation period for Zika virus disease. Emerg Infect Dis 2017;23(5):841–5.
33. Honein MA, Dawson AL, Petersen EE, et al. Birth defects among fetuses and infants of US women with evidence of possible Zika virus infection during pregnancy. JAMA 2017;317(1):59–68.
34. Valdespino-Vázquez MY, Sevilla-Reyes EE, Lira R, et al. Congenital Zika syndrome and Extra-central Nervous system detection of Zika virus in a pre-term newborn in Mexico. Clin Infect Dis 2019;68(6):903–12.
35. Hoen B, Schaub B, Funk AL, et al. Pregnancy outcomes after ZIKV infection in French Territories in the Americas. N Engl J Med 2018;378(11):985–94.
36. Gallo LG, Martinez-Cajas J, Peixoto HM, et al. Another piece of the Zika puzzle: assessing the associated factors to microcephaly in a systematic review and meta-analysis. BMC Public Health 2020;20(1):827.
37. Calvet G, Aguiar RS, Melo ASO, et al. Detection and sequencing of Zika virus from amniotic fluid of fetuses with microcephaly in Brazil: a case study. Lancet Infect Dis 2016;16(6):653–60.
38. Noronha L, Zanluca C, Azevedo ML, et al. Zika virus damages the human placental barrier and presents marked fetal neurotropism. Mem Inst Oswaldo Cruz 2016;111(5):287–93.
39. Poland GA, Ovsyannikova IG, Kennedy RB. Zika vaccine development: current status. Mayo Clin Proc 2019;94(12):2572–86.
40. Stephenson KE, Tan CS, Walsh SR, et al. Safety and immunogenicity of a Zika purified inactivated virus vaccine given via standard, accelerated, or shortened schedules: a single-centre, double-blind, sequential-group, randomised, placebo-controlled, phase 1 trial. Lancet Infect Dis 2020;20(9):1061–70.
41. Vairo F, Haider N, Kock R, et al. Chikungunya: epidemiology, pathogenesis, clinical features, management, and prevention. Infect Dis Clin North Am 2019;33(4): 1003–25.
42. Burt FJ, Chen W, Miner JJ, et al. Chikungunya virus: an update on the biology and pathogenesis of this emerging pathogen. Lancet Infect Dis 2017;17(4):e107–17.

43. Weaver SC, Lecuit M. Chikungunya virus and the global spread of a mosquito-borne disease. N Engl J Med 2015;372(13):1231–9.
44. Mehta R, Gerardin P, de Brito CAA, et al. The neurological complications of chikungunya virus: a systematic review. Rev Med Virol 2018;28(3):e1978.
45. WHO. Chikungunya. WHO. 2020. Available at: https://www.who.int/news-room/fact-sheets/detail/chikungunya. Accessed December 5, 2020.
46. CDC. Chikungunya virus. 2019. Available at: https://www.cdc.gov/chikungunya/geo/index.html. Accessed December 5, 2020.
47. Silva LA, Dermody TS. Chikungunya virus: epidemiology, replication, disease mechanisms, and prospective intervention strategies. J Clin Invest 2017;127(3):737–49.
48. Fritel X, Rollot O, Gerardin P, et al. Chikungunya virus infection during pregnancy, Reunion, France, 2006. Emerg Infect Dis 2010;16(3):418–25.
49. Touret Y, Randrianaivo H, Michault A, et al. [Early maternal-fetal transmission of the Chikungunya virus]. Presse Med 2006;35(11 Pt 1):1656–8.
50. Lenglet Y, Barau G, Robillard PY, et al. [Chikungunya infection in pregnancy: evidence for intrauterine infection in pregnant women and vertical transmission in the parturient. Survey of the Reunion Island outbreak]. J Gynecol Obstet Biol Reprod (Paris) 2006;35(6):578–83.
51. Gérardin P, Barau G, Michault A, et al. Multidisciplinary prospective study of mother-to-child chikungunya virus infections on the island of La Réunion. PLoS Med 2008;5(3):e60.
52. Contopoulos-Ioannidis D, Newman-Lindsay S, Chow C, et al. Mother-to-child transmission of Chikungunya virus: a systematic review and meta-analysis. PLoS Negl Trop Dis 2018;12(6):e0006510.
53. Charlier C, Beaudoin MC, Couderc T, et al. Arboviruses and pregnancy: maternal, fetal, and neonatal effects. Lancet Child Adolesc Health 2017;1(2):134–46.
54. Torres JR, Falleiros-Arlant LH, Dueñas L, et al. Congenital and perinatal complications of chikungunya fever: a Latin American experience. Int J Infect Dis 2016;51:85–8.
55. Villamil-Gómez W, Alba-Silvera L, Menco-Ramos A, et al. Congenital chikungunya virus infection in sincelejo, Colombia: a case series. J Trop Pediatr 2015;61(5):386–92.
56. Ramful D, Carbonnier M, Pasquet M, et al. Mother-to-child transmission of Chikungunya virus infection. Pediatr Infect Dis J 2007;26(9):811–5.
57. Gérardin P, Sampériz S, Ramful D, et al. Neurocognitive outcome of children exposed to perinatal mother-to-child Chikungunya virus infection: the CHIMERE cohort study on Reunion Island. PLoS Negl Trop Dis 2014;8(7):e2996.
58. Waechter R, Ingraham E, Evans R, et al. Pre and postnatal exposure to Chikungunya virus does not affect child neurodevelopmental outcomes at two years of age. PLoS Negl Trop Dis 2020;14(10):e0008546.
59. Barr KL, Vaidhyanathan V. Chikungunya in infants and children: is pathogenesis increasing? Viruses 2019;11(3):294.
60. Gao S, Song S, Zhang L. Recent progress in vaccine development against chikungunya virus. Front Microbiol 2019;10:2881.
61. WHO. Dengue vaccine: WHO position paper - september 2018. Weekly epidemiological record Web site. 2018. Available at: https://apps.who.int/iris/bitstream/handle/10665/274315/WER9336.pdf?ua=1. Accessed December 5, 2020.

62. WHO. Dengue and severe dengue. 2020. Available at: https://www.who.int/en/news-room/fact-sheets/detail/dengue-and-severe-dengue. Accessed December 5, 2020.

63. Centers for disease control and prevention. Dengue. 2020. Available at: https://www.cdc.gov/dengue/index.html. Accessed December 5, 2020.

64. Messina JP, Brady OJ, Golding N, et al. The current and future global distribution and population at risk of dengue. Nat Microbiol 2019;4(9):1508–15.

65. Bhatt S, Gething PW, Brady OJ, et al. The global distribution and burden of dengue. Nature 2013;496(7446):504–7.

66. Rigau-Pérez JG, Clark GG, Gubler DJ, et al. Dengue and dengue haemorrhagic fever. Lancet 1998;352(9132):971–7.

67. Paixão ES, Teixeira MG, Costa MDCN, et al. Dengue during pregnancy and adverse fetal outcomes: a systematic review and meta-analysis. Lancet Infect Dis 2016;16(7):857–65.

68. Murray NE, Quam MB, Wilder-Smith A. Epidemiology of dengue: past, present and future prospects. Clin Epidemiol 2013;5:299–309.

69. Brady OJ, Hay SI. The global Expansion of dengue: How. Annu Rev Entomol 2020;65:191–208.

70. Guo C, Zhou Z, Wen Z, et al. Global epidemiology of dengue outbreaks in 1990-2015: a systematic review and meta-analysis. Front Cell Infect Microbiol 2017; 7:317.

71. FDA. First FDA-approved vaccine for the prevention of dengue disease in endemic regions. 2019. Available at: https://www.fda.gov/news-events/press-announcements/first-fda-approved-vaccine-prevention-dengue-disease-endemic-regions. Accessed December 5, 2020.

72. Skipetrova A, Wartel TA, Gailhardou S. Dengue vaccination during pregnancy - an overview of clinical trials data. Vaccine 2018;36(23):3345–50.

73. Fatimil LE, Mollah AH, Ahmed S, et al. Vertical transmission of dengue: first case report from Bangladesh. Southeast Asian J Trop Med Public Health 2003;34(4):800–3.

74. Chye JK, Lim CT, Ng KB, et al. Vertical transmission of dengue. Clin Infect Dis 1997;25(6):1374–7.

75. Carles G, Talarmin A, Peneau C, et al. [Dengue fever and pregnancy. A study of 38 cases in French Guiana]. J Gynecol Obstet Biol Reprod (Paris) 2000;29(8):758–62.

76. Tan PC, Rajasingam G, Devi S, et al. Dengue infection in pregnancy: prevalence, vertical transmission, and pregnancy outcome. Obstet Gynecol 2008;111(5):1111–7.

77. Phongsamart W, Yoksan S, Vanaprapa N, et al. Dengue virus infection in late pregnancy and transmission to the infants. Pediatr Infect Dis J 2008;27(6):500–4.

78. Sirinavin S, Nuntnarumit P, Supapannachart S, et al. Vertical dengue infection: case reports and review. Pediatr Infect Dis J 2004;23(11):1042–7.

79. Basurko C, Matheus S, Hildéral H, et al. Estimating the risk of vertical transmission of dengue: a prospective study. Am J Trop Med Hyg 2018;98(6):1826–32.

80. Ribeiro CF, Lopes VG, Brasil P, et al. Perinatal transmission of dengue: a report of 7 cases. J Pediatr 2013;163(5):1514–6.

81. Yang J, Zhang J, Deng Q, et al. Investigation on prenatal dengue infections in a dengue outbreak in Guangzhou City, China. Infect Dis (Lond) 2017;49(4):315–7.

82. Keerthy S, Nagesh K. Are we missing neonatal dengue? Indian Pediatr 2019; 56(8):697.

83. Machain-Williams C, Raga E, Baak-Baak CM, et al. Fetal, and neonatal outcomes in pregnant dengue patients in Mexico. Biomed Res Int 2018;2018:9643083.
84. Basurko C, Everhard S, Matheus S, et al. A prospective matched study on symptomatic dengue in pregnancy. PLoS One 2018;13(10):e0202005.
85. Vouga M, Chiu YC, Pomar L, et al. Dengue, Zika and chikungunya during pregnancy: pre- and post-travel advice and clinical management. J Trav Med 2019; 26(8):taz077.
86. Paixão ES, Campbell OM, Teixeira MG, et al. Dengue during pregnancy and live birth outcomes: a cohort of linked data from Brazil. BMJ Open 2019;9(7): e023529.
87. Paixão ES, Teixeira MG, Costa MDCN, et al. Symptomatic dengue during pregnancy and congenital neurologic malformations. Emerg Infect Dis 2018;24(9): 1748–50.
88. Nascimento LB, Siqueira CM, Coelho GE, et al. Symptomatic dengue infection during pregnancy and livebirth outcomes in Brazil, 2007-13: a retrospective observational cohort study. Lancet Infect Dis 2017;17(9):949–56.
89. Pouliot SH, Xiong X, Harville E, et al. Maternal dengue and pregnancy outcomes: a systematic review. Obstet Gynecol Surv 2010;65(2):107–18.
90. Tan L, Wang J, Zeng F, et al. [Analysis of clinical characteristics of the 12 cases of neonatal dengue fever in Guangzhou in 2014 and literatures review]. Zhonghua Er Ke Za Zhi 2015;53(12):943–7.

Chagas Disease

Implementation of Screening to Benefit Mother and Infant

Morven S. Edwards, MD[a],*, Susan P. Montgomery, DVM, MPH[b]

KEYWORDS

- Cardiomyopathy • Chagas disease • Congenital infection • Serologic screening
- *Trypanosoma cruzi*

KEY POINTS

- Chagas disease is underappreciated as a health concern in women in their childbearing years, resulting in potentially fatal cardiac morbidity owing to *Trypanosoma cruzi* infection in women at risk and their children.
- Pregnancy-based serologic screening for *T cruzi* provides the optimal mechanism to identify Chagas disease in at-risk family units because the results will be available at delivery when both mother and infant are in contact with the health care system.
- Treatment of Chagas disease within the first year of life is well tolerated, has a cure rate exceeding 90%, and is highly effective in preventing long-term *T cruzi*–associated cardiac complications.
- Targeted screening, including the cost of treatment with benznidazole, would be cost-effective and would result in $1314 savings per birth and $670 million in lifetime savings per birth-year cohort.

INTRODUCTION

Chagas disease is a vector-borne infection caused by the protozoan parasite, *Trypanosoma cruzi*. Carlos Chagas, working in Brazil in 1909, identified the parasite and its vector, the triatomine bug. He also identified the manifestations of the disease bearing his name.[1] Chagas disease is underappreciated as a health care concern in the United States, in part because the infection usually has occurred years before those affected become residents in the United States. In addition, the acute infection is often asymptomatic. It can cause a mild illness with low-grade fever that does not come to medical attention and does not raise concern for Chagas disease. Without treatment, infection becomes chronic and persists for life.[2] People in the chronic phase can remain

[a] Texas Children's Hospital, Feigin Center, 1102 Bates Avenue, Suite 1120, Houston, TX 77030, USA; [b] Parasitic Diseases Branch, Division of Parasitic Diseases and Malaria, Center Global Health, Centers for Disease Control and Prevention, 1600 Clifton Road, Northeast, Atlanta, GA 30333, USA
* Corresponding author.
E-mail address: morvene@bcm.edu

Clin Perinatol 48 (2021) 331–342
https://doi.org/10.1016/j.clp.2021.03.013   perinatology.theclinics.com
0095-5108/21/© 2021 Elsevier Inc. All rights reserved.

asymptomatic and may remain unaware that they contracted the infection. However, 20% to 30% will develop cardiac and/or gastrointestinal manifestations after years or decades of being asymptomatic.[2,3] Heart failure can result in debilitation and death, and cardiac outcomes from Chagas disease carry a worse prognosis than does heart failure from other causes.[4]

Epidemiology and Transmission

Chagas disease is endemic in Mexico, Central America, and South America. Approximately 300,000 persons in the United States have Chagas disease (**Fig. 1**). Most US residents with Chagas disease acquired infection in Mexico, El Salvador, Guatemala, or Honduras.[5,6] T cruzi is transmitted by infected triatomine bugs, which carry the parasite in their intestinal tracts. Triatomine bugs defecate after taking a blood meal, and transmission occurs when fecal material, containing trypomastigotes of the parasite (**Fig. 2**), is rubbed into a bite wound or the conjunctivae. Transmission also can occur by blood transfusion, organ transplantation, or congenitally.

Chagas disease awareness increased in the United States through implementation of widespread blood donor screening. The first assay for screening blood donations for T cruzi antibody gained Food and Drug Administration (FDA) approval in 2006. Between 2007 and 2019, there were 2462 blood donations confirmed as positive. The highest numbers were from California (890), Florida (325), Texas (199), New York (166), and Virginia (119). All US states, except Hawaii, Wyoming, and South Dakota, had at least 1 confirmed positive blood donation.[7] Blood donor screening and pretransplant screening of donors and recipients of organ transplants have rendered these modes of transmission rare in the United States.

T cruzi is established in southern US states where triatomines transmit the parasite to mammals, typically woodrats, raccoons, and opossums. Although human transmission within the United States has been documented, it is uncommon with fewer than 100 cases to date.[8–10] Chagas disease is reportable in Arizona, Arkansas, Louisiana, Mississippi, Tennessee, Texas, Utah, and Los Angeles County, California.[11]

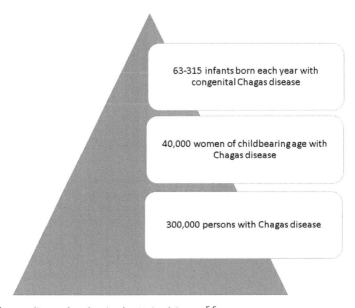

63-315 infants born each year with congenital Chagas disease

40,000 women of childbearing age with Chagas disease

300,000 persons with Chagas disease

Fig. 1. Chagas disease burden in the United States.[5,6]

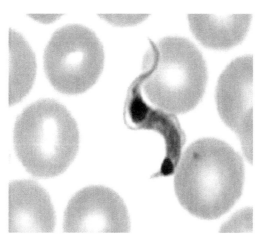

Fig. 2. *T cruzi* trypomastigote in a thin blood smear stained with Giemsa. (*From* Parasites - American Trypanosomiasis (also known as Chagas Disease). Centers for Disease Control and Prevention. Accessed January 6, 2021 at: https://www.cdc.gov/parasites/chagas/.)

Chagas disease contributes substantively to the total US burden of heart disease. The estimated number of people in the United States who have Chagas disease cardiomyopathy is 30,000 to 45,000.[1] Chagas disease–associated cardiomyopathy is clinically similar to non–Chagas disease cardiomyopathy. In a cross-sectional study, 13% of Latin American immigrants in New York City with dilated cardiomyopathy had *T cruzi*–related heart disease.[12] Chagas disease was diagnosed in more than 5% of 327 patients in Los Angeles with conduction abnormalities on electrocardiogram.[13] Right bundle branch block, in particular, is a common early manifestation of Chagas cardiomyopathy. Progression of heart disease can lead to complete heart block, arrhythmias, or embolic phenomena. Death can result from apical aneurysm, heart failure with dilated cardiomyopathy, or ventricular arrhythmias.[14]

An estimated 40,000 women of childbearing age in the United States have Chagas disease.[1] Most of these women acquired infection in an endemic region and are unaware they have an infection that is transmissible congenitally and can cause progressive heart disease, affecting them personally as well as their children. Screening of 4755 Latin American–born adults in Los Angeles County, of whom at least one-half were women of childbearing-age, found a prevalence of Chagas disease of 1.24%, suggesting that there are more than 30,000 people with Chagas disease in Los Angeles County alone and highlighting the magnitude of Chagas disease as a public health concern.[15]

Infants born to women with Chagas disease are at risk for congenital infection, including in the United States. Using the total US birth cohort, *T cruzi* prevalence in home countries of Latin American–born women, and an estimated 1% to 5% transmission, 63 to 315 infected infants are born each year in the United States.[5] The number of *T cruzi*–infected children in the United States with undiagnosed congenital infection was estimated to exceed 2000 over a decade ago.[16]

Congenital transmission occurs during the second or third trimester of pregnancy. Women with Chagas disease can transmit *T cruzi* during sequential pregnancies. Thus, without treatment, each pregnancy carries a risk to the fetus of congenital infection. High maternal parasitic load and human immunodeficiency virus coinfection enhance transmission.[17] Transmission risk continues for women with chronic infection even when they are living in nonendemic regions.[18]

Clinical Relevance to Mother and Infant

Pregnant women with undiagnosed Chagas disease usually have chronic infection contracted before migration to the United States and are unaware that they have *T cruzi* infection. Serologic screening of women from endemic regions benefits both mother and infant.[19,20] Women in the childbearing years diagnosed as having Chagas disease can receive antitrypanosomal treatment after delivery of their infant and completion of breastfeeding.[21] Although treatment of longstanding infection in adults does not reverse existing cardiac damage, treatment may decrease likelihood of Chagas cardiomyopathy.[2] Treatment also prevents transmission of infection to infants during subsequent pregnancies by reducing parasitemia.[22,23]

At birth, 10% to 40% of infants with congenital Chagas disease have signs of infection, such as prematurity, hepatosplenomegaly, and anemia.[24,25] Congenital infection is not associated with malformations because transmission occurs after organ formation is completed. Some of the common and less common clinical features of congenital Chagas disease are shown in **Table 1**.[24,26–28] Common features occur in one-fourth to greater than one-half of affected infants who have signs of infection. Less common features occur in 10% to 25% of affected infants with signs of infection. Presentation with fetal hydrops, ascites, and pericardial effusion in a preterm infant confirmed to have US-acquired congenital infection highlights the potential severity of congenital *T cruzi* infection.[29] Life-threatening manifestations, such as meningoencephalitis or pneumonitis, are not unique to Chagas disease. Disease usually is unrecognized because defining clinical features are lacking and health care clinicians may not suspect the diagnosis. Healthy-appearing congenitally infected infants usually are discharged without evaluation. However, 20% to 30% develop cardiomyopathy or debilitating gastrointestinal manifestations after years or decades of silent infection.[30,31]

Evaluation of Women During Pregnancy

Pregnant women from a Chagas-endemic region should undergo serologic screening for *T cruzi* antibodies through a commercial laboratory. Pregnancy offers the optimal access point for identifying Chagas at-risk family units because delivery is the most likely time for interaction with the health care system.[19] Pregnancy-based screening

Table 1 Clinical features of congenital Chagas disease	
Common Features[a]	**Less Common Features[b]**
Low birth weight	Prematurity
Respiratory distress	Cardiac findings[c]
Hepatomegaly	Meningoencephalitis
Splenomegaly	Neurologic signs
	Edema/anasarca
	Hematologic findings[d]

[a] Observed in 25% or more of infants with signs of infection.
[b] Observed in 10% to 25% of infants with signs of infection.
[c] Includes cardiomegaly, heart failure, arrhythmias.
[d] Includes thrombocytopenia, anemia.

for antibody to *T cruzi* has the advantage that results will be available at delivery. Unfortunately, no single serologic test has high enough sensitivity and specificity to establish the diagnosis. For this reason, diagnosis is based on positive results from 2 or more tests that use different techniques and that detect antibodies to different antigens. Commonly used techniques include enzyme-linked immunosorbent assays and immunofluorescent antibody tests. Confirmatory testing is available through a reference laboratory, such as the Parasitic Diseases Reference Laboratory at the Centers for Disease Control and Prevention (CDC). Requests for confirmatory testing should be coordinated with the respective state health department. A study of 4000 deliveries at 1 Houston hospital, where 85% of mothers cited a Chagas endemic country of origin, found that among 28 women with a positive initial screening test at delivery, 10 had proven chronic Chagas disease by confirmatory testing.[32]

Screening at admission for delivery or screening of neonates offers alternative approaches to identification of women and their infants with Chagas disease. The finding of immunoglobulin G (IgG) antibody to *T cruzi* in cord blood or infant serum is a reflection of the maternal antibody status and indicates that an infant is at risk for congenital infection. A disadvantage to delivery-based screening is that most infants and their mothers, including asymptomatic infants with congenital infection, will have been discharged when results of screening at delivery become available.

Evaluation for Congenital Chagas Disease

Evaluation for suspected congenital Chagas disease should occur as soon as possible after birth. Infants of mothers with a positive *T cruzi* screening serologic test or with confirmed Chagas disease and those with clinical features of Chagas disease require evaluation (**Fig. 3**).[25,33] Serologic testing of maternal blood, if not performed during pregnancy, or of cord blood, is the initial step to determining infant risk. Within the first months of life, the diagnosis relies on detection of motile trypomastigotes through microscopic examination of fresh anticoagulated whole blood or buffy coat, by microscopic examination of Giemsa-stained blood for trypomastigotes, or by polymerase chain reaction (PCR) testing for *T cruzi* DNA in whole blood. This testing is available through the Parasitic Diseases Reference Laboratory at CDC. Infants with an initially positive PCR should undergo repeat testing to exclude contaminating maternal DNA or specimen contamination, each of which is rare. Infants with an initially negative PCR should undergo repeat testing at 4 to 6 weeks of age to confirm absence of infection, as parasitic load increases in the first 1 to 2 months of life. After age 3 months, the parasite is no longer detectable by PCR, and congenital Chagas disease in the first year of life is confirmed by serologic testing (**Fig. 4**). Placentally transferred *T cruzi* antibodies should generally not be detectable after 9 to 12 months of age.[34]

Implications for Family Members of an Index Patient

Diagnosis of Chagas disease in a pregnant woman or newborn infant signals the need to test the woman's other children as well as her parents and siblings. A US-based convenience sample of 189 relatives of 86 Chagas disease patients found a *T cruzi* prevalence of 7.4%.[35] In Catalonia, active surveillance identified 178 siblings of index infants. Testing revealed that 14 (7.8%) siblings also had *T cruzi* infection.[36] Perinatal health care clinicians should consider coordinating follow-up with pediatric caregivers who can provide a pivotal role in providing families with information and testing.

Treatment Options for Mothers Infants and Children

The 2 therapeutics for *T cruzi* are benznidazole and nifurtimox.[2,37] Benznidazole received approval by the FDA for use in children 2 to 12 years of age and is available

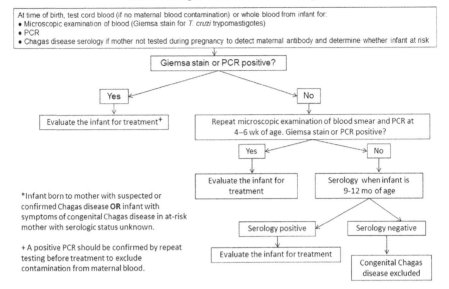

Fig. 3. Steps to establish the diagnosis of congenital Chagas disease in infants younger than 3 months of age. (*From* Congenital Chagas disease. Available at: https://www.cdc.gov/parasites/chagas/health_professionals/congenital_chagas.html. Accessed December 30, 2020.)

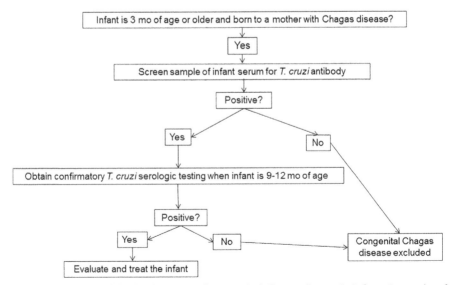

Fig. 4. Steps to establish the diagnosis of congenital Chagas disease in infants 3 months of age or older. (*From* Congenital Chagas disease. Available at: https://www.cdc.gov/parasites/chagas/health_professionals/congenital_chagas.html. Accessed December 30, 2020.)

from www.benznidazoletablets.com/. The total daily dose is 5 to 8 mg/kg/d administered orally in 2 divided doses for a duration of 60 days (**Table 2** provides full prescribing information). Prescribing benznidazole to treat a patient outside of the FDA-approved age range is based on clinical diagnosis and decision by a treating physician.

In August 2020, the FDA approved nifurtimox for the treatment of Chagas disease in pediatric patients from birth to less than 18 years of age and weighing at least 2.5 kg. This indication gained accelerated approval based on the number of treated patients who became IgG antibody negative or who demonstrated a 20% or greater decrease in optical density on *T cruzi* IgG antibody tests. Continued approval for this indication may be contingent on verification and description of clinical benefit in a confirmatory trial or trials. The total daily dose of nifurtimox in pediatric patients is 10 to 20 mg/kg/d administered orally in 3 doses for 60 days for children less than 40 kg and 8 to 10 mg/kg/d administered orally in 3 doses for children greater than 40 kg (**Table 2** provides full prescribing information).

Antiparasitic treatment is recommended for all *T cruzi*–infected infants and children younger than 18 years of age.[37] Treatment is also recommended for all women with chronic disease in the childbearing years who do not have advanced Chagas cardiomyopathy. Adverse effects are common with both drugs but are less frequent and less severe during infancy and childhood than during adulthood.[38] Consultation with an infectious diseases physician is advisable when initiating treatment. Additional information is available at the CDC web site (https://www.cdc.gov/parasites/chagas/health_professionals/tx.html). Questions regarding treatment can be directed to CDC's Parasitic Diseases Inquiries (404-718-4745; e-mail: chagas@cdc.gov).

Table 2
Chagas disease resources

Resource	Content for Health Care Providers
https://www.cdc.gov/parasites/chagas/health_professionals/congenital_chagas.html	**Centers for Disease Control & Prevention:** Information about congenital Chagas disease; algorithms for evaluation of Chagas disease in pregnant women and infants
https://www.chagasus.org	**Chagas Disease Center of Excellence:** General information on Chagas disease
https://LASOCHA.org/en/	**Latin American Society of Chagas:** (LASOCHA) General information on Chagas disease
https://www.uschagasprovidersnetwork.org/	**US Chagas Providers' Network:** Listing of US Chagas disease providers by state; general Chagas disease information
https://www.accessdata.fda.gov/drugsatfda_docs/label/2017/209570lbl.pdf	**Benznidazole prescribing information:** Highlights and full prescribing information for benznidazole
https://www.accessdata.fda.gov/drugsatfda_docs/label/2020/213464s000lbl.pdf	**Nifurtimox prescribing information:** Highlights and full prescribing information for nifurtimox

DISCUSSION

Maternal screening with infant testing and maternal and infant treatment for confirmed Chagas disease would be cost-saving.[19,20] At current costs, targeted screening, including the pricing of benznidazole, would result in savings of $1314 per birth and $670 million in lifetime savings per birth-year cohort.[19,20] Universal screening of all newborns would be similarly cost-saving. An alternate approach to identification of infants with congenital Chagas disease is by newborn screening. The current national US Recommended Uniform Screening Panel (RUSP) for newborn screening detects 35 disorders by point-of-care screening and dried blood spot (DBS) specimens.[39] The RUSP recommends point-of-care screening to identify critical congenital heart defects and hearing loss. Among the 33 disorders on the RUSP identified by DBS screening, those most prevalent are cystic fibrosis, primary congenital hypothyroidism, and sickle cell disease. Based on the expected number of cases per year, congenital Chagas disease is more common than greater than one-half of these 33 disorders, even using the most conservative estimates of the expected number of congenital cases of Chagas disease per year.

Treatment of congenital Chagas disease within the first year of life is always recommended,[37] is well tolerated, has cure rates exceeding 90%, and is highly effective in preventing long-term complications of Chagas disease.[21] In addition, children and adolescents diagnosed with Chagas disease should always receive treatment. Women diagnosed with Chagas disease should receive treatment after delivery and completion of breastfeeding for their own benefit and for protection against *T cruzi* transmission during subsequent pregnancies.

Improving health care clinicians' knowledge of Chagas disease diagnosis, treatment, and prevention is essential to improving Chagas disease outcomes. A survey, tailored for 5 medical specialties, found a general lack of awareness of Chagas disease and knowledge deficits of clinical aspects of the disease.[40] Most US obstetrician-gynecologists had very limited knowledge of Chagas disease.[41] Most Pediatric Infectious Diseases Society members never or rarely considered the diagnosis when caring for infants born to parents from Latin America.[42]

Information that is accurate, practical, and targeted will increase awareness and knowledge of Chagas disease among clinicians.[3] Addressing knowledge gaps will positively affect patient health and will promote congenital transmission screening. Clinicians should be educated as to the outcomes of untreated Chagas disease to understand the importance of screening for and treating of *T cruzi* infection. Improved knowledge should equip clinicians to embrace the feasibility of congenital transmission screening and to engage in efforts to conduct targeted screening and to improve detection and early intervention that will improve outcomes for women, infants, and children infected with *T cruzi*.

CLINICS CARE POINTS

- Pregnant women from a Chagas disease endemic region should undergo serologic screening for *Trypanosoma cruzi* IgG through a commercial laboratory.
- Evaluation for suspected congenital Chagas disease should occur as soon as possible after birth.
- Treatment of congenital Chagas disease in the first year of life has cure rates exceeding 90%.

Best practices

What Is the Current Practice for Chagas Disease Serologic Screening?

- Chronic Chagas disease is rarely considered a diagnostic possibility in US pregnant women who formerly resided in Chagas endemic regions.[41]

- Congenital Chagas disease is not consistently included in the differential diagnosis for infants with signs suggesting a congenital infection.[25]

- Serologic screening for Chagas disease is not integrated into recommended maternal prenatal screening platforms for at-risk women.

What Changes in Current Practice Are Likely to Improve Outcomes?

- Promoting education for perinatal health care clinicians on the risk and impact of Chagas disease to infant and maternal health

- Incorporating *T cruzi* IgG serologic screening into pregnancy testing platforms for at-risk pregnant women or, alternatively, into the US RUSP for newborn screening[19,20,39]

- Providing treatment for women identified as having chronic Chagas disease and for infants with congenital Chagas disease to prevent later development of Chagas cardiomyopathy[37]

Major Recommendations

- Modify electronic medical record formats to prompt order entry for *T cruzi* IgG serologic screening into pregnancy test platforms.

- Conduct studies to demonstrate feasibility of Chagas disease maternal and congenital transmission screening.

- Generate sufficient data to inform organizations that develop guidelines for care of women and infants at risk for Chagas disease to endorse Chagas disease screening in policy statements for maternal and infant care.

Rating for strength of the evidence: Quality of evidence strong; strength of recommendation moderate.

SUMMARY

At least 40,000 women in their childbearing years who are living in the United States have chronic Chagas disease acquired years earlier when they were living in Mexico, Central America, or South America. Most are unaware of their infections and do not know that the infection can cause cardiac damage with a usual onset 10 to 30 years after acquisition and that it can be transmitted congenitally. The risk of congenital transmission is 1% to 5% and, although most infants are asymptomatic at birth, 10% to 40% have signs suggestive of congenital infection and all are at risk for later Chagas cardiomyopathy. Implementation of targeted maternal pregnancy-based screening for *T cruzi* IgG or, alternatively, as a component of newborn screening for congenital infections could benefit both women and their infants. Treatment of acute infant infection affects cure, and treatment of chronically infected women prevents transmission in subsequent pregnancies and reduces the likelihood of development of Chagas cardiomyopathy. Evidence demonstrating feasibility of maternal screening and codifying its benefit to both women and their infants should be a priority so that guidelines endorsing screening are included in policy statements related to maternal and infant care.

DISCLOSURE

M.S. Edwards is the recipient of a personal services agreement from Texas State University. S.P. Montgomery reports no conflict of interest.

REFERENCES

1. Bern C, Messenger LA, Whitman JD, et al. Chagas disease in the United States: a public health approach. Clin Microbiol Rev 2020;33 :e00023-19.
2. Bern C. Antitrypanosomal therapy for chronic Chagas' disease. N Engl J Med 2011;364(26):2527–34.
3. Montgomery SP, Starr MC, Cantey PT, et al. Neglected parasitic infections in the United States: Chagas disease. Am J Trop Med Hyg 2014;90(5):814–8.
4. Shen L, Ramires F, Martinez F, et al. Contemporary characteristics and outcomes in Chagasic heart failure compared with other nonischemic and ischemic cardio-myopathy. Circ Heart Fail 2017;10(11):e004361.
5. Bern C, Montgomery SP. An estimate of the burden of Chagas disease in the United States. Clin Infect Dis 2009;49(5):e52–4.
6. Manne-Goehler J, Umeh CA, Montgomery SP, et al. Estimating the burden of Chagas disease in the United States. PLoS Negl Trop Dis 2016;10(11):e0005033.
7. Chagas Biovigilence Network. Available at: https://www.aabb.org/news-resources/resources/hemovigilance/chagas-biovigilance-network. Accessed December 30, 2020.
8. Cantey PT, Stramer SL, Townsend RL, et al. The United States *Trypanosoma cruzi* infection study: evidence for vector-borne transmission of the parasite that causes Chagas disease among United States blood donors. Transfusion 2012;52(9):1922–30.
9. Dorn PL, Perniciaro L, Yabsley MJ, et al. Autochthonous transmission of *Trypanosoma cruzi,* Louisiana. Emerg Infect Dis 2007;13(4):605–7.
10. Turabelidze G, Vasudevan A, Rojas-Moreno C, et al. Autochthonous chagas disease- Missouri, 2018. MMWR Morb Mortal Wkly Rep 2020;69(7):193–5.
11. Bennett C, Straily A, Haselow D, et al. Chagas disease surveillance activities-seven states, 2017. MMWR Morb Mortal Wkly Rep 2018;67(26):738–41.
12. Kapelusznik L, Varela D, Montgomery SP, et al. Chagas disease in Latin American immigrants with dilated cardiomyopathy in New York City. Clin Infect Dis 2013;57(1):e7–10.
13. Traina MI, Hernandez S, Sanchez DR, et al. Prevalence of Chagas disease in a U.S. population of Latin American immigrants with conduction abnormalities on electrocardiogram. PLoS Negl Trop Dis 2017;11(1):e0005244.
14. Rassi A Jr, Rassi A, Rassi SG. Predictors of mortality in chronic Chagas disease. A systematic review of observational studies. Circulation 2007;115(9):1101–8.
15. Meymandi SK, Forsyth CJ, Soverow J, et al. Prevalence of chagas disease in the Latin American-born population of Los Angeles. Clin Infect Dis 2017;64(9):1182–8.
16. Buekens P, Almendares O, Carlier Y, et al. Mother-to-child transmission of Cha-gas' disease in North America: why don't we do more? Matern Child Health J 2008;12(3):283–6.
17. Gebrekristos HT, Buekens P. Mother-to-child transmission of *Trypanosoma cruzi.* J Pediatr Infect Dis Soc 2014;3(Suppl 1):S36–40.
18. Howard EJ, Xiong X, Carlier Y, et al. Frequency of the congenital transmission of *Trypanosoma cruzi*: a systematic review and meta-analysis. BJOG 2014;121(1):22–33.
19. Perez-Zetune V, Bialek SR, Montgomery SP, et al. Congenital Chagas disease in the United States: the effect of commercially priced benznidazole on costs and benefits of maternal screening. Am J Trop Med Hyg 2020;102(5):1086–9.

20. Stillwaggon E, Perez-Zetune V, Bialek SR, et al. Congenital chagas disease in the United States: cost savings through maternal screening. Am J Trop Med Hyg 2018;98(6):1733–42.

21. Tustin AW, Bowman NM. Chagas disease. Pediatr Rev 2016;37(4):177–8.

22. Murcia L, Simón M, Carrilero B, et al. Treatment of infected women of childbearing age prevents congenital *Trypanosoma cruzi* infection by eliminating the parasitemia detected by PCR. J Infect Dis 2017;215(9):1452–8.

23. Álvarez MG, Vigliano C, Lococo B, et al. Prevention of congenital Chagas disease by benznidazole treatment in reproductive-age women. An observational study. Acta Trop 2017;174:149–52.

24. Freilij H, Altcheh J. Congenital Chagas' disease: diagnostic and clinical aspects. Clin Infect Dis 1995;21(3):551–5.

25. Edwards MS, Stimpert KK, Bialek SR, et al. Evaluation and management of congenital Chagas disease in the United States. J Pediatr Infect Dis Soc 2019; 8(5):461–9.

26. Torrico F, Alonso-Vega C, Suarez E, et al. Maternal *Trypanosoma cruzi* infection, pregnancy outcome, morbidity, and mortality of congenitally infected and non-infected newborns in Bolivia. Am J Trop Med Hyg 2004;70(2):201–9.

27. Blanco SB, Segura EL, Cura EN, et al. Congenital transmission of *Trypanosoma cruzi*: an operational outline for detecting and treating infected infants in north-western Argentina. Trop Med Int Health 2000;5(4):293–301.

28. Messenger LA, Gilman RH, Verastegui M, et al. Toward improving early diagnosis of congenital Chagas disease in an endemic setting. Clin Infect Dis 2017;65(2): 268–75.

29. Centers for Disease Control and Prevention. Congenital transmission of Chagas disease- Virginia, 2010. MMWR Morb Mortal Wkly Rep 2012;61(26):477–9.

30. Lescure F-X, Le Loup G, Freilij H, et al. Chagas disease: changes in knowledge and management. Lancet Infect Dis 2010;10(8):556–70.

31. Bern C, Martin DL, Gilman RH. Acute and congenital Chagas disease. Adv Parasitol 2011;75:19–47.

32. Edwards MS, Rench MA, Todd CW, et al. Perinatal screening for Chagas disease in southern Texas. J Pediatr Infect Dis Soc 2015;4(1):67–70.

33. Congenital chagas disease. Available at: https://www.cdc.gov/parasites/chagas/health_professionals/congenital_chagas.html. Accessed December 30, 2020.

34. Bern C, Verastegui M, Gilman RH, et al. Congenital *Trypanosoma cruzi* transmission in Santa Cruz, Bolivia. Clin Infect Dis 2009;49(11):1667–74.

35. Hernandez S, Forsyth CJ, Flores CA, et al. Prevalence of Chagas disease among family members of previously diagnosed patients in Los Angeles, California. Clin Infect Dis 2019;69(7):1226–8.

36. Basile L, Ciruela P, Requena-Méndez A, et al. Epidemiology of congenital Chagas disease 6 years after implementation of a public health surveillance system, Catalonia, 2010 to 2015. Euro Surveill 2019;24(26):1900011.

37. Bern C, Montgomery SP, Herwaldt BL, et al. Evaluation and treatment of Chagas disease in the United States. A systematic review. JAMA 2007;298(18):2171–81.

38. Altcheh J, Moscatelli G, Moroni S, et al. Adverse events after the use of benznidazole in infants and children with Chagas disease. Pediatrics 2011;127(1): e212–8.

39. Sontag MK, Yusuf C, Grosse SD, et al. Infants with congenital disorders identified through newborn screening-United States, 2015-2017. MMWR Morb Mortal Wkly Rep 2020;69(36):1265–8.

40. Stimpert KK, Montgomery SP. Physician awareness of Chagas disease, USA. Emerg Infect Dis 2010;16(5):871–2.

41. Verani JR, Montgomery SP, Schulkin J, et al. Survey of obstetrician-gynecologists in the United States about Chagas disease. Am J Trop Med Hyg 2010;83(4): 891–5.

42. Edwards MS, Abanyie FA, Montgomery SP. Survey of Pediatric Infectious Diseases Society members about congenital Chagas disease. Pediatr Infect Dis J 2018;37(1):e24–7.

Hepatitis C Virus in Neonates and Infants

Rachel L. Epstein, MD, MSc[a],*, Claudia Espinosa, MD, MSc[b]

KEYWORDS

- Hepatitis C • Infectious disease transmission • Vertical transmission
- Opioid-related disorders • Antiviral therapy • Epidemiology • Transmission • Infant

KEY POINTS

- Hepatitis C virus incidence has increased in pregnant women, with over 29,000 exposed infants born annually in the United States, though this is likely an underestimate.
- All women should be tested for evidence of acute or chronic hepatitis C virus infection in each pregnancy; for those identified, risk factors for perinatal transmission should be assessed before delivery.
- All infants perinatally exposed to hepatitis C virus should be screened for chronic hepatitis C infection.
- Direct-acting antivirals are highly effective, well-tolerated, and now the standard of care for treatment of chronic hepatitis C virus infection in children 3 and older.
- Although direct-acting antivirals are not currently approved during pregnancy, women can be linked to care for treatment after pregnancy and lactation to improve maternal health.

INTRODUCTION

Hepatitis C virus (HCV) remains a major cause of morbidity and mortality worldwide. An estimated 71 million people and 3.26 million children are infected with HCV; all-cause viral hepatitis was responsible for 1.34 million deaths in 2015.[1,2] Injection drug use is the major risk factor for new HCV cases in adults and adolescents; most HCV infections in children are the result of vertical transmission from HCV-infected mothers. In this article, we describe the epidemiology and natural history of hepatitis C infection in pregnant women and infants, review the current recommendations and HCV testing practices in women and infants, suggest a potential algorithm and clinical care pathway to improve HCV testing, and summarize therapeutics for HCV that are approved and are being evaluated.

[a] Department of Medicine, Section of Infectious Diseases, Boston University School of Medicine, 801 Massachusetts Avenue, Crosstown Center 2nd Floor, Boston, MA 02118, USA; [b] Department of Pediatrics, Division of Pediatric Infectious Diseases, Morsani College of Medicine, University of South Florida, 12901 Bruce B Downs Boulevard, Tampa, FL 33612, USA
* Corresponding author.
E-mail address: Rachel.epstein@bmc.org

Clin Perinatol 48 (2021) 343–357
https://doi.org/10.1016/j.clp.2021.03.007
0095-5108/21/© 2021 Elsevier Inc. All rights reserved.

EPIDEMIOLOGY

Although several countries have organized successful campaigns to identify and treat HCV, with 1.75 million new HCV infections each year,[2] much of the world is not on track to meet the World Health Organization (WHO) 2030 HCV elimination goals to reduce new infections by 30% and mortality by 10% by 2020, and by 90% and 65%, respectively, by 2030.[3,4] In the United States, annual acute HCV infections increased from 17,100 cases in 2011 to 50,300 in 2018, with the greatest increase among young adults 20 to 39 years old, including many women of reproductive age.[5] In association with the opioid crisis and a quadrupling of documented opioid use disorder diagnoses among pregnant women in the United States,[6] HCV seroprevalence increased 5-fold from 0.8 per 1000 delivery-hospitalizations in 2000 to 4.1 per 1000 delivery-hospitalizations in 2015.[7] Because the majority of HCV infections in children are due to vertical transmission, increased cases among pregnant women translated to increases in the number of exposed infants each year. National birth certificate data demonstrated an increase to 4.7 cases per 1000 live births in 2017,[8] and increased HCV testing rates in children were also observed among commercial laboratory data in Kentucky and across the United States from 2011 to 2014.[9] Extrapolating from both commercial laboratory testing and national birth data, 29,000 births in 2014 were to women with HCV infection, resulting in 1700 infant infections.[10]

The absence of universal HCV screening or reporting in many countries, coupled with inadequate adherence to testing guidelines, means that the true HCV prevalence can only be estimated. Particularly in countries with only risk-based testing recommendations or who lack the resources or commitment to instate national testing campaigns, many more infections exist than are identified.[11,12] The WHO estimates that only 20% of people worldwide are aware of their chronic HCV infection[2]; those who are unaware likely contribute significantly to transmission. Additionally, laws, stigmatization, and cultural taboos in many areas decrease the reporting of injection drug use, especially during pregnancy, decreasing opportunities for treatment of opioid use disorder, risk factor identification, and subsequent HCV screening.[13–15]

GUIDELINES: HEPATITIS C VIRUS TESTING IN PREGNANT WOMEN

In 2020, both the US Centers for Disease Control and Prevention (CDC) and US Preventative Services Task Force (USPSTF) published updated HCV testing guidance recommending one-time HCV testing for all adults 18 to 79 years old.[16,17] They both recommend initial testing with HCV antibody followed by HCV RNA testing in those who are antibody positive. Positive antibody testing indicates either current or past cleared infection, whereas detection of RNA signifies current hepatitis C infection.

The guidelines differ with regard to testing in pregnancy (**Table 1**). The CDC and the American Association for the Study of Liver Disease/Infectious Diseases Society of America recommend testing all pregnant women for HCV during each pregnancy,[18] if the community HCV prevalence is 0.1% or greater.[16] The USPSTF concluded they did not find sufficient evidence to recommend repeat testing during pregnancy for otherwise low-risk women who had been tested previously. Both the American College of Obstetricians and Gynecologists and the Society for Maternal-Fetal Medicine only recommend testing pregnant women with HCV risk factors in their most recent guidance (see **Table 1**),[19,20] although the American College of Obstetricians and Gynecologists published a statement that they are considering the new CDC and USPSTF guidelines and will release an update after deliberation.[21]

Table 1
HCV testing recommendations during pregnancy

Guiding Body	Recommendation	Year Updated	Source
US Centers for Disease Control and Prevention (CDC)	Test in each pregnancy, except if community prevalence <0.1%	2020	Schillie,[16] 2020
US Preventative Services Task Force (USPSTF)	Test all adults 18–79 years old once in their lifetime, consider in pregnant women <18 y, unclear benefit in low-risk pregnant women who have previously been tested	2020	Owens et al,[17] 2020
American Association for the Study of Liver Disease (AASLD)/ Infectious Diseases Society of America (IDSA)	Test in each pregnancy, ideally at the initial prenatal visit	2018	AASLD-IDSA HCV Guidance Panel,[18] 2018, AASLD-IDSA,[60] 2020
Society for Maternal-Fetal Medicine	Test only if risk factors present, at first prenatal visit, and retest later in pregnancy if ongoing or new risk present	2017	Hughes et al,[20] 2017
American College of Obstetricians and Gynecologists (ACOG)	Test only if risk factors present	2007[a]	ACOG,[19] 2007

[a] The ACOG website states that the organization is currently reviewing the CDC and USPSTF 2020 guidance, after which ACOG will issue updated guidance.[21].

In practice, a number of institutions and 1 US state adopted universal prenatal HCV testing ahead of national guidance. Kentucky initiated statewide universal prenatal HCV testing in July 2018 through legislative action.[22] Data supporting the bill include a report of an earlier implementation of universal HCV screening in a metro area health care system in Kentucky. Among approximately 20,000 women who sought care in the 18 months before and 18 months after the implementation of universal screening, the proportion of HCV seropositive women actually increased (4.3% vs 4.9%; odds ratio, 1.1; 95% confidence interval [CI], 0.9–1.4]). The use of reflex testing also identified significantly more viremic women (both absolute number and proportion of those tested) who were eligible for therapeutic intervention after pregnancy (31/1867 [1.7%] vs 306/9033 [3.4%]; odds ratio, 2.1; 95% CI, 1.4–3.0].[23] Also supporting the failure of risk-based testing to identify women with HCV, a Cincinnati study implemented universal maternal urine drug testing at delivery to assess for intrauterine drug exposure.[24] Given the number of mothers with evidence of substance use at delivery who were not tested for HCV, the authors estimated that 67% of perinatally acquired HCV could be missed owing to a lack of HCV testing in high-risk women and infants only. Modeling studies also predict that universal HCV testing during every pregnancy (even with negative HCV testing before the current pregnancy) is cost effective, and with universal uptake, will result in identification of twice as many HCV-exposed infants compared with risk-based testing alone.[25–27]

CURRENT EVIDENCE: HEPATITIS C VIRUS IN PREGNANCY

Mother-to-child transmission of HCV was recognized even before the virus was identified, but most details of the pathogenesis and mechanism of transmission remain unclear. Most studies of HCV in pregnancy focus on chronic infection because acute hepatitis C infection during pregnancy has been reported infrequently.[28] In chronic infection, transaminases trend down from first to last trimester and increase again postpartum likely owing to immune tolerance and presence of circulating immunosuppressive cytokines synthesized by the placenta.[28,29] HCV viral load on the other hand can either increase in the third trimester and return to baseline levels after delivery[29] or remain stable throughout pregnancy.[30] The effects of pregnancy on HCV disease are variable with some studies documenting worsened necroinflammation and fibrosis in liver biopsies,[28,31] and others describing spontaneous clearance postpartum, associated with the presence of the IL28B-CC allele.[32] Early studies failed to find adverse pregnancy outcomes (miscarriages or other obstetric complications) owing to HCV,[28] but other studies have demonstrated increased risk of maternal gestational diabetes and intrahepatic cholestasis.[33] Reports on infant outcomes are also contradictory, although multiple studies report an increased likelihood of prematurity, congenital abnormalities, low birth weight, small for gestational age births, the need for intensive care, and mechanical ventilation.[28,31,33] One large study that compared outcomes among HCV-infected women and HCV-negative women with and without diagnosed substance use found an increased need for neonatal intensive care and mechanical ventilation in the infants born to women with HCV infection, independent of documented substance use.[33]

VERTICAL TRANSMISSION: PATHOGENESIS

Because HCV is transmitted most effectively through blood, the intrapartum period poses the greatest risk for infant infection. However, an examination of viral sequences in a study of women who transmitted HCV to their neonates revealed that transmission could occur considerably earlier in pregnancy (median time between 24.1 and 36.1 weeks, and as early as 12.8 weeks of gestation).[34] Vertical transmission has been documented only in infants born to viremic mothers, except in the setting of intermittent viremia or in the setting of lower HCV RNA test sensitivity with older testing platforms (eg, branched DNA assays).[35-38] Women with ongoing injection drug use or other HCV risk factors, however, may screen negative in the prepregnancy or early pregnancy periods and their infection may be missed without repeat testing later in pregnancy.[39,40] Presumably these situations represent women who became infected after initial HCV testing; repeat testing during the third trimester should be considered in women with an ongoing risk for acquisition.

VERTICAL TRANSMISSION: RISK FACTORS

A systematic review and meta-analysis including 109 studies calculated the risk of vertical transmission at 5.8% (95% CI, 4.2–7.8) for infants born to women without HIV co-infection, and 10.8% (95% CI, 7.6–15.2) for infants born to mothers co-infected with HIV (adjusted odds ratio, 2.56; 95% CI, 1.50–4.43).[41] However, studies including HIV co-infected mothers adherent to antiretroviral therapy, which might decrease the risk of perinatal HCV infection, have not demonstrated a higher risk of HCV transmission in HIV co-infected mothers.[42] Potential explanations for higher rates of vertical transmission in infants born to HIV co-infected mothers include interference of HIV with HCV-specific humoral and cell-mediated immune responses resulting in higher maternal HCV viral load (and higher viral loads in infected infants).[34,41,43,44] Elevated maternal viral load also correlates with frequent interchange of minor and major viral variants between women and their fetuses[34] and placental changes such as inflammation and altered trophoblast barrier, owing to microhemorrhage, which is more common in women with HIV.[45,46] Vertical transmission is also affected by the number of natural killer cells in the placenta (increased viral cytotoxicity causes a surge of HCV-specific T cells, which increases endogenous interferon, partially explaining the low rates of infection),[47] infection of mononuclear cells (which serve as replication reservoirs),[47–49] and increased genetic variability (increased evasion of host immune response).[50–52]

Obstetric characteristics that may be associated with an increased risk of perinatal transmission include prolonged rupture of membranes during delivery and procedures that increase the chance of maternal–fetal blood transfer (**Table 2**).[30,32,35,36,47,53] Factors that have not been associated with increased risk of perinatal transmission notably include breastfeeding and mode of delivery (see **Table 2**).[35–37,53] HCV RNA has been documented in colostrum or breastmilk, but such detection of HCV has not been associated with infant infection or with maternal viral load.[37] HCV-infected mothers should be counseled that they can breastfeed in the absence of cracked or bleeding nipples or other contraindications to breastfeeding.[54] Women who breastfeed should be advised to regularly check their nipples, and pump and discard the milk if there is cracking or bleeding noted. Prior delivery of an infected infant does not increase the risk for vertical transmission in the current pregnancy.[37]

Table 2	
Factors associated with mother to child transmission of HCV	
Factors Associated with Increased Risk[30,32,36,37,40,42,47,48,78]	
Membrane rupture ≥6 h	
Invasive procedures (eg, amniocentesis)	
Internal fetal monitoring (uterine or fetal scalp)	
Maternal intravenous drug use during pregnancy	
Peripheral mononuclear cells	
Factors not associated with increased risk[35–38,47,53]	
Maternal	Infant
Maternal age	Sex
Parity	Gestational age
Genotype	Birth weight
Transaminases at delivery	Apgar scores
Mode of delivery	Breastfed
Duration of labor	HCV RNA testing of cord blood or peripheral venous sample at birth
Prior affected child	First born
Controversial factors with mixed evidence[30,35,37,42,47,49,55]	
Co-infection with HIV	
High viral load	
Transfer of maternal neutralizing antibody	

GUIDELINES: INFANT HEPATITIS C VIRUS TESTING
Who to Test?

Because HCV testing is now recommended as part of routine prenatal care, maternal HCV status should be reviewed with all other prenatal laboratory tests at the newborn visit to document HCV exposure. Historically, guidelines recommended testing all infants born to HCV seropositive women, given the absence of RNA testing during pregnancy and difficulty ascertaining infection status in the mother. Recommendations for universal maternal testing during each pregnancy, and the increasing use of reflex RNA testing following a positive maternal antibody test translates into a recommendation to test infants born to HCV-infected women only, implying those with detectable RNA suggestive of a current infection (**Table 3**). HCV testing should also be ordered for infants born to HCV seropositive women with an unknown HCV RNA status, and considered for those with an unknown antibody status, particularly in the setting of known or suspected injection drug use, intrauterine opioid exposure, or foster care. In infants born to mothers with unknown HCV antibody status, the detection of maternal antibody at age 3 months or younger suggests exposure.

How and When to Test?

The American Academy of Pediatrics defines the diagnosis of HCV infection in children as the presence of HCV-specific antibodies after age 18 months or 2 positive

Table 3
Testing guidance for HCV-Exposed infants

Guiding Body	Recommendation Who to Test	Recommendation How to Test	Year Updated	Source
US Centers for Disease Control and Prevention (CDC)	Infants born to women with HCV infection	More information needed to balance benefits and costs of earlier RNA test(s)	2020	Schillie,[16] 2020
US Preventative Services Task Force (USPSTF)		No specific mention (Ab recommended in general)	2020	Owens et al,[17] 2020
American Association for the Study of Liver Disease (AASLD)/ Infectious Diseases Society of America (IDSA)		Test with Ab at 18 mo; can consider RNA testing as early as 2 mo of age but recommends against repeated RNA testing	2018	AASLD-IDSA HCV Guidance Panel,[18] 2018
Redbook/American Academy of Pediatrics (AAP)		Test with Ab at 18 mo; can consider RNA	2018	Kimberlin et al,[54] 2018
North American Society for Pediatric Gastroenterology, Hepatology, and Nutrition (NASPGHAN)		testing as early as 1– 2 mo of age if significant maternal anxiety	2012	Mack et al,[56] 2012

Abbreviations: HCV, Hepatitis C virus; Ab, antibody; RNA, ribonucleic acid.

HCV RNA tests on separate dates after age 2 months.[54] Because maternal HCV anti-bodies persist in infants for up to 18 to 24 months,[35,37,55] guidelines recommend ideally waiting until age 18 months or after to test young children (see **Table 3**).[16,18,54,56] A substantial proportion of infants do clear maternal HCV antibody by 12 to 15 months of postnatal age,[39,57] and the majority by age 18 months, although a few may take up to 30 months of age to clear.[37,58] Documentation of the clearance of maternal antibodies is impacted by the type of antibody test used and is delayed in infants born to viremic mothers.[55,59] Some infants also lose maternal antibody just before seroconverting in response to infection.[37] Other markers of infection such as HCV IgM have been considered unreliable,[59] and they are not commercially available. Guidelines differ in that some recommend considering RNA testing as early as 1 to 2 months of age (see **Table 3**).[18,60] Recent data demonstrated that a single RNA test between age 2 and 6 months has a sensitivity and specificity of 100% for diagnosis of chronic HCV infection (95% CI, 87.5–100 and 95% CI, 98.3–100, respectively).[58]

The disadvantages of earlier testing largely lie in cost and additional blood draws, but benefits include decreased parental anxiety and completion of testing before an infant may be lost to follow-up. Numerous studies have unfortunately shown that only 5% to 61% of HCV-exposed infants are adequately tested for HCV infection by age 18 to 30 months or later (**Fig. 1**).[39,58,61–69] One study found that 57% of HCV-exposed infants were lost to follow-up by 3 months of age, all without HCV testing completed, and often without relaying the history of HCV exposure to the transferring pediatrician.[66]

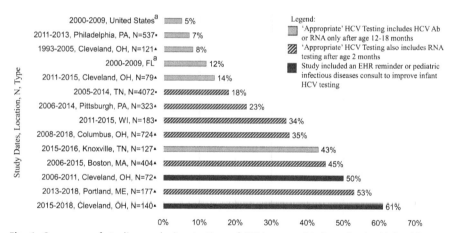

Fig. 1. Summary of studies analyzing testing of HCV-exposed infants in the United States. Each bar represents a separate study or substudy population, with dates, location, total number of HCV-exposed infants meeting study inclusion criteria for characterization of infant HCV testing, and study type. Those followed by an [a] indicate public health reporting data for the proportion of actual cases detected per those expected in Florida and the United States (no number listed as number tested was unknown).[69] Those followed by ■ used either public health reporting combined with commercial laboratory data or Medicaid/administrative claims data,[62,67,68] and those with a ▲ are prospective or retrospective studies from a single institution or health system electronic medical record.[39,58,61,63,64,65,66] Percentages at ends of bars represent the percent of infants appropriately HCV-tested, with definition of appropriate testing color coded as shown (light blue includes testing only after 12 to 18 months, hatched includes also earlier RNA testing, and dark blue solid refers to populations exposed to a testing intervention). Ab, antibody.

New strategies are therefore essential to identify the increasing number of HCV-exposed infants born each year. Multiple institutions have implemented routine screening of infants earlier than 18 months of age. Settings using both antibody and RNA testing before age 18 months have overall higher HCV testing completion rates compared with settings only evaluating infant HCV antibody after 18 months of age (see **Fig. 1**). Multiple programs have implemented successful interventions to expand testing in primary care by pediatricians through education, linkage or ensuring HCV exposure is clearly documented in the electronic health record.[63,70] Other practitioners have created programs to actively link infants to pediatric infectious diseases specialists for testing.[65,71,72] Many primary or subspecialty clinics may not have adequate resources to sustain demand in areas of high HCV prevalence. Based on recommendations and newer RNA testing and follow-up data in infants, we propose an adapted algorithm to guide clinicians in completing infant HCV screening (**Fig. 2**).[58,72] Initiating HCV RNA testing between 2 and 12 months of age will help to minimize loss to follow-up. Doing so at approximately 9 to 12 months of age in conjunction with a well-child visit could minimize extra visits and, when applicable, ordering it simultaneously with anemia or lead screening could also streamline testing to make it more routine and minimize additional blood draws. Many providers find HCV testing in infants challenging owing to phlebotomy logistics (volume requirements, not all pediatric or specialty clinics have phlebotomy on site), and parental acceptance or understanding of the need for additional testing. More research in this area would be

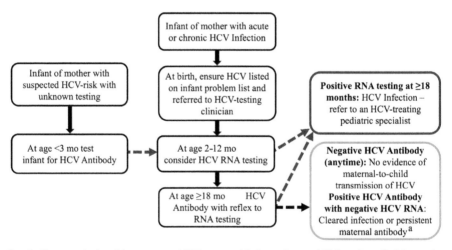

Fig. 2. Proposed algorithm to test HCV-exposed infants by an HCV-testing clinician, who may be primary or specialty care, depending on the health care system, clinician, or family preference. *Black dashed arrow* denotes negative testing, *red dashed arrows* indicate positive HCV RNA testing. Timing suggested by combination of current guidelines, potential concordant timing of RNA with lead/anemia testing, and studies demonstrating poor overall follow-up rates and improved testing rates when earlier HCV RNA testing is used. [a] Can repeat HCV antibody again at age 24 to 30 months to ensure clearance. Ab, antibody; HCV, Hepatitis C virus; RNA, ribonucleic acid. (*Data from* Espinosa C, Jhaveri R, Barritt AS. Unique Challenges of Hepatitis C in Infants, Children, and Adolescents. *Clin Ther.* 2018;40(8):1299-1307 and Gowda C, Smith S, Crim L, Moyer K, Sánchez PJ, Honegger JR. Nucleic Acid Testing for Diagnosis of Perinatally Acquired Hepatitis C Virus Infection in Early Infancy. *Clin Infect Dis.*)

beneficial to help inform clinicians of the risks, benefits, and costs of the different methods and to decrease barriers to completing follow-up.

NATURAL HISTORY AND MONITORING OF HEPATITIS C VIRUS INFECTION IN INFANTS

The monitoring of infants with confirmed HCV infection includes annual liver biochemistries, age-appropriate vaccinations including for hepatitis A and B viruses, and an assessment of disease severity through routine physical examination with noninvasive fibrosis staging modalities (elastography, ultrasound, or serum fibrosis markers).[60] Follow-up of infants from birth up to 5 years usually yields rare to no clinical signs and symptoms of hepatitis.[37] However, most series do report abnormal alanine aminotransferase in most infants intermittently during follow-up.[47] Although significant liver disease and extrahepatic manifestations have been reported in children, significant liver disease in infancy is unlikely.[47,73,74] Neutralizing antibodies are made during the first year of life in infected infants, but they do not provide effective neutralization because HCV can escape the recognition of the host's immune system by mutating within the hypervariable domain (quasi-species).[34,47,50] High viral genetic variability has been associated with progression and poor response to established therapies in small series.[51,75,76] Despite an immature humoral response in infants, activation of innate immunity and interferon production, along with other cytokines, provides immune surveillance, neutralization of infection, and activation of inflammatory response, which might result in clearance of the infant's infection.[47] Spontaneous viral clearance occurs in approximately 25% to 50% of infants with a perinatal infection, usually by 3 years of age.[73] If there are insufficient CD4 and CD8 responses, chronic infection might develop.[47]

TREATMENT

The treatment of HCV-infected infants or pregnant women with established therapies (ribavirin and pegylated interferon) before the approval of direct-acting antiviral agents (DAAs) was not recommended owing to the high risk of serious adverse events, including teratogenicity. Although DAAs have revolutionized HCV treatment in adults, currently there are no approved therapeutic alternatives for infants or pregnant women infected with HCV. A recent phase I clinical trial using ledipasvir/sofosbuvir in HCV-infected pregnant women did, however, show rapid achievement of undetectable HCV viral load and sustained virologic response without significant adverse events.[77] A phase I study with a pangenotypic DAA combination (sofosbuvir/velpatasvir) begun in October 2020 is expected to be completed by June 2023.[38]

DAAs are now approved for children as young as age 3 years for HCV genotypes 1, 4, 5, and 6, and pangenotypic regimens are approved in children age 6 years and older; additional studies are ongoing in younger children.[60] As infants have minimal risk of hepatoxicity before age 3 and high spontaneous clearance rates, DAAs are not expected to be tested or recommended for the treatment of children younger than 3 years of age.

DISCUSSION: FUTURE RESEARCH

We hope the results of treatment trials will support the possibility of treatment during pregnancy, because this is a time that many women are engaged in health care services. Treatment during pregnancy could be a key strategy to both decrease vertical transmission and eliminate maternal infection. Pregnancy is still an opportune time to identify and to link women to care with the possibility of treatment after delivery to improve their own health care and decrease subsequent vertical transmission. More research will be needed to understand how the recent recommendations for universal HCV screening impact care of the maternal–infant dyad.

SUMMARY

Although HCV vertical transmission rates are relatively low,[41] with the increasing incidence of HCV in pregnant women, associated with injection drug use, thousands of HCV-exposed infants are born annually. Knowledge of maternal HCV status can help to guide decisions during delivery and facilitate the identification of at-risk infants, who should undergo evaluation. Testing guidelines for infants born to mothers with HCV infection are not consistent, and testing practices for HCV-exposed infants fall far short of any of these recommendations. DAAs have revolutionized treatment for adults and are now available for children as young as age 3 years. Trials are ongoing to test the safety and efficacy of treating women during pregnancy,[77] and new guidance to test for HCV in each pregnancy could help to improve treatment rates postpartum and prevent vertical transmission to a future child. Pregnancy is a unique opportunity to capture a population that faces many challenges and to initiate evaluation and linkage with the goal of treating women of child-bearing age before future pregnancies. Much work remains, however, to achieve WHO 2030 HCV elimination goals, to determine best testing practices in exposed infants, and to ensure all currently infected infants and children are identified and cured.

CLINICS CARE POINTS

- The US Centers for Disease Control and Prevention now recommend that all women be tested for hepatitis C infection in each pregnancy, unless community prevalence is <0.1%.
- All children born to a mother with hepatitis C infection should be screened by either a hepatitis C antibody test after age 18 months or RNA test after age 2 months.
- Direct acting antiviral agents are now available for children 3 years and older.

DISCLOSURE

Dr R.L. Epstein has nothing to disclose. Dr C. Espinosa has received research funding from Gilead, has participated in advisory board meetings, and has conducted industry-sponsored clinical trials with direct acting agents.

Best Practice Box

What is the current practice for perinatal hepatitis C virus (HCV)?

Best Practice, Guideline, or Care Path Objective(s)
- Test all pregnant women and infants of women with acute or chronic HCV infection for HCV per current guidelines to identify cases and link them to care.
- Avoid invasive procedures during labor that may increase the chance of maternal–fetal blood transfer in women who are known to have acute or chronic HCV infection.
- Vaginal delivery and direct breastfeeding are acceptable in women with acute or chronic HCV infection.

What changes in current practice are likely to improve outcomes?

- The possibility to cure HCV infection in young children with effective, tolerable medications highlights the need to improve diagnostic testing of HCV-exposed infants, to ensure identification of HCV infection and linkage to HCV care.
- Trials of HCV therapy in pregnant women are ongoing, and treatment during pregnancy for both maternal cure and prevention of mother-to-child transmission could be an option in the future.

Is there a clinical algorithm? Yes (see Fig. 2).

Major Recommendations
- Test all pregnant women for HCV,[17] during each pregnancy.[16,18]
- Test all infants born to HCV-infected mothers for HCV antibody after age 18 months; Consider RNA testing after age 2 months.[17,18,54]
- Link children with chronic HCV infection to a clinician for monitoring and treatment with a DAAs approved for their age and genotype.[60]
- Link women with chronic HCV infection to a clinician to initiate therapy after delivery and cessation of breastfeeding.[60]

Bibliographic Source(s). Refs.[16–18,54,60]

REFERENCES

1. Schmelzer J, Dugan E, Blach S, et al. Global prevalence of hepatitis C virus in children in 2018: a modelling study. Lancet Gastroenterol Hepatol 2020;5(4): 374–92.
2. WHO. Global hepatitis report, 2017. World Health Organization; 2017. Available at: http://www.who.int/hepatitis/publications/global-hepatitis-report2017/en/. Accessed November 12, 2020.
3. Hellard M. The global investment case for hepatitis C elimination. Presented at the: EASL; April 10, 2019; Vienna, Austria. Available at: http://www.natap.org/2019/EASL/EASL_37.htm. Accessed April 17, 2019.
4. World Health Organization. Sixty-ninth world health assembly. Draft global health sector strategies. Viral hepatitis, 2016–2021. 2016. Available at: http://apps.who.int/gb/ebwha/pdf_files/WHA69/A69_32-en.pdf. Accessed December 10, 2020.
5. Centers for Disease Control and Prevention. Viral hepatitis surveillance report - United States, 2018 2020. Available at: https://www.cdc.gov/hepatitis/statistics/SurveillanceRpts.htm. Accessed November 12, 2020.
6. Haight SC, Ko JY, Tong VT, et al. Opioid Use disorder documented at delivery hospitalization — United States, 1999–2014. Morb Mortal Wkly Rep 2018; 67(31):845–9.
7. Ko JY, Haight SC, Schillie SF, et al. National trends in hepatitis C infection by opioid Use disorder status among pregnant women at delivery hospitalization — United States, 2000–2015. MMWR Morb Mortal Wkly Rep 2019;68(39):833–8.
8. Rossi RM, Wolfe C, Brokamp R, et al. Reported prevalence of maternal hepatitis C virus infection in the United States. Obstet Gynecol 2020;135(2):387–95.
9. Koneru A, Nelson N, Hariri S, et al. Increased hepatitis C virus (HCV) detection in women of Childbearing age and potential risk for vertical transmission - United States and Kentucky, 2011-2014. MMWR Morb Mortal Wkly Rep 2016;65(28):705–10.
10. Ly KN, Jiles RB, Teshale EH, et al. Hepatitis C virus infection among reproductive-Aged women and children in the United States, 2006 to 2014. Ann Intern Med 2017;(166):775–82.
11. Stasi C, Silvestri C, Voller F. Update on hepatitis C epidemiology: unaware and Untreated infected population could Be the key to elimination. SN Compr Clin Med 2020;1–8. https://doi.org/10.1007/s42399-020-00588-3.

12. Doyle JS, Scott N, Sacks-Davis R, et al. Treatment access is only the first step to hepatitis C elimination: experience of universal anti-viral treatment access in Australia. Aliment Pharmacol Ther 2019;49(9):1223–9.

13. Elms N, Link K, Newman A, et al. Need for women-centered treatment for substance use disorders: results from focus group discussions. Harm Reduct J 2018;15. https://doi.org/10.1186/s12954-018-0247-5.

14. Angelotta C, Weiss CJ, Angelotta JW, et al. A moral or medical problem? The relationship between legal penalties and treatment practices for opioid Use disorders in pregnant women. Womens Health Issues 2016;26(6):595–601.

15. Gressler LE, Shah S, Shaya FT. Association of Criminal statutes for opioid Use disorder with prevalence and treatment among pregnant women with commercial insurance in the United States. JAMA Netw Open 2019;2(3). https://doi.org/10.1001/jamanetworkopen.2019.0338.

16. Schillie S. CDC recommendations for hepatitis C screening among adults — United States, 2020. MMWR Recomm Rep 2020;69. https://doi.org/10.15585/mmwr.rr6902a1.

17. Owens DK, Davidson KW, Krist AH, et al. Screening for hepatitis C virus infection in adolescents and adults: US preventive Services Task Force recommendation statement. JAMA 2020. https://doi.org/10.1001/jama.2020.1123.

18. AASLD-IDSA HCV Guidance Panel. Hepatitis C guidance 2018 update: AASLD-IDSA recommendations for testing, managing, and treating hepatitis C virus infection. Clin Infect Dis 2018;67(10):1477–92.

19. American College of Obstetricians and Gynecologists. ACOG practice Bulletin No. 86: viral hepatitis in pregnancy. Obstet Gynecol 2007;110(4):941–56.

20. Hughes BL, Page CM, Kuller JA. Society for maternal-fetal medicine (SMFM) Consult series #43: hepatitis C in pregnancy: screening, treatment and management. Am J Obstet Gynecol 2017. https://doi.org/10.1016/j.ajog.2017.07.039.

21. American College of Obstetricians and Gynecologists. Screening for hepatitis C virus infection 2020. Accessed November 14, 2020. Available at: https://www.a-cog.org/en/Clinical/Clinical Guidance/Practice Advisory/Articles/2020/04/Screening for Hepatitis C virus infection.

22. Adams J. AN ACT relating to screening for hepatitis C.. 2018. Available at: https://apps.legislature.ky.gov/record/18rs/sb250.html. Accessed December 10, 2020.

23. Rose M, Myers J, Evans J, et al. Hepatitis C virus risk-based Vs. Universal screening among pregnant women: implementation and cost-effectiveness analysis. Hepatology 2018;68(S1):1–183.

24. Protopapas S, Murrison LB, Wexelblatt SL, et al. Addressing the disease burden of vertically-acquired hepatitis C virus (HCV) infection among opioid-exposed infants. Open Forum Infect Dis 2019. https://doi.org/10.1093/ofid/ofz448.

25. Tasillo A, Eftekhari Yazdi G, Nolen S, et al. Short-term effects and long-term cost-effectiveness of universal hepatitis C testing in prenatal care. Obstet Gynecol 2019;133(2):289–300.

26. Chaillon A, Rand EB, Reau N, et al. Cost-effectiveness of universal hepatitis C virus screening of pregnant women in the United States. Clin Infect Dis 2019;69(11):1888–95.

27. Chaillon A, Wynn A, Kuchner T, et al. Cost-Effectiveness of Antenatal rescreening among pregnant women for hepatitis C in the United States. Hepatology 2020;72(S1):962A.

28. Floreani A. Hepatitis C and pregnancy. World J Gastroenterol 2013;19(40):6714–20.

29. Paternoster DM, Santarossa C, Grella P, et al. Viral load in HCV RNA-positive pregnant women. Am J Gastroenterol 2001;96(9):2751–4.

30. Dibba P, Cholankeril R, Li AA, et al. Hepatitis C in pregnancy. Dis Basel Switz 2018;6(2). https://doi.org/10.3390/diseases6020031.

31. Money D, Boucoiran I, Wagner E, et al. Obstetrical and neonatal outcomes among women infected with hepatitis C and their infants. J Obstet Gynaecol Can 2014;36(9):785–94.

32. Hashem M, Jhaveri R, Saleh DA, et al. Spontaneous viral load decline and subsequent clearance of chronic hepatitis C virus in postpartum women correlates with favorable interleukin-28B gene allele. Clin Infect Dis 2017;65(6):999–1005.

33. Pergam SA, Wang CC, Gardella CM, et al. Pregnancy complications associated with hepatitis C: data from a 2003–2005 Washington state birth cohort. Am J Obstet Gynecol 2008;199(1):38.e1-e9.

34. Fauteux-Daniel S, Larouche A, Calderon V, et al. Vertical transmission of hepatitis C virus: variable transmission Bottleneck and evidence of midgestation in Utero infection. J Virol 2017;91(23). https://doi.org/10.1128/JVI.01372-17.

35. Syriopoulou V, Nikolopoulou G, Daikos GL, et al. Mother to child transmission of hepatitis C virus: rate of infection and risk factors. Scand J Infect Dis 2005;37(5): 350–3.

36. Dal Molin G, D'Agaro P, Ansaldi F, et al. Mother-to-infant transmission of hepatitis C virus: rate of infection and assessment of viral load and IgM anti-HCV as risk factors. J Med Virol 2002;67(2):137–42.

37. Mast EE, Hwang L-Y, Seto DSY, et al. Risk factors for perinatal transmission of hepatitis C virus (HCV) and the natural history of HCV infection acquired in infancy. J Infect Dis 2005;192(11):1880–9.

38. Dore GJ, Kaldor JM, McCaughan GW. Systematic review of role of polymerase chain reaction in defining infectiousness among people infected with hepatitis C virus. BMJ 1997;315(7104):333–7.

39. Epstein RL, Sabharwal V, Wachman EM, et al. Perinatal transmission of hepatitis C virus: defining the Cascade of care. J Pediatr 2018;203:34–40.e1.

40. Resti M, Azzari C, Galli L, et al. Maternal drug use is a preeminent risk factor for mother-to-child hepatitis C virus transmission: results from a multicenter study of 1372 mother-infant pairs. J Infect Dis 2002;185(5):567–72.

41. Benova L, Mohamoud YA, Calvert C, et al. Vertical transmission of hepatitis C virus: systematic review and meta-analysis. Clin Infect Dis 2014;59(6):765–73.

42. Conte D, Fraquelli M, Prati D, et al. Prevalence and clinical course of chronic hepatitic C virus (HCV) infection and rate of HCV vertical transmission in a cohort of 15,250 pregnant women. Hepatol Baltim Md 2000;31(3):751–5.

43. Le Campion A, Larouche A, Fauteux-Daniel S, et al. Pathogenesis of hepatitis C during pregnancy and childhood. Viruses 2012;4(12):3531–50.

44. Polis CB, Shah SN, Johnson KE, et al. Impact of maternal HIV coinfection on the vertical transmission of hepatitis C virus: a meta-analysis. Clin Infect Dis 2007; 44(8):1123–31.

45. Chandwani S, Greco MA, Mittal K, et al. Pathology and human immunodeficiency virus expression in placentas of seropositive women. J Infect Dis 1991;163(5): 1134–8.

46. Prasad MR, Honegger JR. Hepatitis C virus in pregnancy. Am J Perinatol 2013; 30(2). https://doi.org/10.1055/s-0033-1334459.

47. Wen JW, Haber BA. Maternal-fetal transmission of hepatitis C infection: what is so special about babies? J Pediatr Gastroenterol Nutr 2014;58(3):278–82.

48. Azzari C, Moriondo M, Indolfi G, et al. Higher risk of hepatitis C virus perinatal transmission from drug user mothers is mediated by peripheral blood mononuclear cell infection. J Med Virol 2008;80(1):65–71.

49. Resti M, Jara P, Hierro L, et al. Clinical features and progression of perinatally acquired hepatitis C virus infection. J Med Virol 2003;70(3):373–7.

50. Moradpour D, Penin F, Rice CM. Replication of hepatitis C virus. Nat Rev Microbiol 2007;5(6):453–63.

51. Escobar-Gutiérrez A, Soudeyns H, Larouche A, et al. Vertical transmission of hepatitis C virus: a tale of multiple outcomes. Infect Genet Evol J Mol Epidemiol Evol Genet Infect Dis 2013;20:465–70.

52. Cruz-Rivera M, Carpio-Pedroza JC, Escobar-Gutiérrez A, et al. Rapid hepatitis C virus divergence among chronically infected individuals. J Clin Microbiol 2013; 51(2):629–32.

53. Cottrell EB, Chou R, Wasson N, et al. Reducing risk for mother-to-infant transmission of hepatitis C virus: a systematic review for the U.S. Preventive Services Task Force. Ann Intern Med 2013;158(2):109–13.

54. Kimberlin DW, Brady MT, Jackson MA, et al. Hepatitis C. In: Kimberlin DW, editor. Red Book 2018-2021 report of the Committee on infectious diseases. 31st edition. Grove Village (IL): American Academy of Pediatrics; 2018. p. 431. Available at: https://redbook.solutions.aap.org/chapter.aspx?sectionid=189640105& bookid=2205. Accessed August 2, 2018.

55. Ferrero S, Lungaro P, Bruzzone BM, et al. Prospective study of mother-to-infant transmission of hepatitis C virus: a 10-year survey (1990-2000). Acta Obstet Gynecol Scand 2003;82(3):229–34.

56. Mack CL, Gonzalez-Peralta RP, Gupta N, et al. NASPGHAN practice guidelines: diagnosis and management of hepatitis C infection in infants, children, and adolescents. J Pediatr Gastroenterol Nutr 2012;54(6):838–55.

57. Bal A, Petrova A. Single clinical practice's report of testing initiation, antibody clearance, and transmission of hepatitis C virus (HCV) in infants of chronically HCV-infected mothers. Open Forum Infect Dis 2016;3(1). https://doi.org/10. 1093/ofid/ofw021.

58. Gowda C, Smith S, Crim L, et al. Nucleic acid testing for diagnosis of perinatally acquired hepatitis C virus infection in early infancy. Clin Infect Dis 2020. https:// doi.org/10.1093/cid/ciaa949.

59. Thomas SL, Newell ML, Peckham CS, et al. Use of polymerase chain reaction and antibody tests in the diagnosis of vertically transmitted hepatitis C virus infection. Eur J Clin Microbiol Infect Dis 1997;16(10):711–9.

60. AASLD-IDSA. Recommendations for testing, managing, and treating hepatitis C. HCVGuidelines.org. 2020. Available at: https://www.hcvguidelines.org/. Accessed December 14, 2020.

61. Chappell CA, Hillier SL, Crowe D, et al. Hepatitis C virus screening among children exposed during pregnancy. Pediatrics 2018;e20173273. https://doi.org/ 10.1542/peds.2017-3273.

62. Kuncio DE, Newbern EC, Johnson CC, et al. Failure to test and identify perinatally infected children born to hepatitis C virus-infected women. Clin Infect Dis 2016; 62(8):980–5.

63. Hojat LS, Greco PJ, Bhardwaj A, et al. Using preventive health Alerts in the electronic health record improves hepatitis C virus testing among infants perinatally exposed to hepatitis C. Pediatr Infect Dis J 2020;39(10):920–4.

64. Bell R, Wolfe I, Cox D, et al. Hepatitis C screening in mothers and infants exposed to opioids. Hosp Pediatr 2019. https://doi.org/10.1542/hpeds.2018-0225.

65. Abughali N, Maxwell JR, Kamath AS, et al. Interventions using electronic medical records improve follow up of infants born to hepatitis C virus infected mothers. Pediatr Infect Dis J 2014;33(4):376–80.
66. Towers CV, Fortner KB. Infant follow-up postdelivery from a hepatitis C viral load positive mother. J Matern Fetal Neonatal Med 2019;32(19):3303–5.
67. Watts T, Stockman L, Martin J, et al. Increased risk for mother-to-infant transmission of hepatitis C virus among Medicaid recipients — Wisconsin, 2011–2015. MMWR Morb Mortal Wkly Rep 2017;66. https://doi.org/10.15585/mmwr.mm6642a3.
68. Lopata SM, McNeer E, Dudley JA, et al. Hepatitis C testing among perinatally exposed infants. Pediatrics 2020;145(3). https://doi.org/10.1542/peds.2019-2482.
69. Delgado-Borrego A, Smith L, Jonas MM, et al. Expected and actual case Ascertainment and treatment rates for children infected with hepatitis C in Florida and the United States: epidemiologic evidence from statewide and nationwide surveys. J Pediatr 2012;161(5):915–21.
70. Cave B, Sanders K, Moser S, et al. Working toward elimination of hepatitis C: the Kentucky hepatitis Academic mentorship program. Clin Liver Dis 2020;16(3):123–6. https://doi.org/10.1002/cld.1028.
71. Epstein R, Moloney C, Pelton S. Engaging Mother-Infant Dyads in Hepatitis C Care Through Perinatal Pediatrics Infectious Diseases Consultation. Presented at the: International Network of Hepatitis in Substance Users (INHSU) 2019 Annual Meeting; September 13, 2019; Montreal, CA.
72. Espinosa C, Jhaveri R, Barritt AS. Unique challenges of hepatitis C in infants, children, and adolescents. Clin Ther 2018;40(8):1299–307.
73. Espinosa CM, Jhaveri R. Update on the management of hepatitis B and C infections in the neonatal period. Semin Perinatol 2018;42(3):185–90.
74. Squires James E, Balistreri William F. Hepatitis C virus infection in children and adolescents. Hepatol Commun 2017;1(2):87–98.
75. Farci P, Quinti I, Farci S, et al. Evolution of hepatitis C viral quasispecies and hepatic injury in perinatally infected children followed prospectively. Proc Natl Acad Sci U S A 2006;103(22):8475–80.
76. Morishima C, Polyak SJ, Ray R, et al. Hepatitis C virus-specific immune responses and quasi-species variability at baseline are associated with nonresponse to antiviral therapy during advanced hepatitis C. J Infect Dis 2006;193(7):931–40.
77. Chappell CA, Scarsi KK, Kirby BJ, et al. Ledipasvir plus sofosbuvir in pregnant women with hepatitis C virus infection: a phase 1 pharmacokinetic study. Lancet Microbe 2020;1(5):e200–8.
78. Azzari C, Resti M, Moriondo M, et al. Vertical transmission of HCV is related to maternal peripheral blood mononuclear cell infection. Blood 2000;96(6):2045–8.

The Role of Breast Milk in Infectious Disease

Laura S. Madore, MD*, Donna J. Fisher, MD

KEYWORDS

- Human milk • Breastfeeding • Infectious disease • Contamination
- Misadministration

KEY POINTS

- Human milk has many advantageous anti-infective and immunologic properties, making it the ideal nutritional source to optimize the well-being of infants.
- There are certain infectious circumstances where breast milk feedings should be withheld or strict precautions followed; however, these are rare events.
- Contamination and misadministration when handling human milk is a safety concern, especially when caring for vulnerable preterm infants, but there are ways to minimize these occurrences.

BACKGROUND

Human milk is the preferred nutritional source for all infants, especially ill and premature neonates, owing to the many well-established short- and long-term benefits that human milk provides. One of the major benefits of human milk is its protection against different pathogens and infectious illnesses. The American Academy of Pediatrics thus recommends exclusive breastfeeding for the first 6 months of life for all infants.[1] Despite protecting against disease, human milk can, in rare instances, also be the source of transmission of infection to the neonate. Whether owing to maternal illness, human milk mishandling, or misadministration, there is the potential for inadvertent exposure to certain pathogens that can place the neonate at risk. This review describes the potential of human milk to transmit infection to the neonate and discuss ways to reduce these occurrences in the hospital-based setting. Alternatively, it also reviews the many anti-infective benefits that human milk has to offer, which far outweigh any potential risks.

University of Massachusetts Medical School-Baystate, 759 Chestnut Street, Springfield, MA 01199, USA
* Corresponding author.
E-mail address: Laura.MadoreMD@baystatehealth.org

Clin Perinatol 48 (2021) 359–378
https://doi.org/10.1016/j.clp.2021.03.008
0095-5108/21/© 2021 Elsevier Inc. All rights reserved.

BREAST MILK ANTI-INFECTIVE PROPERTIES

Although this section focuses on the prevention of rare transmissible pathogens through human milk, it cannot be overstated that human milk, through numerous mechanisms, is protective against infectious diseases of bacterial, viral, and parasitic origin. Human milk contributes to the infant's immune function by promoting the growth of nonpathogenic flora, decreasing colonization with enteropathogens, and enhancing the development of mucosal barriers. Human milk can provide the passage of immune cells and other anti-infective proteins and enzymes.[2] Human milk is not sterile and consists of normal gut flora (such as Bifidobacteria and lactobacilli) that help to populate the developing neonatal gut microbiota, which confers gut protection and health.

Although macronutrients of human milk are generally thought to provide nutritional benefits to the neonate, each also helps protect against disease processes. Milk lipids, for instance, inactive numerous pathogens in vitro.[3] Milk proteins are an important source of bioactive components and the building blocks of anti-infective properties that all confer immunity and anti-infective protection to the neonate.[4] Human milk oligosaccharides are indigestible carbohydrates that are abundant in human milk. They act as prebiotics, forming the necessary substrates for the replenishment of native intestinal microflora and are inhibitory against some pathologic bacteria. Human milk oligosaccharides have also been shown to provide protection against numerous viruses.[5]

Other important entities, such as immunoglobulins (eg, secretory IgA), functioning immune cells (eg, neutrophils, macrophages, and lymphocytes), lactoferrin, lysozyme, cytokines, and other anti-inflammatory factors aid in the development of the immature immune system and confer antimicrobial properties to the breast milk–fed infant.[6] A study from Australia found that human milk leukocytes increased significantly from baseline in a mother's milk in response to her infected infant, suggesting that a mother's mammary gland can respond directly to an acute neonatal infection.[7]

In a dose-dependent manner, human milk decreases the rates of certain chronic illnesses and decreases the rates of respiratory infections, otitis media, and gastroenteritis, as well as decreases the risk for late-onset sepsis and the risk of necrotizing enterocolitis in premature infants.[1,2] The many innate benefits of breast milk make it superior to infant formula, especially for premature infants who are at a greater risk of invasive infections. Mother's own milk is preferred over donor milk because the pasteurization process required for the inactivation of microbial contaminants and the multiple freeze–thaw cycles required for transport minimizes many of the anti-infective properties and nutritional components of the donor milk.[8] However, in situations where mother's expressed milk is not available, donor milk is preferred to formula in the preterm population.[1] Processes should be in place to support lactation via improved multidisciplinary and societal supports and increase access to donor milk when mother's own milk is not an option.

TRANSMITTED INFECTIONS AND HUMAN MILK

This article focuses on the most common pathogens that can be transmitted rarely through human milk or direct breastfeeding. It is important to understand that human milk is just one of the many potential vehicles for postnatal transmission of infections and excluding other more common mechanisms (eg, caregivers, environment, invasive interventions in a hospital setting) can be challenging. Additionally, human milk can help to prevent or ameliorate illness owing to the many benefits discussed elsewhere in this article. Therefore, human milk administration should only be discontinued in very rare circumstances as outlined elsewhere in this discussion.

All neonatal units should have policies in place to address infection-related precautions and contraindications to breastfeeding. The development of these policies should be via a multidisciplinary approach involving neonatologists, pediatric infectious disease physicians, infection control specialists, and epidemiologists. In specific or rare cases, decisions regarding breastfeeding safety should be made in consultation with an infectious disease specialist. We review how human milk feeding is impacted by infections transmitted through various modes, and take a deeper dive into specific infectious agents.

Airborne Diseases

In cases where mothers have active diseases that are transmitted through the airborne route, such as measles, varicella, disseminated zoster, and tuberculosis (TB), infants may need to be separated from their mothers temporarily, until deemed noninfectious. During separation, infants can receive mother's expressed milk because the potential route of transmission is via the mother's airborne droplets and not her expressed milk, as long as there are no active lesions on the breast (such as with varicella zoster [VZV] or TB), in which case the milk expressed from the affected side should be discarded. Direct breastfeeding may resume when all of the following conditions have been met: the infectious period is over, any active breast lesions healed, and, in the case of measles, after infant has received immunoglobulin.[9]

Droplet Diseases

Pathogens transmitted through larger respiratory droplets such as adenovirus, diphtheria, influenza, Haemophilus spp, mumps, mycoplasma, Neisseria spp, pertussis, other respiratory viruses such as respiratory syncytial virus, coronaviruses, rubella, and Streptococcus spp are not shed in human milk and, thus, an infant can continue to receive expressed milk from a woman with one of these infections.[9] Breastfeeding should be continued as long as proper precautions are in place, such as meticulous hand hygiene and surgical mask donning while contagious.

Contact Diseases

Contact precautions (gloves and gown) are used for diarrheal diseases, multidrug-resistant organisms, staphylococcal skin and soft tissue infections, and viral skin infections. The use of expressed breast milk and breastfeeding is acceptable in most situations where contact precautions are, recommended except when the breast is affected directly by active, open skin lesions, in which case breastfeeding and expressed milk feedings from the affected breast can be resumed once the lesions have healed.[10]

Table 1 presents breastfeeding issues for selected maternal infections that are transmitted by contact and/or droplets but not necessarily transmitted through human milk.

COMMON VIRAL INFECTIONS

The transmission of viral infections through breast milk is well documented for HIV, cytomegalovirus (CMV), and human T-lymphotropic virus (HTLV) (**Table 2**). Exposure to small amounts of virus in human milk multiple times a day over the period of breastfeeding (months to years) likely contributes to transmission from a breastfeeding

Table 1
Maternal infections that impact infant breastfeeding but are not transmissible in human milk

Organism	Predominant Modes of Transmission	Usual Timing of Infant Infection	Impact of Maternal Infection on the Breastfed Infant
Bacillus anthracis (anthrax)	Contact with skin eschar (airborne if bioterror event)	NA	Separate infant from infected mother and no BF/EBM from affected breast until 48 h after appropriate treatment
Candida species	Contact	Postnatal	Express milk, and can BF from unaffected side while mother and infant receive treatment
HSV-1 or HSV-2	Contact	Postnatal	No BF/EBM from affected breast until lesions healed but infant can BF/receive EBM from unaffected breast; must cover lesions
Mycobacterium tuberculosis	Airborne	Postnatal	Separate infant from mother with active pulmonary disease until completed 2 wk of treatment; infant can receive EBM during this time, except when TB mastitis present
Staphylococcus aureus	Contact	Postnatal	No BF/EBM if uncontained draining or open breast lesions but pumping/dumping encouraged; BF/EBM from unaffected side allowed when lesions covered
Treponema pallidum (syphilis)	Blood and body fluids, skin lesion contact	Congenital/perinatal	If syphilitic lesions on breast/nipple then avoid BF/EBM until treated and lesions healed, otherwise no contraindication to BF/EBM
Primary varicella (chickenpox)	Airborne and contact	Postnatal/perinatal	Isolate separately from mother if possible until lesions crusted; can receive EBM. Keep lesions covered. Provide varicella zoster immunoglobulin to high-risk infants
Varicella-zoster virus (shingles)	Contact and droplet	Postnatal	Avoid contact with lesions-keep covered; if lesions on breast, no BF/EBM on affected side until crusted over but can BF from unaffected side

Abbreviations: BF, breastfeeding; EBM, expressed breast milk; NA, not applicable.

Table 2
Pathogens associated with human milk transmission

Pathogen	Transmissible via Human Milk?	Human Milk Feedings Contraindicated?
HIV	Yes	Yes, contraindicated when safe feeding alternatives exist
Hepatitis B virus	Yes	No, transmission risk low especially after neonatal administration of recommended immunoglobulin and vaccine
Hepatitis C virus	No, but theoretical transmission if woman is viremic and if nipples are cracked and bleeding	No, unless cracked and bleeding nipples
CMV	Yes—risk of clinically significant infection in neonate is variable	No, although can be considered in high-risk infant (premature, immunocompromised, etc) with primary maternal infection
Human T-cell lymphotropic virus type I or type II	Yes	Yes, contraindicated when safe alternatives exist
Viral hemorrhagic fevers (eg, Ebola)	Yes	Yes, contraindicated in suspected or active disease

woman to her infant. The subsequent sections address the more common viral illnesses for which human milk ingestion may pose a risk for transmission.

HIV

HIV may be detected in both cell-free and cell-associated portions of human milk. Many studies have shown that the rate of transmissibility is associated with maternal viral load and is drastically decreased in women who are virologically suppressed on highly active antiretroviral therapy. Maternal receipt of antiretroviral therapy is likely to decrease the levels of free HIV in human milk, but the presence of cell-associated virus (intracellular HIV DNA) may remain and may continue to pose a transmission risk.[10]

In settings where alternatives are available, it is not recommended for HIV-infected mothers to breastfeed or provide their expressed milk under any circumstances.[9,11] This practice is an important component of preventing mother-to-child transmission. However, in settings where potable water and formula are not readily available, infants who are not breastfed are at an increased risk of morbidity and mortality owing to malnutrition and infectious diseases, and thus breastfeeding may outweigh the risk of potentially acquiring HIV. In these settings, compliance with maternal antiretroviral therapy and exclusive breastfeeding has been associated with lower rates of acquiring HIV compared with mixed feedings of formula and human milk.[12]

Cytomegalovirus

Postnatally acquired CMV rarely results in clinically significant disease in full-term infants owing to a more developed immune system and the acquisition of transplacental maternal antibodies; however, in premature and immunocompromised neonates, CMV can range from mild disease to clinically significant disease manifesting as hepatitis, pneumonitis, and a sepsis-like picture with leukopenia, thrombocytopenia, and possibly death.[13,14]

Postnatal CMV can be acquired via personal contact, saliva, or human milk from a seropositive woman during a primary or reactivated infection.[15] Rates of transmission from the milk of CMV IgG–positive mothers to preterm neonates ranges from 6% to 58%, with the median rates of symptomatic disease being 3.7% and severe disease 0.7%, with the more immature infants being greatest at risk.[16] Freeze–thaw cycling may decrease viral titers and pasteurization may eliminate CMV viral particles from human milk14,16, however, these treatments must be weighed against the simultaneous concern of reducing important anti-infective properties of the milk. Although breastfeeding is not contraindicated, whether to continue or discontinue providing human milk from a known CMV seropositive mother to her premature infant is debated, and must be weighed carefully, taking into consideration the immune benefits of human milk.

Hepatitis B Virus

Chronic hepatitis B virus (HBV) infection develops in 90% of infants infected before or during birth. If infected after birth, about 30% develop chronic HBV, which can manifest as chronic active infection, chronic persistent hepatitis, cirrhosis, and a later risk of hepatocellular carcinoma.[9]

HBV can be found in breast milk from a chronically infected mother, but the risk of transmission is low, and HBV infection is not considered a contraindication to breastfeeding.[17] In this situation, the benefits of human milk outweigh the theoretical risk of transmission. Furthermore, infants born to women who are hepatitis B surface antigen positive should receive HBV immunoglobulin and the first dose of monovalent HBV vaccine within 12 hours of birth, per standard guidelines.[9,17] Breastfeeding need not be delayed during this time.

Hepatitis C Virus

Chronic hepatitis C virus (HCV) infection results in the same potential sequelae as does HBV, and develops in more than 75% of infected adults. Limited data suggest a more indolent course in children with chronic infection and cirrhosis occurring less often with most cases being asymptomatic.[9] HCV has been detected in human milk, but there have been no documented cases of human milk transmission from an infected woman to a neonate via human milk feeding, except with HIV coinfection. In the United States, women who have cracked or bleeding nipples, especially when high HCV loads are present, are advised to temporarily refrain from breastfeeding or feeding human milk expressed from the affected side.[9] Otherwise, women with HCV infection are encouraged to breastfeed or express human milk, with the understanding that there may be a theoretical risk of transmission.

Human T-Lymphotropic Virus

Although uncommon in women born in the United States and not routinely screened for in pregnant mothers, women who are HTLV type I or II infected should not breastfeed or provide expressed milk.

HTLV type I is associated with the development of malignant neoplasms and neurologic disorders among adults and is endemic in Japan, the Caribbean, and parts of South America and Africa. Early life transmission is associated with higher risks of leukemia. Studies suggest that infant transmission occurs primarily through breastfeeding.[18] Although the freezing and thawing of expressed human milk may decrease infectivity, currently it is not recommended that HTLV-I–seropositive women breastfeed or provide expressed breast milk if a viable alternative (eg, formula or donor milk) is available.[1,9]

HTLV type II is a retrovirus that causes chronic ataxia and other multisystem illnesses. It has been detected among American and European injection drug users and some American Indian/Alaska Native groups. HTLV-II has been detected in human milk and maternal–infant transmission has been documented, but few data are available.[18] Thus, similar to HTLV-I, it is not recommended that HTLV-II seropositive women breastfeed or provide expressed milk.[1,9]

Herpes simplex virus

Herpes simplex virus (HSV) types I and II cause severe perinatal infections and, less frequently, prenatal and postnatal infections. HSV infections in infants attributed to maternal HSV breast lesions have been documented, but there has been no evidence to support HSV transmission in human milk.[9] Breastfeeding or expressing milk in the absence of breast lesions is appropriate in women experiencing an HSV infection when contact precautions are followed, including covering the lesions, remaining clothed or gowned, and careful handwashing. Feeding breast milk, directly or expressed, from the affected breast is contraindicated until lesions healed.[19]

Varicella Zoster

Primary VZV infection as chicken pox and reactivation as zoster or shingles has been associated with neonatal varicella infections. Postnatal transmission occurs primarily through respiratory droplets and contact with skin lesions. VZV DNA and antibodies have been identified in breast milk, but there have been no data to support the transmission of VZV or attenuated vaccine virus through human milk ingestion.[9] In VZV-exposed infants, VZV immunoglobulin should be given to those deemed at high risk, to include immunocompromised, premature, or development of maternal primary VZV infection within 5 days before or 2 days after delivery.[1,9] If a lactating woman develops VZV, the American Academy of Pediatrics and the Centers for Disease Control and Prevention (CDC) recommend that the infant be isolated separately until the maternal vesicles have dried, despite infant VZV immunoglobulin administration.[1,19] Infant can receive expressed milk as long as the lesions are covered and the breast pump avoids vesicles.[9] Others suggest mother–infant separation can harm successful breastfeeding and thus may not be warranted if lesions can be covered adequately.[20] If a lactating woman is exposed to VZV, varicella vaccine can be administered and human milk feeding can continue.

With varicella reactivation or shingles, breastfeeding can continue as long as the lesions do not involve the breast and are covered. If there is breast involvement in the area where the infant's mouth may contact a lesion, avoid breastfeeding or supplying expressed milk from the affected side until the lesion is crusted is appropriate.[19]

Other Viruses

Viral hemorrhagic fevers (eg, Ebola virus) are a deadly and highly contagious group of viruses that are transmitted via blood and body fluids, including breast milk; thus, breastfeeding in confirmed or suspected maternal cases is contraindicated. Viruses detected in low levels in human milk but do not pose a contraindication to breastfeeding include hepatitis A virus, rubella, West Nile virus, and Zika virus. In these instances, transmission to an infant is extremely uncommon, and benefits of breastfeeding are felt to outweigh the risks.[9,21,22] There is no evidence for transmission through human breast milk of any of the following: parvovirus B19, respiratory syncytial virus, severe acute respiratory syndrome novel coronavirus 1 (SARS-CoV 1), and Dengue virus. See the "Emerging Infections" section elsewhere in this article, which addresses SARS-Co-V 2 and human milk feeding.

BACTERIAL INFECTIONS

Transmission of bacterial organisms from mother to child through human milk is relatively rare compared with other more common routes of transmission (eg, perinatal or contact exposures). Bacteria are present in human milk and pumping or other methods of expressing milk are not sterile procedures. The innate antibacterial and anti-infective properties of human milk decrease the opportunity for transmission of pathogens to the neonate. In select maternal systemic infections, mastitis with open or draining lesions, or breast/nipple lesions, women may be advised to replace direct breastfeeding with expression of human milk, select an unaffected breast for direct breastfeeding or human milk expression, or express but not feed their milk to their neonate. There are no data to support the routine culturing of milk for the presence of bacteria, viruses, or other organisms.[23,24]

Escherichia coli

E coli is a common cause of neonatal systemic bacterial infection as well as urinary tract infections and bacteremia in infants and is ubiquitous in the environment. It is generally thought that breast milk is not a source of neonatal *E coli* infection owing to its anti-infective properties[25]; however, there has been recent documentation of an outbreak in a Japanese neonatal intensive care unit (NICU) likely attributed to contaminated unpasteurized milk sharing, which is not a recommended or routine practice.[26] If a woman has an *E coli* infection, breastfeeding can continue as long as proper contact precautions are maintained.

Haemophilus influenzae

H influenza type b (Hib) infections have decreased significantly owing to widespread vaccination. There is no evidence of Hib transmission through human milk, and human milk ingestion may actually prevent oropharyngeal infant Hib colonization.[27] If a breastfeeding woman has invasive Hib disease, then chemoprophylaxis is indicated for all household members, especially the incompletely or partially immunized infant.[9] Given that Hib is spread via respiratory droplets, the continuation of breastfeeding with careful masking and hand hygiene is appropriate.

Staphylococcus Species

Staphylococcus aureus is the most common etiology associated with soft tissue and musculoskeletal infections in children and colonizes up to half of all healthy children. Both methicillin-susceptible and methicillin-resistant *S aureus* are associated with health care–associated colonization and infection, with difficulty in eradication and treatment, especially with methicillin-resistant *S aureus*. Postnatal contact with family members, health care workers, and contaminated surfaces or equipment are the likely source of colonization and invasive infection in the heath care setting.[9] *S aureus* is also one of the most common causes of mastitis in lactating women. Per the CDC recommendations, continued breastfeeding while being treated for staphylococcal mastitis is generally encouraged to promote drainage and infection resolution. Additionally, there are no data to support staphylococcal bacteria transmissibility via human milk. If, however, there is purulent drainage or open skin lesions on the breast that are unable to be contained by covering, or the infant is premature or at risk for invasive infections, then expressing and discarding milk from affected breast is warranted while continuing to breastfeed from unaffected side.[19]

Coagulase-negative staphylococcal infection is a common cause of late-onset disease in premature, low birth weight infants who require invasive devices for monitoring or therapy, prolonged antibiotic use, and prolonged hospitalization. There is no evidence to support that a coagulase-negative staphylococcal infection is transmitted via human milk and, given the anti-infective properties of human milk, breastfeeding and expressed human milk are encouraged.

Group B Streptococcus (GBS; Streptococcus agalactiae) is transmitted primarily during delivery and remains the most common cause of neonatal early-onset sepsis despite intrapartum maternal prophylaxis significantly decreasing the early-onset disease burden. GBS infection is also a significant cause of neonatal late-onset sepsis. Although there is evidence that GBS can colonize human milk, it remains unclear if this is an infection source or a marker of heavier colonization load.[28] Routine culturing of the breast or human milk and therapy to eradicate colonization have not proven beneficial. Based on the available data, continuation of breast milk feedings should be encouraged owing to its anti-infective properties, although some investigators suggest that, in recurrent episodes of late-onset GBS disease in the preterm neonate, cessation of maternal breast milk feedings may be considered until the disease is resolved.[29]

Listeria
Listeria monocytogenes is a food-borne illness, and infection during pregnancy infrequently results in stillbirth, premature delivery, or severe disease in the neonate through perinatal acquisition. No published information documents transmission of L monocytogenes through human milk; thus, breastfeeding or the use of expressed breast milk from an infected individual is not contraindicated.

Chlamydia
Chlamydial infection is the most frequent sexually transmitted disease in the United States. Perinatal infection acquired from passage through the birth canal of an infected woman results in neonatal conjunctivitis and pneumonitis. Specific secretory IgA has been identified in colostrum and breast milk, but there is no evidence for transmission through human milk.[24]

Gonorrhea
Neisseria gonorrhea is transmitted during passage through the birth canal and infrequently from postnatal contact with an infected person. Transmissions of N gonorrhea via human milk have not been documented. Breastfeeding can continue while an infected woman is treated with ceftriaxone.[24]

Tuberculosis
Postnatal exposure through aerosolized droplets or droplet nuclei by a family member with active pulmonary TB is possible or, rarely, from a breastfeeding woman with TB mastitis. When a breastfeeding woman has active pulmonary disease, it is recommended to start isoniazid prophylaxis in her infant and separate until a minimum of 2 weeks of appropriate treatment and no longer contagious, per American the Academy of Pediatrics and CDC recommendations.[1,19] There have been no documented cases of transmission of TB through breast milk other than with TB mastitis; thus, an infant can receive expressed milk during separation as long as there is no documented

TB mastitis and proper precautions in place (eg, mask and sterile equipment while pumping). With asymptomatic TB, separation of the infant is not indicated and breast-feeding can be continued.[9]

Brucella Species

Mothers with untreated brucellosis should not breastfeed or provide expressed milk to their infants until their infection is eradicated.[1,19,30]

OTHER INFECTIONS

Various other organisms are mentioned in discussions of breastfeeding and infection, a few selected organisms are reviewed here.

Lyme Disease

Borrelia burgdorferi is the spirochete that causes Lyme disease, a multisystem disease presenting in various stages, and is primarily arthropod-borne and -transmitted. Although *B burgdorferi* DNA has been reported in breast milk, there is no evidence for illness in the infant or transmission of the spirochete to the infant through breast milk.[31]

Candidal Infections

Candida can readily colonize most infants without producing significant illness, but can also be associated with invasive disease in hospitalized neonates. Mucocutaneous candidal disease is the most common form of illness in infants, causing thrush and diaper rash. Invasive candidal infection occurs primarily in individuals with altered immunity or altered skin or mucosal barriers and after the use of broad-spectrum antibiotics. Transmission occurs through direct contact, including breastfeeding.[24] With either maternal candidal mastitis or neonatal oral candidiasis, the simultaneous treatment of both conditions may be considered. Nursing directly from the unaffected breast and milk expression from the affected side is generally advised, with continuation of expressed milk feedings in otherwise healthy neonates.

Toxoplasmosis

Toxoplasma gondii is a protozoan associated with a congenital syndrome manifest by severe central nervous system and ocular sequelae. Postnatal neonatal infection is usually asymptomatic or can present as mild disease. *T gondii* has been transmitted through maternal milk in animal models, but this finding has not been demonstrated in human milk.[32] Breastfeeding and expressed human milk may be provided during maternal toxoplasmosis infection.

Syphilis

Treponema pallidum is a spirochete that is generally contracted as a sexually transmitted disease and can cause multisystem disease in stages similar to Lyme disease. Postnatal infection may occur in the infant through contact with open lesions or secretions from an infected person. There is no evidence for transmission of *T pallidum* in human milk in the absence of breast or nipple lesions.[24] In the rare circumstance that syphilitic lesions involve the breast or nipples, then direct breastfeeding or providing milk expressed from the affected breast should be avoided until maternal treatment has been completed and the lesions have healed.

Botulism

There is no evidence that *Clostridium botulinum,* its spores or its toxin can be transmitted through human milk; there may be a protective effect of human milk against the development of infant botulism.[24]

EMERGING INFECTIONS: HUMAN MILK AND SEVERE ACUTE RESPIRATORY SYNDROME NOVEL CORONAVIRUS 2

Early in the SARS-CoV-2 pandemic, several studies from Wuhan, China, assessed the transmission of SARS-CoV-2 from nursing mothers to their infants. There were a few instances of transmission, although it is unclear if human milk and/or contact through breastfeeding was the source of positive viral tests.[33,34] As the pandemic progressed, more data have accumulated about the risk of human milk as a source of transmission.[35] A few case reports cite the detection of SARS-CoV-2 RNA in expressed human milk; however, the viability and transmissibility of detected virus were not described. In 1 study, samples of expressed milk from 1 of 2 mildly symptomatic women with confirmed SARS-CoV-2 had viral RNA detected on days 4 to 7 of illness, but this study did not test for viable virus.[36] In another report, viral RNA was detected from the expressed milk of a mildly symptomatic SARS-CoV-2–positive mother intermittently over 10 days, but viable virus was not demonstrated; her infant did test positive and was only mildly symptomatic with a cough.[37]

Forty-nine case reports or series published through June 2020 found that human milk-fed versus formula-fed infants acquired coronavirus disease 2019 (COVID-19) at similar rates (4.7% vs 5.3%).[38] A US study assessing donated human milk from 18 SARS-CoV-2–positive women, 17 of whom were symptomatic, found no detectable replication-competent virus from any human milk sample, including 1 sample from which viral RNA was detected.[39] This report supports the very low risk of clinically significant transmission of SARS-CoV-2 from mothers with COVID-19 to their infant via human milk.

Additionally, there is evidence to suggest that human milk can provide immune protection. A case report of a SARS-CoV-2 polymerase chain reaction–positive, mildly symptomatic mother with an unaffected breastfed newborn had both IgG to and IgA to SARS-CoV-2 detectable in her expressed milk.[40] A recent study of 15 human milk samples (8 SARS-CoV-2 polymerase chain reaction–positive and COVID-19-recovered donors; 7 untested but COVID-19–suspected donors) exhibited significant specific IgA reactivity to the full SARS-CoV-2 spike protein in all samples and a majority exhibited significant IgA, secretory Ab, IgG, and/or IgM binding to the receptor-binding domain.[41]

Although additional research is needed regarding the immune response to SARS-CoV-2 in human milk, the feeding of human milk should be encouraged, either via direct breastfeeding or via expressed human milk if direct breastfeeding is not possible. Standard infection prevention guidelines should be followed for handling and cleaning of pumping and the corresponding apparatus, containers of expressed milk, and storage.[19] There is no recommended postexposure prophylaxis or testing of a neonate who receives human milk from a COVID-19 positive woman, whether planned or accidental administration, because there is no evidence of transmissible viable virus in human milk.

MATERNAL VACCINATION DURING LACTATION

Lactating nonpregnant women may be immunized similarly to other nonpregnant adults because there is no evidence to support the presence of live virus vaccine in human milk, with the exception of yellow fever vaccine. Lactation is a precaution for yellow fever vaccine administration owing to 3 serious adverse events in breastfeeding neonates after recent yellow fever vaccination of their mothers. However, if travel to an endemic area is unavoidable or an outbreak occurs, a lactating woman should be vaccinated against yellow fever.[9]

Data are being accrued on the safety of mRNA COVID-19 vaccines in lactating women, the impact on milk production and excretion, and the effects on the breastfed infant. Recently, antibody transfer into the breastmilk of lactating women 1 week after initial dose of mRNA COVID-19 vaccination has been demonstrated suggesting the possibility of passive protection to the breastfed infant after maternal vaccination.[42] The mRNA vaccines are not presumed to be a risk to an infant receiving human milk per the CDC, the Society of Maternal-Fetal Medicine, and other national and international orginzations.[43,44]Thus, COVID-19 vaccination of lactating women should not be delayed and human milk feeding should be continued.

SPECIAL CONSIDERATIONS: DONOR MILK

Many NICUs provide donor human milk for infants in whom mother's own milk is unavailable or in low supply. Recent studies have demonstrated numerous benefits of providing donor milk as opposed to formula to preterm infants to prevent acute and long-term adverse events.[45,46] For this reason, the use of donor milk and the number of human milk banks worldwide are increasing. Most US hospitals procure pasteurized donor milk from nonprofit milk banks affiliated with the Human Milk Banking Association of North America or from several for-profit commercial milk banks. These milk banks have established strict policies for health screening and blood serologic testing of donor women (primarily for HIV, HTLV, syphilis, and hepatitis B and C) as well as for the safe collection, storage, shipping, handling, pooling, and pasteurization of milk.[47,48] Although it is still possible for donor milk to be contaminated with infectious agents, pasteurization is highly effective in rendering viruses and most bacteria inert.[49] Furthermore, bacteriologic screening is performed after pasteurization and those batches with abundant bacterial loads are discarded. There have been no reported cases of infant illness attributed to improper screening, handling or shipping by donor banks, although there was a report of 3 *Pseudomonas*-related deaths in preterm infants at a single NICU that were attributed to improper donor milk preparation at the receiving hospital.[50]

In contrast, informal direct milk sharing from other mothers or from the internet is not considered safe and, therefore, not recommended.[19] Owing to minimal oversight, the chances of contamination with organisms and other substances or intentional dilution for the purposes of monetary gain, informal direct human milk sharing is strongly discouraged.

BREAST MILK HANDLING CONSIDERATIONS

The safe collection and proper storage of expressed human milk is invaluable to the health of the recipient infant. Whether from the biological mother or from human donors through an established human milk bank, hospitals with nurseries and those that provide care to infants and children must have processes in place for safe collection, handling, storage, and administration of human milk to infants.

When handling expressed milk in the health care setting, there are multiple opportunities for exposure to both pathogenic and nonpathogenic organisms. Once contaminated, human milk provides the substrate and environment supporting microbial growth. Infant feedings, both human milk and formula, have been linked to sepsis and necrotizing enterocolitis.[51–53] Therefore, it is imperative that proper hygiene and sanitation of workspace and equipment, use of sterile additives, and maintaining appropriate storage conditions and administration techniques be applied with human milk and formula preparation and administration.

Hand Hygiene

Hand hygiene is by far the most important aspect of infection prevention in the NICU. Handwashing is recommended before and after handling or preparing an individual's milk, and immediately if visibly soiled. Handwashing is preferred over hand sanitizers because these are not as effective against spores, norovirus, and other select contaminants.[54,55] Compliance with proper handwashing should be monitored and re-education undertaken on a routine basis for all staff members handling milk. Gloves should be worn at appropriate times to prevent hand soiling, but owing to the possibility of contamination, donning gloves should not replace proper handwashing. Hospitals should use policies limiting artificial nails, long natural nails, chipped or cracked polish, and hand jewelry for all staff and families, because these items have been linked to gram-negative bacteria, staphylococcal species, and yeast outbreaks in NICUs.[54] Additionally, pumping mothers should be instructed on proper hand hygiene when expressing or handling their milk.[19,55]

Workplace and Equipment Considerations

Policies and staff education should be in place to ensure appropriate cleaning, sanitizing and/or sterilizing of milk handling areas and equipment needed for milk preparation.[56] Many health care facilities use the Hazard Analysis Critical Control Point principles to build their practices and policies. A separate work space for milk handling that is distinct from the patient care area (eg, mixing room or milk room) and dedicated, trained staff to handle human milk and milk mixing (eg, milk technicians) are essential.[55] The episodes that were attributed to the *Pseudomonas*-related deaths of 3 preterm infants were associated with contaminated equipment used in measuring human milk,[50] highlighting the extreme outcomes that can result from inadequate cleaning. Additionally, women expressing human milk should be instructed on the proper cleaning procedures for their pumping and collection supplies.

Human Milk Additives

Human milk is insufficient to support the optimal growth and bone health in the premature infant; thus, nutritional supplementation of expressed human milk with bovine- or human milk-derived additives.[1] The US Food and Drug Administration regulates the manufacturing, distribution, and recall of infant formulas and most human milk additives. Additives should be inspected visually for integrity (intact seal, undamaged container or package, normal-appearing product) and should not be used past the expiration date. They should be stored unopened and per manufacturer's recommendations, usually in a low humidity, room temperature-controlled area.[57]

Liquid formula additives and preparations are sterile; however, powdered additives and formulas are not leading to greater potential for contamination. Therefore, liquid formulations should preferably be used for at-risk populations per the CDC recommendations.[57] This recommendation followed a cluster of fatal *Cronobacter sakazakii* infections attributed to contaminated powdered formula.[58] Additionally, powdered fortifier has been shown to inactive some of human milk's innate antibacterial activity.[59] Owing to the potential risk and the concern for underreporting, ready-to-feed human milk additives are preferred over powdered additives and formulations.

Human Milk Storage and Administration

In general, expressed human milk and prepared human milk should be stored in glass or food-grade plastic containers with tight-fitting lids, or in plastic bags designed specifically for human milk storage. Each container should be labeled with the infant's full name, medical record number, the date and time of expression, and the inclusion of additives, if relevant. The temperatures of refrigerators and freezers used for human milk storage should be monitored with access only to clinical staff.[55] Freshly expressed human milk may be refrigerated at 4°C for up to 96 hours, or frozen for up to 6 months; thawed human milk must be kept refrigerated and administered within 24 hours.[60]

No more than a 24-hour supply should be prepared at one time, and prepared feedings should be dispensed in single-dose units to the clinical area.[61] Heating prepared human milk may impact the immunologic and nutritional components; thus, it is recommended to warm to no higher than body temperature using acceptable methods (warm water baths, heating units, or bead baths).[48,61] There is a suggested maximum 4-hour hang time for neonates receiving prepared human milk with recommended feeding tube changes.[55] Feeding tube colonization is possible, either from the feed itself or from retrograde reflux from the infant, and has been associated with feeding intolerance and necrotizing enterocolitis.[53] Transpyloric feeding tubes pose an additional risk because they bypass the protective acidic gastric secretions that can help to neutralize pathogenic organisms.[53,55]

Human Milk Misadministration

Despite having established protocols in place, human milk misadministration events occur within the hospital setting with an incidence ranging from 1 error for every 10,000 feeding opportunities[62] to 0.7 errors per month in 1 NICU study conducted over a 10-year period.[63] Errors can occur for multiple reasons, including mislabeling and not following procedures to ensure appropriate human milk administration.

Infectious risks from a single misadministered feeding of human milk are very minimal. When evaluating risk, the gestational and chronologic age of the infant, and the health and infectious status of the donor woman (the woman whose human milk was inadvertently administered to the wrong infant) as well as the recipient woman (the woman whose infant received an incorrect human milk feeding), should be explored. The more common infectious agents that are transmissible via human milk with potential adverse health outcomes, as shown in **Table 2**, include HIV, hepatitis B and C viruses, and CMV.[9]

Although exposure to another woman's milk can cause a great deal of anxiety and may have a notable nonclinical impact (eg, lack of trust in care team), the infectious risk to the recipient infant is almost negligible.[64] As soon as the error is recognized, the feeding should be discontinued, and both families should be informed and reassured about the extremely low risk of pathogen transmission. Current CDC recommendations no longer require the donor or recipient mother to undergo serologic tests for HIV or hepatitis B and C,[19] although in high-risk situations this testing may be considered. The costs of any screening should be covered by the institution as part of the risk management and mitigation of error policy. Testing neonates is discouraged, because this practice does not address the theoretic transmission risk. Questions to ask donor mother are expression time and handling of the misadministered breast milk, including the presence of cracked or bleeding nipples, and willingness to share recent infectious disease history and medication use with the other family and the care team. A discussion with the family of the recipient infant should include reassurance of the minimal risk of infectious disease transmission, information about the misadministered milk, and pertinent medical information that the donor mother is willing to share.[19] To the extent feasible, the confidentially of both mothers must be maintained. Ongoing psychosocial support for the families and staff should be offered, and discussions with the families should be documented per each institution's policy.

Prevention of Future Errors and Exposures

Many human process errors can be the cause of human milk misadministration in the hospital setting. These often involve the misidentification or mislabeling of the bottle, but occasionally a mother is misidentified. A recent report describes an infant being given to the wrong mother for direct breastfeeding.[65] A study found that more than 75% of human milk misadministration errors happened during evening and night shifts.[66] Other types of errors with human milk misadministration are rare but potentially more serious, such as mistaken intravenous administration of human milk.[67]

A root cause analysis should be pursued in all cases so that measures can be implemented to prevent future occurrences. A review of current policies and procedures, along with re-education of staff is warranted. Potential causal factors, including but not limited to overcrowding, increased patient to staff ratios, and nonadherence to the verification of identity, should be addressed. Large nursery services have determined that hiring human milk technicians to assist with storage, labeling, handling, fortifying, and dispensing expressed human breast milk is cost effective, because it decreases errors, improves quality, and enhances family satisfaction.[68] Point-of-care human milk bar code scanners as check point systems have been implemented in many facilities to prevent misadministration. Bar-coded labels are given to mothers to label their expressed milk bottles for storage and, at the time of feeding, the milk and the designated neonate's identity band should be scanned.[69] Human milk administration errors are preventable and may be addressed by reinforcing the understanding that expressed human milk is a biological product and although the clinical consequences of misadministration are minimal, the psychosocial impact is tremendous.

SUMMARY

Owing to the many advantages of human milk, including its anti-infective and immunologic properties, human milk feeding should be encouraged and supported, except in rare circumstances. Noninfectious contraindications to human milk feeding include active maternal illicit substance abuse, certain maternal medications, and infant galactosemia. Infectious contraindications to direct or expressed human milk feeding include maternal infection with HIV, HTLV, Ebola virus, untreated brucellosis, and active breast lesions (eg, HSV, TB mastitis) from the affected side only. The safety of human milk through the prevention of contamination and misadministration should be reinforced by policies and practices that support the perception that human milk is a biological fluid. In instances where human milk feeding is not indicated, counseling of the family and offering safe feeding alternatives should be undertaken.

CLINICS CARE POINTS

- Human milk should be promoted as the ideal source of nutrition for all infants due to its multitude of benefits, which include its many anti-infective and immunologic properties that help improve overall health. Mother's own milk is superior to donor milk or formula, especially for the vulnerable preterm population.

- There are rare instances when breast milk feedings should be withheld. Infectious-related contraindications are maternal HIV, HTLV, viral hemorrhagic fevers, and untreated brucellosis; avoidance of milk from affected breast is recommended with certain active breast lesions (eg, HSV, TB mastitis) and cracked/bleeding nipples with Hepatitis C. The CDC and AAP Red Book, as well as peer-reviewed research, are quality resources to help guide clinicians in these situations.
- Contamination and misadministration of human milk is possible in the hospital setting which can put infants at risk. Evidence-based practices and policies regarding the safe handling of human milk should be in place to minimize these occurrences.
- In the vast majority of cases, the benefits of mother's milk feeding far outweigh any potential yet rare risks of infectious illness passed to an infant through breastfeeding. Support for lactating mothers should be optimized to help initiate and maintain supply.

Best practices

What is the current practice for human milk feeding and infection prevention?

Best Practice/Guideline/Care Path Objective(s)
   Human milk feedings should be promoted for all infants due its multitude of benefits, with consideration for the rare yet possible occurrence of contamination through certain maternal infections or milk mishandling. Practices and policies should be in place to minimize these potential risks to help maintain human milk's natural anti-infective properties.

What changes in current practice are likely to improve outcomes?

There have been no major advances in this area other than building evidence of the natural immunologic benefits of mother's own milk. Centers that support safe administration of human milk feeding are likely to have improved neonatal outcomes.

Is there a Clinical Algorithm? If so, please include [either create your own, use from article or search from an Elsevier application] See Table 2 for pathogens associated with human milk transmission.

Major Recommendations

Promotion of the safe administration of mother's own milk to all infants and avoidance of human milk in only rare, evidence-based situations where risks outweigh benefits

Rating for the Strength of the Evidence

Moderate

Bibliographic Source(s): This is important list current sources relevant to evidence

Reference numbers: [1,19]

DISCLOSURE

All above authors have no commercial or financial conflicts of interest.
   Funding: All above authors declare no funding sources.

REFERENCES

1. American Academy of Pediatrics. Policy Statement. Breastfeeding and the use of human milk. Pediatrics 2012;129(3):e827–41.
2. Hill DR, Newburg DS. Clinical applications of bioactive milk components. Nutr Rev 2015;73(7):463–76.
3. Isaacs CE, Litov RE, Thormar H. Antimicrobial activity of lipids added to human milk, infant formula, and bovine milk. J Nutr Biochem 1995;6(7):362–6.

4. Lonnerdal B. Human milk proteins: key components for the biological activity of human milk. Adv Exp Med Biol 2004;554:11–25.

5. Morozov V, Hansman G, Hanisch FG, et al. Human milk oligosaccharides as promising antivirals. Mol Nutr Food Res 2018;62(6):e1700679.

6. Chirico G, Marzollo R, Cortinovis S, et al. Antiinfective properties of human milk. J Nutr 2008;138(9):1801S–6S.

7. Hassiotou F, Hepworth AR, Metzger P, et al. Maternal and infant infections stimulate a rapid leukocyte response in breastmilk. Clin Transl Immunol 2013;2(4):e3.

8. Peila C, Moro GE, Bertino E, et al. The effect of holder pasteurization on nutrients and biologically-active components in donor human milk: a review. Nutrients 2016;8(8):477.

9. American Academy of Pediatrics Committee on Infectious Diseases. Red book: 2018-2021 report of the committee on infectious diseases. Itasca (IL): American Academy of Pediatrics; 2018.

10. Gaillard P, Fowler MG, Dabis F, et al. Use of antiretroviral drugs to prevent HIV-1 transmission through breast-feeding: from animal studies to randomized clinical trials. J Acquir Immune Defic Syndr 2004;35(2):178–87.

11. Committee on Pediatric AIDS. Infant feeding and transmission of human immunodeficiency virus in the United States. Pediatrics 2013;131(2):391–6.

12. World Health Organization. Guidelines on HIV and infant feeding: principles and recommendations for infant feeding in the context of HIV and a summary of evidence. Geneva (Switzerland): World Health Organization; 2010.

13. Lawrence RM. Cytomegalovirus in human breast milk: risk to the premature infant. Breastfeed Med 2006;1(2):99–107.

14. Hamprecht K, Goelz R. Postnatal cytomegalovirus infection through human milk in preterm infants: transmission, clinical presentation, and prevention. Clin Perinatol 2017;44(1):121–30.

15. Hamprecht K, Witzel S, Maschmann J, et al. Rapid detection and quantification of cell free cytomegalovirus by a high-speed centrifugation-based microculture assay: comparison to longitudinally analyzed viral DNA load and pp67 late transcript during lactation. J Clin Virol 2003;28:303–16.

16. Kurath S, Halwachs-Baumann G, Müller W, et al. Transmission of cytomegalovirus via breast milk to the prematurely born infant: a systematic review. Clin Microbiol Infect 2010;16(8):1172–8.

17. Shi Z, Yang Y, Wang H, et al. Breastfeeding of newborns by mothers carrying hepatitis B virus: a meta-analysis and systematic review. Arch Pediatr Adolesc Med 2011;165(9):837–46.

18. Carneiro-Proietti ABF, Amaranto-Dimasio CF, Leal-Horiguchi RHC, et al. Mother-to-Child transmission of Human T-cell lymphotopic viruses-1/2" what we know, and what are the gaps in understanding and preventing this route of infection. Journ Peds Infect Dis Soc 2014;(3):S24–9.

19. Centers for Disease Control and Prevention. Breastfeeding. Available at: www.cdc.gov/breastfeeding. Accessed February 26 2021.

20. Sendelbach DM, Sanchez PJ. Varicella, influenza: not necessary to separate mother and infant. Pediatrics 2012;130(2):e464.

21. Hinckley AF, O'Leary DR, Hayes EB. Transmission of West Nile virus through human breast milk seems to be rare. Pediatrics 2007;119(3):e666–71.

22. Centers for Disease Control and Prevention. Zika virus transmission in infants and children. Available at: www.cdc.gov/zika/prevention/transmission-methods.html. Accessed December 14, 2020.

23. Schanler RJ, Fraley JK, Lau C, et al. Breastmilk cultures and infection in extremely premature infants. J Perinatol 2011;31(5):335–8.
24. Riordan J, Wambach K. Breastfeeding and human lactation. 4th edition. Sudbury (MA): Jones and Bartlett Publishers; 2010.
25. Lawrence RM, Lawrence RA. Breast milk and infection. Clin Perinatol 2004; 31(3):501.
26. Nakamura K, Kaneko M, Abe Y, et al. Outbreak of extended-spectrum β-lactamase-producing Escherichia coli transmitted through breast milk sharing in a neonatal intensive care unit. J Hosp Infect 2016;92(1):42–6.
27. Hokama T, Sakamoto R, Yara A, et al. Incidence of Haemophilus influenzae in the throats of healthy infants with different feeding methods. Pediatr Int 1999;41(3): 277–80.
28. Poupolo KM, Lynfield R, Cummings JJ. Committee on fetus and newborn, committee on infectious diseases. management of infants at risk for Group B streptococcal disease. Pediatrics 2019;144(2):e20191881.
29. Zimmermann P, Gwee A, Curtis N. The controversial role of breast milk in GBS late-onset disease. J Infect 2017;74(Suppl 1):S34–40.
30. Bhatnagar A, Khera D, Singh K, et al. Acquired Brucella bacteraemia in a young infant. BMJ Case Rep 2017;2017. bcr2016217522.
31. Schmidt BL, Aberer E, Stockenhuber C, et al. Detection of Borrelia burgdorferi DNA by polymerase chain reaction in the urine and breast milk of patients with Lyme borreliosis. Diagn Microbiol Infect Dis 1995;21(3):121–8.
32. Remington JS, McLeod K, Thulliez P, et al. Toxoplasmosis. In: Remington JS, Klein JO, editors. Infectious diseases of the fetus and newborn infant. Philadelphia: Saunders; 2001. p. p205–346.
33. Zhang Zj, Yu XJ, Fu T, et al. Novel coronavirus infection in newborn babies under 28 days in China. Eur Respir J 2020;8:00697–2020.
34. Liu W, Wang Q, Zhang Q, et al. Coronavirus disease 2019 (COVID-19) during pregnancy: a case series 2020. Available at: www.preprints.org/manuscript/202002.0373/v1. Accessed November, 2020.
35. Kimberlin DW, Puopolo KM. Breast milk and COVID-19: what do We know? Clin Infect Dis 2021;72(1):131–2.
36. Groß R, Conzelmann C, Müller JA, et al. Detection of SARS-CoV-2 in human breastmilk. Lancet 2020;395(10239):1757–8.
37. Tam P, Ly K, Kernich M, et al. Detectable severe acute respiratory syndrome coronavirus 2(SARS-CoV-2) in human breast milk of a mildly symptomatic patient with coronavirus disease. 2019 (COVID-19). Clin Infect Dis 2021;72(1):128–30.
38. Walker KF, ODonoghue K, Grace N, et al. Maternal transmission of SARS-COV-2 to the neonate, and possible routes for such transmission: a systematic review and critical analysis. BJOG 2020;127(11):1324–36.
39. Chambers C, Krogstad P, Bertrand K, et al. Evaluation for SARS-CoV-2 in breast milk from 18 infected women. JAMA 2020;324(13):1347–8.
40. Dong Y, Chi X, Hai H, et al. Antibodies in the breast milk of a maternal woman with COVID-19. Emerg Microbes Infect 2020;9(1):1467–9.
41. Fox A, Marino J, Amanat F, et al. Robust and specific secretory IgA against SARS-CoV-2 detected in human milk. iScience 2020;23(11):101735.
42. Baird JK, Jensen SM, Urba WJ, et al. SARS-CoV-2 antibodies detected in human breast milk post-vaccination. medRxiv 2021 Mar 10. Accessed April 14, 2021.
43. ACIP COVID-19 vaccines work group. Available at: http://www.cdc.gov/vaccines/acip/meetings/%20downloads/slides-2020-12/slides-12-12/COVID-03-Mbaeyi.pdf. Accessed December 14, 2020.

44. SMFM statement on COVID vaccination in pregnancy. Available at: www.smfm.
    org/publications/339-society-formaternal-fetal-medicine-smfm-statement-sars-
    cov-2-vaccination-in-pregnancy. Accessed December 14, 2020.
45. Corpeleijn WE, de Waard M, Christmann V, et al. Effect of donor milk on severe
    infections and mortality in very low-birth-weight infants. The early nutrition study
    randomized clinical trial. JAMA Pediatr 2016;170(7):654–61.
46. O'Connor DL, Gibbins S, Kiss A, et al. Effect of supplemental donor human milk
    compared with preterm formula on neurodevelopment of very low-birth-weight in-
    fants at 18 month-A randomized clinical trial. JAMA 2016;316(18):1897–905.
47. Committee on Nutrition; Section on Breastfeeding; Committee of Fetus and
    Newborn. Donor human milk for the high-risk infant: preparation, safety, and us-
    age options in the United States. Pediatrics 2017;139(1):e20163440.
48. Human Milk Banking Association of North America. Best Practice for Expressing,
    Storing and Handling Human Milk in Hospitals, Homes and Child Care Settings.
    4th Ed. Fort Worth, TX: HMBANA; 2019.
49. Czank C, Prime DK, Hartmann B, et al. Retention of the immunological proteins of
    pasteurized human milk in relation to pasteurizer design and practice. Pediatr
    Res 2009;66(4):374–9.
50. Geisinger provides update on neonatal intensive care Unit at Geisinger medical
    center. 2019. Available at: www.geisinger.org/sites/nicu-update. Accessed
    December 1, 2020.
51. Smith SL, Serke L. Case report of sepsis in neonates fed expressed mother's milk.
    J Obstet Gynecol Neonatal Nurs 2016;45(5):699–705.
52. Weems MF, Dereddy NR, Arnold SR. Mother's milk as a source of Enterobacter
    cloacae sepsis in a preterm infant. Breastfeed Med 2015;10(10):503–4.
53. Mehall JR, Kite CA, Saltzman DA, et al. Prospective study of the incidence and
    complications of bacterial contamination of enteral feeding in neonates.
    J Pediatr Surg 2002;37(8):1177–82.
54. Boyce JM, Pittet D, Healthcare Infection Control Practices Advisory Committee.
    HICPAC/SHEA/APIC/IDSA hand hygiene Task Force. Guideline for hand hygiene
    in health-care settings. MMWR Recomm Rep 2002;51(RR-16):1–CE4.
55. Pediatric Nutrition Dietetic Practice Group. Infant and pediatric feedings: guide-
    lines for preparation of human milk and formula in health care facilities. 3rd edi-
    tion. Chicago, IL: Academy of Nutrition and Dietetics; 2019.
56. Rutala WA, Weber DJ. Healthcare infection control practices advisory committee,
    CDC. Guideline for Disinfection and Sterilization in Healthcare facilities 2008.
    Available at: www.cdc.gov/infectioncontrol/guidelines/disinfection. Accessed
    November 6, 2020.
57. WHO. Safe preparation, storage and handling of powdered infant formula. 2007.
    Available at: www.who.int/foodsafety/publications/powdered-infant-formula/en.
    Accessed November 6, 2020.
58. U.S. Centers for Disease Control and Prevention. Enterobacter sakazakii infec-
    tions associated with the Use of powdered infant formula. MMWR 2002;51:
    298–300.
59. Chan GM, Lee ML, Rechtman DJ. Effects of a human milk-derived human milk
    fortifier on the antibacterial actions of human milk. Breastfeed Med 2007;2(4):
    205–8.
60. Slutzah M, Codipilly CN, Potak D, et al. Refrigerator storage of expressed human
    milk in the neonatal intensive care unit. J Pediatr 2010;156(1):26–8.
61. Boullata JI, Carrera AL, Harvey L, et al. ASPEN safe practices for enteral nutrition
    therapy Task Force, American Society for Parenteral and Enteral Nutrition. ASPEN

safe practices for enteral nutrition therapy. J Parenter Enteral Nutr 2017;41(1): 15–103.

62. Drenckpohl D, Bowers L, Cooper H. Use of the six sigma methodology to reduce incidence of breast milk administration errors in the NICU. Neonatl Netw 2007; 26(3):161–6.

63. Wolford SR, Smith C, Harrison MLL. A retrospective two year study of breast milk error prevention in the neonatal intensive care unit. Neonatal Intensive Care 2013; 226(2):41–2.

64. Warner BB, Sapsford A. Misappropriated human milk: fantasy, fear, and fact regarding infectious risk. Newborn Infant Nurs Rev 2004;4:56–61.

65. Sauer CW, Marc-Aurele K. Parent misidentification leading to the breastfeeding of the wrong baby in a neonatal intensive care unit. Am J Case Rep 2016;17:574–9.

66. Zeilhofer UB, Frey B, Zandee J, et al. The role of critical incident monitoring in detection and prevention of human breast milk confusions. Eur J Pediatr 2009; 168(10):1277–9.

67. Doring M, Brenner B, Handgretinger R, et al. Inadvertent intravenous administration of maternal breast milk to a six week old infant: a case report and review of the literature. BMC Res Notes 2014;7:17.

68. Oza-Frank R, Kachoria r, Dail J, et al. A quality improvement project to decrease human milk errors in the NICU. Pediatrics 2017;139(2):e20154451.

69. Dougherty D, Nash A. Bar coding from breast to baby: a comprehensive breast milk management system for the NICU. Neonatal Netw 2009;28(5):321–8.

Antibiotic Stewardship for the Neonatologist and Perinatologist

Sophie Katz, MD, MPH[a], Ritu Banerjee, MD, PhD[a], Hayden Schwenk, MD, MPH[b],*

KEYWORDS

- Stewardship • Antibiotic • Diagnostic • Sepsis • Neonatal intensive care unit

KEY POINTS

- The overuse and misuse of antibiotics in the neonatal intensive care unit is associated with adverse outcomes.
- Neonatal intensive care unit antibiotic stewardship programs can safely decrease unnecessary antibiotic use.
- Stewardship targets in the neonatal intensive care unit include optimizing the diagnosis and management of sepsis and necrotizing enterocolitis, surgical prophylaxis, and the use of diagnostic tests.

INTRODUCTION

Antibiotics are the most commonly prescribed medications in neonatal intensive care units (NICUs) worldwide.[1] Point prevalence surveys demonstrate that the percent of hospitalized neonates receiving antibiotics in NICUs in the United States has declined, from roughly 40% in 2000 to 23% in 2017.[2,3] However, antibiotic use is common among preterm infants, the vast majority of whom receive antibiotics within the first few days of life and many times thereafter during prolonged hospitalizations.[4,5]

Antibiotic use rates vary substantially across NICUs, suggesting that there are opportunities to standardize and optimize antibiotic prescribing.[3] Across a large network of California NICUs with similar burdens of infection, antibiotic use varied 40-fold[6] and did not correlate with rates of proven infection or necrotizing enterocolitis (NEC).[7] A substantial proportion of neonatal antibiotic treatment reflects overuse or misuse in the form of inappropriately broad or narrow spectra, prolonged duration, and unnecessary therapy for nonbacterial etiologies. Given their immature and developing

[a] Vanderbilt University Medical Center, 1161 21st Avenue, Nashville, TN 37232, USA; [b] Center for Academic Medicine, Pediatric Infectious Diseases, Mail code 5660, 453 Quarry Road, Stanford, CA 94304, USA
* Corresponding author.
E-mail address: hschwenk@stanford.edu
Twitter: @StanfordPedsASP (H.S.)

Clin Perinatol 48 (2021) 379–391
https://doi.org/10.1016/j.clp.2021.03.009
0095-5108/21/© 2021 Elsevier Inc. All rights reserved.
perinatology.theclinics.com

microbiome, neonates may be especially susceptible to antibiotic-associated adverse outcomes, including NEC[4,8,9] and metabolic, immunologic, and developmental disorders.[8–11]

The implementation of NICU antibiotic stewardship programs (ASPs) has demonstrated that antibiotic use can be decreased without detrimental clinical outcomes in this high-risk population.[12] Because neonates differ from older children in their vulnerability to infection, unique clinical syndromes, pathogen distribution, frequent antibiotic exposure, and drug metabolism, NICU stewardship initiatives and metrics may differ from those used in other hospital units. In this review, we highlight common clinical syndromes in the NICU that represent opportunities for antibiotic stewardship and review the evidence for successful stewardship interventions and implementation strategies in the NICU.

STEWARDSHIP TARGETS
Sepsis

Neonatal sepsis is a syndrome associated with hemodynamic changes and other clinical manifestations resulting in significant morbidity and mortality and is often caused by bacterial, viral, or fungal infections. Depending on the age of onset and timing of the episode, neonatal sepsis is classified as either early-onset sepsis (EOS; ≤72 hours of life) or late-onset sepsis (LOS; >72 hours of life). The signs and symptoms of neonatal sepsis are nonspecific and overlap with those of noninfectious conditions, resulting in the frequent overuse of antibiotics for the management of possible or rule out sepsis. NICU stewardship efforts related to neonatal sepsis include predictive models to assess risk of EOS, appropriate diagnosis and management of culture-negative sepsis, and decreasing empiric vancomycin use.

Early-onset sepsis
An area of active research is the development and validation of sepsis calculators to better predict EOS using combinations of maternal risk factors, laboratory assessments, and physical examination findings.[13–15] Perhaps the most promising and widely used calculator was developed for infants 34 weeks of gestation or greater using maternal and infant data from more than 600,000 livebirths occurring at 14 hospitals from 1993 to 2007.[14] The neonatal population was risk stratified into 3 groups: treat with antibiotics empirically (4.1% of all live births; 60.8% of all EOS cases; sepsis incidence of 8.4/1000 live births), observe and evaluate (11.1% of births; 23.4% of cases; 1.2/1000), and continued observation without antibiotics (84.8% of births; 15.7% of cases; 0.11/1000). In a retrospective cohort study of 204,485 infants, the use of the EOS calculator was associated with a decrease in blood culture orders and empiric antibiotic administration in the first 24 hours without any change in the incidence of adverse clinical outcomes.[16] A meta-analysis of 13 studies demonstrated that, compared with conventional antibiotic management strategies, the application of the EOS calculator was associated with less empiric antibiotic therapy and without missed EOS.[17]

Late-onset sepsis
Standardizing the criteria for the evaluation of possible LOS and the need to initiate antibiotics is an additional stewardship target. A single-center quasiexperimental study using a multidisciplinary team approach to the development of local guidelines for common infections, with a focus on NICU prospective audit and feedback[18] included a unit-wide educational effort and quarterly stewardship team meetings. A pediatric clinical pharmacist attended patient care rounds and the ASP performed daily prospective audit and feedback. Significant decreases were seen in LOS

evaluation and prescription events per 100 NICU days of clinical service during their 5-year study period, with an average decrease of 2.65 LOS evaluations per NICU clinician per year.

Because coagulase-negative staphylococcal species and *Staphylococcus aureus* are commonly associated with LOS, vancomycin is often used for empiric therapy in infants with suspected LOS. In settings with a low prevalence of methicillin-resistant *S aureus*, narrower therapy (ie, nafcillin or oxacillin) may be a reasonable alternative. One retrospective cohort study including 2 NICUs evaluated the impact of vancomycin use guidelines on antibiotic use and infection-related morbidity or mortality and found significant decreases in vancomycin use without an increase in adverse events.[19] A recent single-center study used a quality improvement framework to develop key drivers and interventions, including physician education, antibiotic time outs, clinical pathway development, and daily prospective audits and feedback.[20] Vancomycin use decreased from 112 to 38 days of therapy per 1000 patient-days and vancomycin-associated acute kidney injury declined from 1.4 to 0.1 events per 1000 patient-days.

Finally, it should be noted that current blood culture techniques continuously detect low levels of bacterial growth, so bacteremia is detected within 36 hours in more than 90% of infections without antibiotic pretreatment.[21] Shortening the duration of empiric therapy to 36 hours in infants with rapid clinical improvement has the potential to greatly decrease unnecessary antibiotic use in uninfected preterm infants.

Culture-negative sepsis

Culture-negative sepsis is often diagnosed in infants with signs and symptoms that are compatible with sepsis, but with a negative microbiologic evaluation and without a focus of infection.[22] The morbidity and mortality associated with neonatal sepsis and mistrust of available microbiologic data as being falsely negative often results in the continuation of antibiotics despite negative cultures. A prospective cohort study in 2 NICUs found that the use of antibiotics for culture-negative infections contributed to more antibiotic use than episodes with positive cultures.[23]

Potential interventions for culture-negative sepsis include standardization of the diagnosis and empiric antibiotic therapy duration. There is evidence that a 5-day course for empiric treatment of culture-negative sepsis is not associated with worse outcomes compared with longer treatment durations and in 1 study was associated with a significant decrease in antibiotic days of therapy per 1000 patient-days (343.2 in the baseline period vs 252.2 in the intervention period).[12]

Necrotizing Enterocolitis

NEC is a devastating illness that is associated with increased risk of death as well as significant morbidity, including intestinal strictures, short bowel syndrome, neurodevelopmental delay, and growth impairment.[24] Recent data from the Vermont Oxford Network suggest that the incidence and mortality rate of NEC among very low birth weight infants are both decreasing, with an overall incidence of 6% in 2017 and a 4.1% decrease in all-cause mortality between 2006 and 2017.[25] However, mortality rates among infants with NEC remain significantly higher than among infants without NEC.

The pathophysiology underlying NEC has not yet been elucidated fully, but is thought to be related to a combination of intestinal immaturity, bacterial colonization, breakdown of the gut barrier with bacterial translocation, inflammation, disrupted intestinal perfusion, and intestinal injury.[26] Reported risk factors include prematurity, low birth weight, formula feeding,[27] and both antenatal[28] and postnatal antibiotic exposure.[24,29] Studies linking perinatal antibiotic exposure to NEC have been conflicting, with results suggesting no impact on the risk of NEC,[30] an increased risk for NEC (particularly with the use of specific antibiotic classes or prolonged antibiotic courses),[4,9,31] and in some studies, a protective effect of early antibiotic exposure.[32,33] It is likely that the impact of antibiotic exposure on the risk for NEC depends on the age of the neonate when antibiotics are administered,[32] their spectrum of activity,[31] and the duration of therapy.[4,31]

Although the evidence linking antibiotic exposure to NEC is conflicting, observational studies have demonstrated decreases in the rate of NEC after the implementation of antibiotic stewardship strategies. A multifaceted quality improvement initiative that included decreased use of cefotaxime, early use of ampicillin, and the discontinuation of ampicillin in infants with negative blood cultures led to a significant decrease in NEC in a large neonatal network.[34] Another single-center quality improvement effort decreased antibiotic exposure via mandatory review of antibiotics at 36 hours, noninitiation of antibiotics in low-risk infants, and discontinuing antibiotic therapy in well-appearing infants with a negative blood culture and a reassuring C-reactive protein (CRP). With this bundle, they achieved their lowest ever rate of NEC (1.4%).[35] Additional prospective studies would be helpful to better understand whether nuances in the timing, choice, and duration of antibiotic exposure differentially impact the risk for NEC.

To date, there is no definitive evidence to support the use of a particular antibiotic regimen or duration of therapy for infants with NEC. The optimal empiric agent(s) would cover bacteria that have been implicated in the disease process, preserve beneficial bacteria important to sustaining a normal microbiota, be simple to administer, and be associated with a low rate of toxicity. Various regimens have been studied, including monotherapy with piperacillin–tazobactam or a carbapenem, and various combinations of ampicillin, cefotaxime, ceftazidime, gentamicin, vancomycin, metronidazole, and clindamycin. A recent single-center, retrospective review of antibiotic regimens administered to infants with surgical NEC identified 22 different preoperative and 15 different postoperative antibiotic regimens.[36] Ampicillin, gentamicin, and metronidazole was the most common preoperative and postoperative regimen, administered for an average duration of 10.6 days and 6.6 days, respectively. Another single-center retrospective study identified 14 different antibiotics administered in 20 distinct combinations for the management of NEC.[37] As has been reported in other similar series, no single regimen seemed to be associated with superior outcomes. In a univariate analysis that did not control for other patient factors, there was no difference in outcomes between infants who received fewer than 10 days of ampicillin, gentamicin, and metronidazole versus those who were treated for more than 10 days.

Recommendations from the Infectious Diseases Society of America (IDSA) and the Surgical Infection Society include one of the following regimens: ampicillin, gentamicin, and metronidazole; ampicillin, cefotaxime, and metronidazole; or meropenem.[38,39] There is no advantage to double anaerobic coverage and such redundant combinations (eg, meropenem and metronidazole) should be avoided. They also suggest that 7 to 10 days of therapy is adequate once source control is achieved. Clinicians should consider the local microbiology of their NICU when constructing empiric antibiotic regimens for NEC. Given the spectrum of disease and potential need for surgical intervention, neonatologists should collaborate with infectious disease specialists, surgeons, and pharmacists when developing institution-specific decisions regarding the approach to the management of infants with NEC.

Antibiotic Prophylaxis in Surgery

There are relatively few data regarding the incidence of surgical site infection (SSI) and potentially modifiable risk factors, including perioperative antibiotic prophylaxis, among hospitalized neonates. Data from 1 retrospective study at a level III NICU reported an SSI incidence of 12% with no discernible differences in perioperative antibiotic exposure between infants who did and did not develop an SSI.[40] In the absence of data to guide consensus regarding perioperative antibiotic prophylaxis in the neonatal population, most practices are institution specific. As a result, there is significant heterogeneity in the use of antibiotics among infants born with surgical conditions.[41–43]

A retrospective review of patients with uncomplicated gastroschisis across 5 hospitals identified variability in both the antibiotic choice (ampicillin and gentamicin vs cefotaxime and metronidazole) and duration (mean 10–15 days) after primary closure or closure after silo reduction.[42] Another single center reported the use of 6 different postoperative antibiotics for a range of 1 to 14 days among a cohort of infants with abdominal wall defects.[43] Importantly, preoperative antibiotic use is a notable contributor to antibiotic exposure in the NICU, particularly for infants with abdominal wall defects and congenital diaphragmatic hernias, despite low rates of infection in the early postnatal period among infants with these surgical conditions.[41–43]

Potential opportunities for antibiotic stewardship among neonates undergoing surgical procedures include withholding perioperative antibiotics for designated clean procedures,[44] standardizing and shortening courses of postoperative antibiotics,[43,45–47] and limiting preoperative antibiotics to infants with evidence of clinical illness or in whom another reason for antibiotic administration may exist.[41,42] There is no clear evidence that antibiotics need to be continued beyond 24 hours postoperatively, with 1 single-center, retrospective study finding no difference in the rates of SSI within 30 days of procedure, between neonates who received 24 hours or less of postoperative antibiotics versus those who received more than 24 hours of antibiotics after abdominal surgery.[47] A multidisciplinary effort at 1 hospital led to the creation of a standardized approach to perioperative antibiotics, including a single preoperative dose of piperacillin-tazobactam within 1 hour before the surgical incision and prompt discontinuation of antibiotics within 72 hours postoperatively.[46] Infants with perinatally recognized surgical conditions did not receive postnatal antibiotics unless there was evidence of or risk factors for infection, and empiric antibiotics were discontinued if cultures were negative at 48 hours. Compliance with perioperative and postnatal recommendations during the postintervention period was high, with a statistically significant decrease in antibiotic exposure. There was also a decrease in SSI rates within 30 days between the preintervention and postintervention periods. Another hospital included in their gastroschisis protocol a recommendation to discontinue antibiotics within 48 hours after the initial surgical intervention (either primary closure or silo placement), unless there was another clinical indication to continue antibiotic therapy.[45] Among all patients, the frequency of antibiotic discontinuation within 48 hours improved from 50% in the preintervention period to 76% in the postintervention period. Importantly, there were no documented infections among the cohort of infants whose antibiotics were discontinued within 48 hours of silo placement.

Diagnostic Stewardship

Diagnostic stewardship supports antibiotic stewardship efforts.[48,49] Diagnostic stewardship involves ordering the right test for the right patient at the right time, as well as interpreting the test result correctly.[48] Appropriate use and interpretation of infectious disease testing can enable clinicians to make accurate diagnoses and provide timely antibiotic therapy, while reducing antibiotic overuse and misuse.

Blood cultures are one of the most commonly obtained laboratory tests in the NICU. However, blood culture yield depends on obtaining an adequate volume of blood for a neonate's weight, the use of appropriate sterile technique to reduce contamination, and collection before the administration of antibiotics to optimize organism detection. In the NICU, the recommended volume for blood cultures is a minimum of 1 mL, which may be challenging in low birth weight infants. Clinicians should be aware that the positivity rate of blood cultures declines with decreasing blood volume, especially for low-burden bacteremia, which occurs frequently in patients with sepsis.[50,51] Inadequately low blood volumes are also associated with higher recovery rates of blood culture contaminants.[52] Blood cultures are the gold standard for diagnosing sepsis, but clinicians must ensure that appropriate volumes of blood are collected before antibiotic administration to optimize the usefulness of this diagnostic test.

Clinicians increasingly rely on biomarkers like CRP and procalcitonin (PCT) to aid in the diagnosis of neonatal sepsis, but studies are mixed regarding the accuracy of these tests to predict neonatal infection. A meta-analysis of 22 studies compared CRP performance with the gold standard of blood culture and found that CRP had a sensitivity of 62% and a specificity of 74% for detecting LOS. The authors concluded that CRP alone was not sufficient to detect LOS and would have missed 152 infections and erroneously diagnosed 156 patients with sepsis.[53] PCT is more specific than CRP for bacterial infection and can facilitate antibiotic de-escalation in adults and older children with pneumonia or sepsis.[54,55] In a multicenter, randomized controlled trial in Europe, neonates older than 34 weeks gestational age admitted with EOS were randomized to have PCT-guided antibiotic decision-making versus standard of care.[56] The study enrolled more than 1700 infants and found that the PCT group had a 10-hour decrease in antibiotic therapy compared with the standard of care group, with no difference in rates of reinfection or death. Notably, in the PCT arm, 25% of physicians did not adhere to the PCT protocol.[56] Thus, although the use of PCT may be a promising strategy to support early and safe antibiotic de-escalation in the NICU, coupling PCT testing with compliance measures may be needed to improve adherence with testing and treatment algorithms.

Syndromic, molecular diagnostics for simultaneous detection of viral and bacterial pathogens from respiratory and cerebrospinal fluid have become widely available and are quickly becoming the standard of care in many institutions. The clinical impact of syndromic multiplex polymerase chain reaction panels in the NICU has not been quantified and requires additional research. In a single-center prospective cohort study, NICU patients were evaluated weekly for viral respiratory tract infection from birth until hospital discharge by collecting nasal swabs for testing with the eSensor RVP (Genmark Dx, Carlsbad, CA).[57] Investigators found that 5 of 74 infants (7%) had detection of a respiratory virus that was presumed to be hospital acquired. In 2 additional single-center prospective cohort studies of infants admitted to the NICU for the evaluation of sepsis, molecular detection of a respiratory virus occurred in 8% and 6% of evaluations.[58,59] The use of molecular methods in these studies detected higher than anticipated prevalence of respiratory viral infections in the NICU, but whether routine use of these diagnostics will alter antibiotic management of high-risk infants warrants further study.

The usefulness of the multiplex meningitis/encephalitis panel (Biofire, Inc, Salt Lake City, UT) in the NICU is even less clear.[60] The multiplex meningitis/encephalitis panel, like other molecular approaches, has the potential to detect bacterial organisms that do not grow in culture owing to antibiotic pretreatment.[61] However, it may not add value over routine cerebrospinal fluid testing like bacterial culture and monoplex polymerase chain reaction for herpes simplex virus. Because most molecular diagnostics are highly sensitive and can often detect nonpathogenic organisms, they should be used only in infants with appropriate symptoms and a high pretest probability of true infection, with a specimen submitted for routine bacterial culture, and must always be interpreted within the clinical context. Future studies should evaluate the clinical impact and cost effectiveness of implementing molecular syndromic testing in the NICU.

IMPLEMENTATION

Suggested frameworks for the implementation of ASPs have been developed by the Centers for Disease Control and Prevention as well as the IDSA and the Society for Healthcare Epidemiology of America.[62,63] Of particular importance in the development of NICU-specific ASPs is the need for collaboration between multiple specialties, including neonatology, infectious diseases, and surgery, and several disciplines, including physician attendings, physician trainees, nurses, and pharmacists. The importance of input from physicians and pharmacists embedded in the NICU to help develop, prioritize, and deploy interventions cannot be overemphasized. Because the patterns and drivers of antibiotic use may be unit specific, buy-in and leadership support from NICU providers are essential to programmatic success.[64]

A variety of approaches have been used to steward antibiotics in the NICU. Although the use of preauthorization and prospective audit and feedback have been identified as priority interventions by the Centers for Disease Control and Prevention and the IDSA/Society for Healthcare Epidemiology of America, much of the published

Table 1	
Antibiotic stewardship targets in the NICU	
Target	**Strategies**
EOS	Use of a sepsis calculator to identify at-risk infants
	Use of biomarkers to decrease antibiotic duration
LOS	Develop clinical guidelines to standardize diagnosis and treatment
	Based on local epidemiology, consider empiric use of nafcillin/oxacillin, rather than vancomycin
	Prospective audit and feedback to identify opportunities for antibiotic optimization
	Use of antibiotic time outs to reevaluate empiric therapy and need for ongoing antibiotics
Culture-negative sepsis	Standardized approach to diagnosis, including appropriate blood culture volumes
	Standardized duration of therapy (eg, 5 d)
NEC	Develop protocols that decrease antibiotic exposure, and thereby the risk of NEC, whenever possible
	Establish institutional approach to antibiotic treatment and duration of therapy
	Avoid antibiotic regimens with redundant anaerobic activity
Perioperative prophylaxis	Avoid perioperative antibiotic prophylaxis for clean procedures
	Standardize and/or shorten postoperative antibiotic courses
	Limit preoperative antibiotic exposure for neonates with surgical conditions (eg, congenital diaphragmatic hernia)
Diagnostic stewardship	Obtain appropriate volume blood cultures
	Use biomarkers to improve the negative predictive value of sterile cultures and reduce antibiotic exposure

literature regarding NICU-specific stewardship has focused on the use of clinical practice guidelines, either as a stand-alone effort or as part of a multifaceted approach.[18–20,65–68] Prospective audits and feedback have also been shown to reduce antibiotic use in the NICU.[18,20,65,66,69,70] There are relatively little published data on the efficacy of preauthorization strategies in the NICU, although a few studies reported improved antibiotic susceptibility profiles following implementation of formulary restrictons.[71–73] Several interventions have leveraged the electronic health record to improve antibiotic use. For example, the addition of automatic stop dates to electronic orders has been shown to reduce unnecessarily prolonged empiric or condition-specific antibiotic courses.[12,67,71] Multicenter quality improvement initiatives, led by groups like the Vermont Oxford Network and the California Perinatal Quality Care Collaborative, have also been important in identifying and addressing opportunities for improved antibiotic use in the NICU.[74–76] Other strategies include the use of antibiotic time-outs,[20] improved diagnostics,[66] and provider education.[65,69]

SUMMARY

Antibiotic use is common in NICUs and there is increasing awareness that inappropriate antibiotic use in the neonatal population is associated with adverse outcomes. Common clinical syndromes in the NICU that represent opportunities for antibiotic stewardship include sepsis, NEC, and perioperative prophylaxis (**Table 1**). Strategies for the implementation of antibiotic stewardship in the NICU include diagnostic stewardship, guideline development, and prospective audit and feedback, and should be implemented with multidisciplinary collaboration. Areas for future research include prospective studies evaluating antibiotic exposure as a risk factor for NEC and other complications, clinical impact and cost effectiveness of implementing molecular syndromic testing in the NICU, and best practices around implementation of antibiotic stewardship in the NICU setting.

CLINICS CARE POINTS

- Neonatologists are encouraged to develop and implement antibiotic stewardship interventions in collaboration with surgeons, infectious disease specialists, pharmacists, nurses, and other NICU providers.

- NICUs with low rates of MRSA should consider the use of vancomycin-sparing regimens (eg, nafcillin/oxacillin + gentamicin) for the empiric treatment of neonates with LOS.

- For infants with suspected sepsis, consider limiting antibiotic durations to 5 days for those who clinically improve with negative cultures.

- The narrowest spectrum antibiotic regimen should be given for the shortest duration to minimize the risk of NEC.

- Infants with surgical conditions should receive antibiotics only if there is a clinical indication and perioperative antibiotic prophylaxis should be discontinued within 24 to 48 hours of most surgeries.

- NICUs are encouraged to develop policies and procedures that ensure blood cultures of adequate weight-based volume are appropriately and optimally collected.

- A variety of strategies have been used to improve antibiotic prescribing in the NICU, including guideline development and prospective audit and feedback. ASPs should work with members of the NICU team and infection preventionists to identify unit-specific, high-priority targets.

Best practices

What is the current practice for optimizing antibiotic use in the neonatal intensive care unit?

- Antibiotic use is common in the neonatal intensive care unit (NICU).
- NICU-specific antibiotic stewardship interventions have been shown to safely decrease unnecessary antibiotic use.
- Although not specific to the neonatal population, evidence-based guidelines for implementing an antibiotic stewardship program exist.
- Clinical practice guidelines, prospective audit and feedback, and preauthorization strategies have been shown to improve the quality of antibiotic prescribing in the NICU.

What changes in current practice are likely to improve outcomes?

- Development of multidisciplinary, NICU-specific antibiotic stewardship programs.
- Empiric antibiotic regimens should be based on local epidemiology and recommend the use of narrow spectrum agents whenever possible.
- In collaboration with surgeons, NICU-specific perioperative antibiotic prophylaxis guidelines should be developed to prevent unnecessarily prolonged or broad spectrum postoperative antibiotic courses.
- Review of diagnostic strategies, such as blood culture practices, to ensure the right test is ordered for the right patient at the right time and that the results are interpreted correctly.

Major Recommendations

- Given the density and variability of antibiotic prescribing in the NICU, the development of NICU-specific antibiotic stewardship targets and strategies is imperative.
- NICU antibiotic stewardship programs should be multidisciplinary and include stakeholders from the neonatology, infectious diseases, and surgery. Representation should be cross-disciplinary and include physicians, nurses, and pharmacists.
- Based on published experience, the development of clinical practice guidelines, use of prospective audit and feedback, and diagnostic stewardship strategies are potential approaches to the implementation of antibiotic stewardship in the NICU.

Summary Statement

- The appropriateness of antibiotic prescribing in the NICU can be improved with antibiotic and diagnostic stewardship interventions that target common neonatal syndromes, including sepsis, necrotizing enterocolitis, and surgical conditions.

Bibliographic Sources: Refs.[22,62,63,64,67]

DISCLOSURE

The authors have nothing to disclose.

REFERENCES

1. Krzyzaniak N, Pawlowska I, Bajorek B. Review of drug utilization patterns in NICUs worldwide. J Clin Pharm Ther 2016;41:612–20.
2. Grohskoph L, Huskins W, Sinkowitz-Cochran R, et al. Use of antimicrobial agents in United States neonatal and pediatric intensive care patients. Pediatr Infec Dis J 2005;24:766–73.
3. Dantuluri K, Griffith H, Thurm C, et al. Variability of antibiotic use in neonatal intensive care units in the United States. Washington, DC: In: 2019: Presented at ID-Week October 4, 2019.

4. Cotten CM, Taylor S, Stoll B, et al. Prolonged duration of initial empirical antibiotic treatment is associated with increased rates of necrotizing enterocolitis and death for extremely low birth weight infants. Pediatrics 2009;123(1):58–66.

5. Flannery DD, Ross RK, Mukhopadhyay S, et al. Temporal trends and center variation in early antibiotic use among premature infants. JAMA Netw Open 2018; 1(1):e180164.

6. Schulman J, Dimand R, Lee H, et al. Neonatal intensive care unit antibiotic use. Pediatrics 2015;135.

7. Schulman J, Profit J, Lee H, et al. Variations in neonatal antibiotic use. Pediatrics 2018;142:e20180115.

8. Ting J, Synnes A, Roberts A, et al. Association between antibiotic use and neonatal mortality and morbidities in very low-birth-weight infants without culture-proven sepsis or necrotizing enterocolitis. JAMA Ped 2016;170:1181–7.

9. Kuppala V, Meinzen-Derr J, Morrow A, et al. Prolonged initial empirical antibiotic treatment is associated with adverse outcomes in premature infants. J Pediatr 2011;159:720–5.

10. Cox LM, Yamanishi S, Sohn J, et al. Altering the intestinal microbiota during a critical developmental window has lasting metabolic consequences. Cell 2014; 158(4):705–21.

11. Olszak T, An D, Zeissig S, et al. Microbial exposure during early life has persistent effects on natural killer T cell function. Science 2012;336(6080):489–93.

12. Cantey JB, Wozniak PS, Pruszynski JE, et al. Reducing unnecessary antibiotic use in the neonatal intensive care unit (SCOUT): a prospective interrupted time-series study. Lancet Infect Dis 2016;16(10):1178–84.

13. Puopolo KM, Draper D, Wi S, et al. Estimating the probability of neonatal early-onset infection on the basis of maternal risk factors. Pediatrics 2011;128(5): e1155–63.

14. Escobar GJ, Puopolo KM, Wi S, et al. Stratification of risk of early-onset sepsis in newborns >/= 34 weeks' gestation. Pediatrics 2014;133(1):30–6.

15. Capin I, Hinds A, Vomero B, et al. Are early-onset sepsis evaluations and empiric antibiotics mandatory for all neonates admitted with respiratory distress? Am J Perinatol 2020.

16. Kuzniewicz MW, Puopolo KM, Fischer A, et al. A quantitative, risk-based approach to the management of neonatal early-onset sepsis. JAMA Pediatr 2017;171(4):365–71.

17. Achten NB, Klingenberg C, Benitz WE, et al. Association of use of the neonatal early-onset sepsis calculator with reduction in antibiotic therapy and safety: a systematic review and meta-analysis. JAMA Pediatr 2019;173(11):1032–40.

18. Nzegwu NI, Rychalsky MR, Nallu LA, et al. Implementation of an antimicrobial stewardship program in a neonatal intensive care unit. Infect Control Hosp Epidemiol 2017;38(10):1137–43.

19. Chiu CH, Michelow IC, Cronin J, et al. Effectiveness of a guideline to reduce vancomycin use in the neonatal intensive care unit. Pediatr Infect Dis J 2011;30(4): 273–8.

20. Hamdy RF, Bhattarai S, Basu SK, et al. Reducing vancomycin use in a level IV NICU. Pediatrics 2020;146(2):e20192963.

21. Mukhopadhyay S, Sengupta S, Puopolo KM. Challenges and opportunities for antibiotic stewardship among preterm infants. Arch Dis Child Fetal Neonatal Ed 2019;104(3):F327–32.

22. Zachariah P, Saiman L. Expanding antimicrobial stewardship strategies for the NICU: management of surgical site infections, perioperative prophylaxis, and culture negative sepsis. Semin Perinatol 2020;151327.
23. Wirtschafter DD, Padilla G, Suh O, et al. Antibiotic use for presumed neonatally acquired infections far exceeds that for central line-associated blood stream infections: an exploratory critique. J Perinatol 2011;31(8):514–8.
24. Nino DF, Sodhi CP, Hackam DJ. Necrotizing enterocolitis: new insights into pathogenesis and mechanisms. Nat Rev Gastroenterol Hepatol 2016;13(10):590–600.
25. Han SM, Hong CR, Knell J, et al. Trends in incidence and outcomes of necrotizing enterocolitis over the last 12years: a multicenter cohort analysis. J Pediatr Surg 2020;55(6):998–1001.
26. Alganabi M, Lee C, Bindi E, et al. Recent advances in understanding necrotizing enterocolitis. F1000Res 2019;8.
27. Quigley M, Embleton ND, McGuire W. Formula versus donor breast milk for feeding preterm or low birth weight infants. Cochrane Database Syst Rev 2019; 7:CD002971.
28. Weintraub AS, Ferrara L, Deluca L, et al. Antenatal antibiotic exposure in preterm infants with necrotizing enterocolitis. J Perinatol 2012;32(9):705–9.
29. Cotten CM. Modifiable risk factors in necrotizing enterocolitis. Clin Perinatol 2019; 46(1):129–43.
30. Greenberg RG, Chowdhury D, Hansen NI, et al. Prolonged duration of early antibiotic therapy in extremely premature infants. Pediatr Res 2019;85(7):994–1000.
31. Raba AA, O'Sullivan A, Semberova J, et al. Are antibiotics a risk factor for the development of necrotizing enterocolitis-case-control retrospective study. Eur J Pediatr 2019;178(6):923–8.
32. Berkhout DJC, Klaassen P, Niemarkt HJ, et al. Risk factors for necrotizing enterocolitis: a prospective multicenter case-control study. Neonatology 2018;114(3): 277–84.
33. Li Y, Shen RL, Ayede AI, et al. Early use of antibiotics is associated with a lower incidence of necrotizing enterocolitis in preterm, very low birth weight infants: the NEOMUNE-NeoNutriNet cohort study. J Pediatr 2020;227:128–34.e2.
34. Ellsbury DL, Clark RH, Ursprung R, et al. A multifaceted approach to improving outcomes in the NICU: the pediatrix 100 000 babies campaign. Pediatrics 2016;137(4):e20150389.
35. Makri V, Davies G, Cannell S, et al. Managing antibiotics wisely: a quality improvement programme in a tertiary neonatal unit in the UK. BMJ Open Qual 2018;7(2):e000285.
36. Blackwood BP, Hunter CJ, Grabowski J. Variability in antibiotic regimens for surgical necrotizing enterocolitis highlights the need for new guidelines. Surg Infect (Larchmt) 2017;18(2):215–20.
37. Murphy C, Nair J, Wrotniak B, et al. Antibiotic treatments and patient outcomes in necrotizing enterocolitis. Am J Perinatol 2020;37(12):1250–7.
38. Mazuski JE, Tessier JM, May AK, et al. The surgical infection society revised guidelines on the management of intra-abdominal infection. Surg Infect (Larchmt) 2017;18(1):1–76.
39. Solomkin JS, Mazuski JE, Bradley JS, et al. Diagnosis and management of complicated intra-abdominal infection in adults and children: guidelines by the Surgical Infection Society and the Infectious Diseases Society of America. Clin Infect Dis 2010;50(2):133–64.
40. Clements KE, Fisher M, Quaye K, et al. Surgical site infections in the NICU. J Pediatr Surg 2016;51(9):1405–8.

41. Keene S, Murthy K, Pallotto E, et al. Acquired infection and antimicrobial utilization during initial NICU hospitalization in infants with congenital diaphragmatic hernia. Pediatr Infect Dis J 2018;37(5):469–74.
42. Lusk LA, Brown EG, Overcash RT, et al. Multi-institutional practice patterns and outcomes in uncomplicated gastroschisis: a report from the University of California Fetal Consortium (UCfC). J Pediatr Surg 2014;49(12):1782–6.
43. Ravikumar C, Mitchell IC, Cantey JB. Antibiotic utilization and infection among infants with abdominal wall defects. Pediatr Infect Dis J 2020;39(12):1116–20.
44. Williams K, Lautz T, Hendrickson RJ, et al. Antibiotic prophylaxis for pyloromyotomy in children: an opportunity for better stewardship. World J Surg 2018;42(12): 4107–11.
45. Gilliam EA, Vu K, Rao P, et al. Minimizing variance in gastroschisis management leads to earlier full feeds in delayed closure. J Surg Res 2020;257:537–44.
46. Walker S, Datta A, Massoumi RL, et al. Antibiotic stewardship in the newborn surgical patient: a quality improvement project in the neonatal intensive care unit. Surgery 2017;162(6):1295–303.
47. Vu LT, Vittinghoff E, Nobuhara KK, et al. Surgical site infections in neonates and infants: is antibiotic prophylaxis needed for longer than 24 h? Pediatr Surg Int 2014;30(6):587–92.
48. Messacar K, Parker S, Todd J, et al. Implementation of rapid molecular infectious disease diagnostics: the role of diagnostic and antimicrobial stewardship. J Clin Microbiol 2017;55:715–23.
49. Patel R, Fang F. Diagnostic stewardship: opportunity for a laboratory-infectious diseases partnership. Clin Infect Dis 2018;67:799–801.
50. Dien Bard J, McElvania TeKippe E. Diagnosis of bloodstream infections in children. J Clin Microbiol 2016;54:1418–24.
51. Connell T, Rele M, Cowley D, et al. How reliable is a negative blood culture result? Volume of blood submitted for culture in routine practice in a children's hospital. Pediatrics 2007;119:891–6.
52. Kellogg J, Ferrentino F, Goodstein M, et al. Frequency of low-level bacteremia in infants from birth to two months of age. Pediatr Infec Dis J 1997;16:381–5.
53. Brown J, Meader N, Wright K, et al. Assessment of C-reactive protein diagnostic test accuracy for late-onset infection in newborn infants A systematic review and meta-analysis. JAMA Ped 2020;174:260–8.
54. Katz S, Crook J, Gillon J, et al. Use of a procalcitonin-guided antibiotic treatment algorithm in the pediatric intensive care unit. Pediatr Infec Dis J 2020;40(4): 333–7.
55. de Jong E, van Oers J, Beishuizen A, et al. Efficacy and safety of procalcitonin guidance in reducing the duration of antibiotic treatment in critically ill patients: a randomised, controlled, open-label trial. Lancet Infect Dis 2016;16:819–27.
56. Stocker M, van Herk W, El Helou S, et al. Procalcitonin-guided decision making for duration of antibiotic therapy in neonates with suspected early-onset sepsis: a multicentre, randomised controlled trial (NeoPIns). Lancet 2017;390:871–81.
57. Poole C, Camins B, Prichard M, et al. Hospital-acquired viral respiratory infections in neonates hospitalized since birth in a tertiary neonatal intensive care unit. J Perinatol 2019;39:683–9.
58. Cerone J, Santos R, Tristram D, et al. Incidence of respiratory viral infection in infants with respiratory symptoms evaluated for late-onset sepsis. J Perinatol 2017; 37:922–6.
59. Ronchi A, Michelow I, Chapin K, et al. Viral respiratory tract infections in the neonatal intensive care unit: the VIRIoN-I study. J Pediatr 2014;165:690–6.

60. Dantuluri K, Konvinse K, Crook J, et al. Human herpesvirus 6 detection during the evaluation of sepsis in infants using the FilmArray meningitis/encephalitis panel. J Pediatr 2020;223:204–6.e1.

61. Arora H, Asmar B, Salimnia H, et al. Enhanced identification of Group B Streptococcus and Escherichia coli in young infants with meningitis using the Biofire Filmarray Meningitis/Encephalitis panel. Pediatr Infec Dis J 2017;36:685–7.

62. CDC. Core Elements of hospital antibiotic stewardship programs. Atlanta, GA: US Department of Health and Human Services, CDC; 2019. Available at: https://www.cdc.gov/antibiotic-use/core-elements/hospital.html.

63. Barlam TF, Cosgrove SE, Abbo LM, et al. Implementing an antibiotic stewardship program: guidelines by the infectious diseases society of America and the society for Healthcare Epidemiology of America. Clin Infect Dis 2016;62(10):e51–77.

64. Cantey JB. Optimizing the use of antibacterial agents in the neonatal period. Paediatr Drugs 2016;18(2):109–22.

65. Lee KR, Bagga B, Arnold SR. Reduction of broad-spectrum antimicrobial use in a tertiary children's hospital post antimicrobial stewardship program guideline implementation. Pediatr Crit Care Med 2016;17(3):187–93.

66. Ting JY, Paquette V, Ng K, et al. Reduction of inappropriate antimicrobial prescriptions in a tertiary neonatal intensive care unit after antimicrobial stewardship care bundle implementation. Pediatr Infect Dis J 2019;38(1):54–9.

67. McPherson C, Liviskie C, Zeller B, et al. Antimicrobial stewardship in neonates: challenges and opportunities. Neonatal Netw 2018;37(2):116–23.

68. Karlowicz MG, Buescher ES, Surka AE. Fulminant late-onset sepsis in a neonatal intensive care unit, 1988-1997, and the impact of avoiding empiric vancomycin therapy. Pediatrics 2000;106(6):1387–90.

69. McCarthy KN, Hawke A, Dempsey EM. Antimicrobial stewardship in the neonatal unit reduces antibiotic exposure. Acta Paediatr 2018;107(10):1716–21.

70. Thampi N, Shah PS, Nelson S, et al. Prospective audit and feedback on antibiotic use in neonatal intensive care: a retrospective cohort study. BMC Pediatr 2019; 19(1):105.

71. Lu C, Liu Q, Yuan H, et al. Implementation of the smart use of antibiotics program to reduce unnecessary antibiotic use in a neonatal ICU: a prospective interrupted time-series study in a developing country. Crit Care Med 2019;47(1):e1–7.

72. Murki S, Jonnala S, Mohammed F, et al. Restriction of cephalosporins and control of extended spectrum beta-lactamase producing gram negative bacteria in a neonatal intensive care unit. Indian Pediatr 2010;47(9):785–8.

73. Calil R, Marba ST, von Nowakonski A, et al. Reduction in colonization and nosocomial infection by multiresistant bacteria in a neonatal unit after institution of educational measures and restriction in the use of cephalosporins. Am J Infect Control 2001;29(3):133–8.

74. Ho T, Buus-Frank ME, Edwards EM, et al. Adherence of newborn-specific antibiotic stewardship programs to CDC recommendations. Pediatrics 2018;142(6): e20174322.

75. Dukhovny D, Buus-Frank ME, Edwards EM, et al. A collaborative multicenter QI initiative to improve antibiotic stewardship in newborns. Pediatrics 2019;144(6): e20190589.

76. Schulman J, Benitz WE, Profit J, et al. Newborn antibiotic exposures and association with proven bloodstream infection. Pediatrics 2019;144(5):e20191105.

Immunization in the Neonatal Intensive Care Unit

Dustin D. Flannery, DO, MSCE[a,b], Kelly C. Wade, MD, PhD, MSCE[a,b],*

KEYWORDS

- Immunization • Vaccines • Vaccine-preventable diseases • Prematurity
- Neonatal intensive care unit

KEY POINTS

- Premature infants are at high risk for critical illness caused by vaccine-preventable diseases.
- Premature infants have adequate response to vaccines when offered at chronologic age, regardless of birth weight or gestational age, with the exception of the first dose of hepatitis B vaccine.
- Rotavirus vaccine is safe and effective in preterm infants and recent studies have not shown transmission of rotavirus vaccine virus strains among hospitalized patients.
- Vaccine education is critical for parents of infants hospitalized in the neonatal intensive care unit.
- Infants discharged from the neonatal intensive care unit with complete vaccination have higher rates of vaccination during childhood.

INTRODUCTION

Neonates are at high risk for infections, including vaccine-preventable diseases. Transfer of maternal antibodies during pregnancy, particularly in the third trimester, offers significant protection. Maternal vaccination is now routinely used as a strategy to protect newborns from influenza and pertussis. Premature infants are among the most vulnerable populations because they have decreased epithelial and mucosal defense mechanisms, immature innate and cellular immune responses, and reduced opportunities for maternal transfer of antibodies in third trimester. Slow pathogen recognition, lower cytokine and complement levels, and smaller pools of circulating white blood

Funding: Dr D.D. Flannery receives grant funding from the Agency for Healthcare Research and Quality (K08HS027468), the Children's Hospital of Philadelphia, and from 2 research contracts from the Centers for Disease Control and Prevention, all unrelated to the current article.
[a] Department of Pediatrics, Newborn care at Pennsylvania Hospital, 800 Spruce Street, Philadelphia, PA 19107, USA; [b] Division of Neonatology, Children's Hospital of Philadelphia, 3401 Civic Center Boulevard, Philadelphia, PA 19104, USA
* Corresponding author.
E-mail address: kelly.wade@pennmedicine.upenn.edu

cells all contribute to the increased risk of infections with viruses and bacteria.[1,2] In prospective studies, a history of prematurity is an independent risk factor for severe infections or infectious complications caused by vaccine-preventable infections such as pertussis, pneumococcus, and rotavirus (RV).[3–6]

Timely vaccination of premature infants at the same chronologic age as full-term infants, regardless of gestational age (GA) or birth weight (BW), confers important protection. The 1 exception to this chronologic-age rule is for hepatitis B virus (HBV) vaccination. Despite the immunogenicity of vaccination in premature infants, many remain inadequately vaccinated when discharged from the neonatal intensive care unit (NICU). Reasons for incomplete vaccination rates at NICU discharge are complex.

This article reviews critical advances in immunization strategies designed to protect neonates receiving ongoing hospital care in the NICU. This protection starts with maternal vaccination to optimize maternal antibody transfer to the fetus. It reviews vaccinations offered during the first months after birth and highlights considerations for infants receiving intensive care. It then explores special considerations for neonatal immunizations that contribute to incomplete vaccination rates at NICU discharge, including the core knowledge of proven immunogenicity in extremely premature infants, review of adverse event data, quality improvement strategies that promote vaccination, and communication strategies for vaccine hesitancy.

MATERNAL VACCINATION FOR NEWBORN PROTECTION

Maternal vaccination is an ideal strategy to provide early protection for newborns while protecting the pregnant and postpartum woman and fetus from serious disease. Opportunities for maternal vaccination occur before pregnancy, during pregnancy, and in the postpartum period (**Table 1**).

Prepregnancy

Vaccines received before pregnancy, including during childhood and adolescence, allow protection of the woman and fetus through transplacental transfer of maternal antibodies. Women of childbearing age should receive vaccines according to the Centers for Disease Control and Prevention (CDC) Advisory Committee on Immunization Practices (ACIP) immunization schedules, including a yearly seasonal influenza vaccine.[7] Accurate vaccine records can facilitate preconception and pregnancy vaccine counseling. Preconception determination of rubella immunity is ideal to allow measles-mumps-rubella (MMR) vaccine administration to prevent congenital rubella syndrome.[8] MMR is a live-virus vaccine; therefore, women should avoid becoming pregnant until 1 month after MMR vaccination because of theoretic risks to an exposed fetus.[7]

During Pregnancy

Recommendations regarding vaccination during pregnancy continue to evolve in light of understanding of the dynamics of transplacental antibody transfer, vaccine safety during pregnancy, and neonatal protection. At present, 2 vaccines are routinely recommended during every pregnancy: influenza and combined tetanus-diphtheria–acellular pertussis (Tdap).[9] These vaccines are safe when administered during pregnancy and are associated with a reduction in maternal infection-attributable illness, increased BW, decrease in premature birth, and reduction in fetal death and neonatal illness.[8,10]

Pregnant and postpartum women and newborns are at increased risk of severe influenza complications and attributable mortality. Influenza vaccine is recommended

Table 1
Highlights of vaccination practices in the neonatal intensive care unit

Vaccination Timepoint	Highlights
Maternal vaccination	• Influenza and Tdap vaccination are recommended during every pregnancy • Higher maternal antibody concentrations correlate with higher fetal titers and longer protection after birth • Transplacental antibody transfer increases in third trimester such that, at term, fetal antibody concentrations exceed those in the mother • Premature infants miss some of this transplacental transfer and are at higher risk of infection • Influenza vaccination protects mother and baby from severe influenza-related illness and hospitalization • Pertussis vaccination helps prevent pertussis-related illness and hospitalization in young infants, which can be fatal • Infants are not eligible for pertussis vaccination until 2 mo and influenza vaccination until 6 mo of age
Newborn HBV vaccine	• HBV vaccine is immunogenic and effective shortly after birth • Postexposure prophylaxis (HBV vaccine and HBIG) prevents >90% perinatal HBV infection • Nine out of 10 newborns with perinatal HBV infection develop chronic HBV infection and many develop chronic liver disease such as cirrhosis and liver cancer in early childhood • HBV vaccine prevents perinatal transmission as well as child-to-child and household transmission after the perinatal period • HBV vaccination schedule depends on infant BW and maternal HBsAg status • To achieve higher rate of seropositivity, premature infants (BW<2000 g) whose mothers are HBsAg negative can receive their first dose of HBV vaccine at 1 mo of age and then complete the 3-dose series
Infant immunization series (2-mo, 4-mo, and 6-mo vaccines: DTaP, IPV, Hib, PCV)	• Premature infants miss the essential in utero transfer of maternal antibody; therefore, these immunizations are critical • Vaccines are administered at chronologic age without regard to GA or BW (HBV is the exception) • Premature infants can respond effectively to vaccines • Vaccines are typically well tolerated in premature infants; adverse events may occur (apnea, fever, and decreased feedings) but are usually transient and self-limited • Vaccines should be discussed with parents and caregivers early in hospital course to allow time for education and answering their questions • Although diphtheria, tetanus, and polio are rare in developed countries, these vaccines also prevent more common infections such as pneumonia, pertussis, and meningitis
RV vaccine	• RV vaccine is the only live-attenuated virus recommended for young infants starting at 2 mo • Maximum age limits for the first and last dose of vaccine are designed to minimize the risk of intussusception • Vaccine is often administered to age-eligible infants at time of discharge from the NICU • Recent studies have not shown patient-to-patient transmission in the hospital setting

Abbreviations: DTaP, diphtheria, tetanus, acellular pertussis vaccine; HBIG, hepatitis B immune globulin; HBsAg, hepatitis B surface antigen; Hib, *Haemophilus influenzae* type b; IPV, inactivated poliovirus; PCV, pneumococcal conjugate vaccine; Tdap, tetanus, diphtheria, acellular pertussis vaccine.

during each pregnancy and the inactivated vaccine is preferred.[9] The timing of influenza vaccination during pregnancy to optimize maternal and newborn benefit is not well established; early vaccination may protect women from severe influenza, but later vaccination in the third trimester offers higher antibody transfer to fetus.[11] Current recommendations are for pregnant women to be prioritized for influenza vaccination during any stage of pregnancy.[9] Influenza vaccine during pregnancy has an estimated vaccine effectiveness of 40% against maternal influenza-associated hospitalization during pregnancy and 46% to 63% against confirmed influenza infection in infants born to immunized women.[12–14]

Pertussis booster vaccination, in the form of Tdap, is the second critical vaccination during each pregnancy. Pertussis (whooping cough) can cause severe respiratory infection in newborns, which may be fatal. A Tdap booster is recommended between the 27th and 36th week of gestation of every pregnancy in order to maximize third trimester transplacental antibody transfer to protect against pertussis in very young infants.[9] Tdap vaccine during pregnancy leads to a 78% to 90% decreased risk of pertussis infection in young infants, with an estimated vaccine effectiveness of 58% to 94% against pertussis-related infant hospitalization and 95% against pertussis-related infant death.[15,16]

Live vaccines are generally contraindicated during pregnancy because of the theoretic risk to the fetus.[9] Vaccines specifically contraindicated during pregnancy include MMR vaccine, live (intranasal) influenza vaccine, and varicella vaccine.[9] Human papilloma virus vaccine is not a live-virus vaccine but administration is not generally recommended during pregnancy. Yellow fever, oral typhoid fever, and Japanese encephalitis vaccines are also usually contraindicated unless travel to an endemic area is necessary and benefits are determined to outweigh risks.[9]

Postpregnancy

After delivery, administration of vaccines may be indicated for women who were found to be nonimmune in pregnancy. If influenza and/or Tdap vaccine were not administered during pregnancy, maternal administration in the immediate postpartum period is recommended to prevent newborn exposure. Most routine vaccines are safe for breastfeeding women and their newborns.[9] Postpartum vaccination is particularly recommended for women nonimmune to rubella or varicella. Live viruses in vaccines are usually not excreted in human milk and therefore breastfeeding is not a contraindication to MMR vaccination.[17] Notably, both smallpox and yellow fever vaccines are generally contraindicated during breastfeeding because of risk of neonatal transmission or associated acute neurotropic disease, unless travel to an endemic area is necessary and the benefit of receipt of vaccine outweighs the risk.[9]

Other Family/Household Members

In addition to pregnant and postpartum women, other household members and infant caretakers should ensure they have received all recommended vaccines, including pertussis and the yearly seasonal influenza vaccine, to decrease the risk of newborn exposure.[18] Influenza and pertussis are highly contagious and easily spread through respiratory droplets. Protection after influenza vaccine or Tdap booster typically takes at least 2 weeks; therefore, these vaccines are ideally administered at least 2 weeks before delivery or exposure to a newborn to ensure ample time for antibody production.[18] Some neonatal centers and pediatric offices offer these vaccines on site as an effective means of increasing vaccination rates of family members of this vulnerable population.[19–21] Health care workers are required to be vaccinated to protect their patients.

NEONATAL/INFANT VACCINATION

Vaccination of neonates and infants prevents serious infections (see **Table 1**). Most vaccines are administered by chronologic age, regardless of BW or GA. The exception to this rule is HBV vaccine, which is administered based on BW and maternal hepatitis B status. Controversy exists regarding the administration of live oral RV vaccine among infants who remain hospitalized, and recommendations are evolving.

Hepatitis B Virus

Without postexposure prophylaxis, the CDC estimates that 40% of infants born to mothers with HBV develop chronic HBV infection.[22] Transmission of HBV through bodily fluids most often occurs during delivery; in utero transmission is rare.[23] Nine out of 10 newborns with perinatal infection develop chronic HBV, which can lead to chronic liver disease such as cirrhosis and hepatocellular carcinoma as early as age 6 years.[23–25] Prevention of perinatal HBV relies on maternal screening for hepatitis B surface antigen (HBsAg) during each pregnancy and postexposure prophylaxis for eligible newborns.

Newborn hepatitis B virus vaccine

The first HBV vaccine was licensed in 1982, after the discovery that antibodies to HBsAg confer immunity, and was the first vaccine to prevent cancer.[24] HBV monovalent vaccine is considered the newborn vaccine because it is the only vaccine routinely recommended by the ACIP for newborns. This recommendation is endorsed by the American Academy of Pediatrics (AAP), American Academy of Family Physicians, and American College of Obstetricians and Gynecologists.[23,26,27] At present, the available HBV recombinant vaccines include a single-antigen formulation, which is recommended before 6 weeks of age, and in combination with other vaccines for administration after 6 weeks of age.

HBV vaccine is the only vaccine where BW is taken into account when determining timing of administration. For infants born to mothers who are HBsAg negative, those with BW greater than or equal to 2000 g who are medically stable receive HBV vaccine within 24 hours of birth, whereas those with BW less than 2000 g receive the vaccine at 1 month of age or before hospital discharge, whichever occurs first (**Table 2**). In 2017, the time frame changed to within 24 hours in an effort to prevent the ~1000 cases of perinatal HBV infection that still occur annually in the United States.[22,26,28] The BW cutoff of 2000 g serves as a surrogate marker for prematurity and the delay in vaccination allows for a higher seropositive response among premature infants (see **Table 2**).[27]

Postexposure prophylaxis to prevent perinatal hepatitis B virus infection

Prevention of perinatal HBV infection depends on screening women for HBV during every pregnancy and the administration of postexposure prophylaxis to their infants. If a pregnant woman is HBsAg positive, both HBV vaccine and hepatitis B immune globulin (HBIG) should be administered within 12 hours of birth regardless of BW; these infants require HBsAg and hepatitis B surface antibody testing at 9 to 12 months of age (see **Table 2**). If maternal HBsAg status is unknown at the time of birth, immediate management includes early HBV vaccination and expedited maternal testing; the timing of HBIG depends on infant BW and maternal test result (see **Table 2**). Administration of both hepatitis B vaccine and HBIG in the immediate newborn period prevents perinatal HBV transmission in more than 90% of infants; a randomized controlled trial of infants born to HBsAg-positive mothers found only 6% of treated infants became HBsAg positive versus 88% of infants who received neither vaccine nor

Table 2
Hepatitis B vaccination recommendations for newborns

Maternal HBsAg Status	Birth Weight	Recommendations[a]
HBsAg negative	≥2000 g	Administer vaccine within 24 h of birth (if medically stable)
	<2000 g	Administer vaccine at chronologic age 1 mo or hospital discharge if earlier
HBsAg positive	≥2000 g	Administer vaccine and HBIG within 12 h of birth[b]
	<2000 g	Administer vaccine and HBIG within 12 h of birth[b,c]
HBsAg unknown[d]	≥2000 g	Administer vaccine within 12 h and determine maternal HBsAg status within 7 d; administer HBIG if she is positive or remains unknown by 7 d
	<2000 g	Administer vaccine and HBIG within 12 h of birth[c]

[a] Use monovalent HBV vaccine for doses administered before age 6 weeks; combination vaccine products are not recommended before 6 weeks.
[b] Test infant for HBsAg and hepatitis B surface antibody at age 9 to 12 months. If HBV series is delayed, test 1 to 2 months after final dose.
[c] Administer 3 additional doses of vaccine (total of 4 doses) beginning at age 1 month.
[d] Determine maternal HBsAg status as soon as possible.
   Adapted from Recommended Child and Adolescent Immunization Schedule for ages 18 years or younger, United States, 2021. Centers for Disease Control. Available at: https://www.cdc.gov/vaccines/schedules/hcp/imz/child-adolescent.html. Accessed April 13, 2021.

HBIG.[23,29] The HBV vaccine alone is 75% effective against perinatally acquired infection.[23,24] Because the effectiveness of immunoprophylaxis is directly related to the duration of time between perinatal virus exposure and administration of vaccine and HBIG, it is imperative that immunoprophylaxis is administered in an expedited fashion (see **Table 2**).[23] Vaccine response does not vary appreciably with concomitant HBIG administration.[22]

Hepatitis B virus vaccination series during infancy
The routine HBV vaccination series includes 3 doses at 0, 1 to 2, and 6 months.[27] If an infant did not receive the newborn dose within 24 hours, then the first dose is still recommended to be administered as soon as feasible. The minimum interval between doses 1 and 2 is 4 weeks. Infants born weighing less than 2000 g who receive a vaccine before 24 hours of age may not have an adequate immune response and should therefore receive a vaccine at 1 month of age and continue the series for a total of 4 immunizations (see **Table 2**). The minimum age for the final dose (third or fourth depending on scenario) is 24 weeks of age, and the minimum intervals between doses are 4 weeks for dose 1 to 2, 8 weeks for dose 2 to 3 or 4, and 16 weeks between dose 1 and 3 or 4.[27] Up to 95% of infants develop protective antibodies after completing a 3-dose series.[23,24] Although 3 doses are recommended for most newborns, administration of 4 doses may occur when combination vaccines are used beyond the newborn period.

Priority and impact of hepatitis B virus vaccination
A 68% decrease in HBV infection prevalence among children was observed within 10 years of initiation of universal HBV vaccination in the United States in 1991.[30] In a population-based Thai study, the age-standardized rates for childhood liver cancer for vaccinated versus nonvaccinated children aged 5 years and older were significantly lower at 0.24 and 0.95 per million, respectively.[31] Although the HBV vaccine prevents chronic infection and cancer, there is a long delay between newborn intervention and future prevention of chronic HBV, which can lead to a perception of low priority for early vaccination.[24,32] The strategy of universal early vaccination within

24 hours is designed to further decrease perinatal transmission, which can occur in infants born to women with unknown, undocumented, or a change in HBV status during pregnancy. In addition, the birth dose of vaccine also provides early protection against child-to-child or household transmission after the perinatal period.[22–24] The alternative strategy of selective vaccination only for infants born to infected women is not currently recommended in the United States because most newborns would remain unprotected during early infancy and therefore would be at increased risk of infection and subsequent severe, chronic liver disease and malignancy, even in low-prevalence regions.[24,32]

Diphtheria, Tetanus, Pertussis, Haemophilus influenzae Type b, Pneumococcus, and Poliovirus

Administration by chronologic age

The 2-month, 4-month, and 6-month infant vaccination series, including diphtheria, tetanus, and acellular pertussis (DTaP); *Haemophilus influenzae* type b (Hib); pneumococcal conjugate (PCV13); and inactivated poliovirus (IPV) vaccines, are recommended at chronologic age regardless of prematurity or BW (see **Table 1**). These vaccines are commonly administered to infants who remain in the NICU for 2 months or longer; HBV and RV vaccines are discussed separately. Premature infants are particularly vulnerable to vaccine-preventable diseases such as pertussis, pneumonia, and meningitis, but have adequate immune responses when vaccinated at 2 months' chronologic age and beyond. Therefore, the ACIP recommends that premature infants receive the standard vaccination schedule according to chronologic age, regardless of BW and GA, with the exception of HBV vaccine.[27] Therefore, infants born at 23 weeks' GA generally follow the same schedule, based on chronologic age, as a full-term infants. Premature infants do not typically require additional doses of vaccines.

Vaccine timing and catch-up

The ACIP provides a yearly update regarding immunization practices and recommended schedules.[27] This guidance also discusses minimum age, minimal interval between doses, and specifically addresses catch-up schedules for incompletely immunized infants and children. The minimum age for DTaP, Hib, PCV13, and IPV vaccines is 6 weeks.[27] In most circumstances, a 4-week interval is sufficient between vaccine doses for catch-up immunizations. Booster vaccines are recommended at older ages to ensure seroprotection and promote longer-lasting immunity. At 6 months of age, infants can receive their first influenza vaccine. At 12 to 15 months, additional doses of DTaP, Hib, and PCV13 vaccines are recommended along with initiation of vaccines for MMR, varicella, and hepatitis A.[33]

Combination vaccines

Combination vaccines decrease the need for multiple inoculations by combining multiple antigens. The safety and efficacy of combination vaccines are evaluated in randomized controlled trials compared with individual vaccine components.[34] Combination vaccines are equally immunogenic and have similar side effect profiles. Various brands of combination vaccines exist and, although they are interchangeable for the purposes of HBV protection, the overall interchangeability of acellular pertussis-containing combination vaccines has yet to be determined.[23] In the largest retrospective study available (N = 14,000 premature infants), combination vaccines were not associated with an increase in postvaccination sepsis evaluations or escalation in respiratory support.[35]

Rotavirus Vaccine

RV is a leading cause of severe gastroenteritis in infants worldwide. Two live-attenuated RV oral vaccines were US Food and Drug Administration (FDA) approved from 2006 to 2008. RV1[36] is a monovalent, live-attenuated human virus oral vaccine that provides immunity using a 2-dose regimen at 2 and 4 months, including safety and efficacy in infants as young as 27 weeks' GA.[37] RV5[38] is a pentavalent live-attenuated, human-bovine reassortant vaccine that provides immunity using a 3-dose regimen at 2, 4, and 6 months, including safety and efficacy in infants as young as 25 weeks' GA. Administration of either vaccine begins at 6 to 8 weeks of age, with subsequent doses at least 4 weeks apart. Since implementation of RV vaccination, sustained reductions of 50% to 90% in RV-associated gastroenteritis hospitalization have been shown in the United States and Europe compared with the prevaccine era.[39,40] Unvaccinated young infants less than 42 days of age have also experienced sustained reduction in RV-associated hospitalizations, presumably through herd protection.[41] Despite this success, questions remain regarding the risk of intussusception and how to improve low rates of vaccination among hospitalized very premature infants given the theoretic risk of in-hospital transmission.

Age of administration and intussusception

Initial vaccination at a young age, ideally 6 to 12 weeks, offers early protection against severe RV gastroenteritis, when the risk of intussusception is lowest. RV vaccination is the only immunization licensed with maximum age limits for administration. The maximum age of the first dose is up to 14 weeks 6 days (104 days) and the maximum age of the final dose varies from 24 weeks (RV1) to 32 weeks of age (RV5).[27] These age limits attempt to minimize the risk of intussusception, a rare but serious condition that has been associated with many viral infections. Among infants less than 36 months of age, the incidence of intussusception is estimated to be 22 to 33 per 100,000 person-years, with a peak around 5 to 8 months of age.[42–44] The first RV vaccine (RRV-TV Rotashield) was withdrawn from the market in 1999 for an increased attributable risk of intussusception, estimated to occur in 1 in 10,000 vaccinated infants. Risk is highest after the first dose and when the first dose is administered after 90 days of age.[45] At present, the licensed vaccines, RV1 and RV5, have no increased risk for intussusception in large placebo-controlled trials.[46–48] However, postmarketing studies using large databases continue to show a small increased risk, with an estimated 1 to 6 additional cases per 100,000 vaccinated infants.[49] The small increased rate after the first dose may be mitigated by lower intussusception rate within the first year of age.[50] There does not seem to be an increased risk of intussusception when the first dose is administered at less than 90 days of age.[51] The benefit of reduced severe RV gastroenteritis-associated hospitalizations vastly outweighs the small risk of intussusception.

Importance of rotavirus vaccine for premature infants

RV vaccination is recommended for premature infants whose risk of severe viral gastroenteritis is greater than that of full-term infants.[27,51] Overall safety and efficacy are similar in premature infants compared with term infants when vaccination occurs at chronologic age with the first dose administered at 6 to 12 weeks (maximum age 14 weeks 6 days).[37] Immunization is associated with a greater than 90% decrease in RV-associated hospitalizations in normal-BW, low-BW, and very-low-BW infants alike.[52] Seroconversion has been shown in a small number of vaccinated premature infants with a history of bowel resection, including those with intestinal failure.[53,54] Although the oral route is preferred, the vaccine can be administered through a nasogastric feeding tube followed by administration of a small volume of liquid.

A challenge to the age-limited licensing of RV vaccines in hospitalized infants is the theoretic risk of patient-to-patient transmission of the live, but attenuated, RV vaccine virus. The ACIP recommends age-eligible RV vaccination at the time of hospital discharge.[55] However, without in-hospital administration, infants hospitalized beyond 104 days of age would become age ineligible. In a large American NICU, 63% of very-low-BW infants did not receive the RV vaccine at discharge, primarily because of age ineligibility.[56] These unvaccinated and often medically fragile infants remain at risk for complications of native RV infections; in 2017, an RV outbreak in a subacute pediatric care facility affected nearly all residents, most of whom were unvaccinated or incompletely vaccinated, and led to 1 death.[57] This report highlights the importance of in-hospital RV vaccination among infants with prolonged hospitalizations.[58]

Rotavirus vaccine shedding and viral transmission

Following both RV1 and RV5 administration, shedding of attenuated virus may be detected in the stools of recipient infants, with higher rates following RV1 than RV5.[36,38,59] Following RV1 administration, a placebo-controlled trial in twin pairs detected in-home transmission in 18% (15 out of 80 twin pairs), of whom none of the placebo recipients were symptomatic and 4 placebo recipients showed seroconversion.[60] With RV5, shedding and risk of horizontal transmission are complicated by the finding of reassortment among pentavalent vaccine strains.[61] Such reassortant RV strains could be associated with changes in virulence and diarrheal illness. There is 1 case report of transmission of a vaccine-derived double-reassortant strain to an older, unvaccinated sibling who developed gastroenteritis and required emergency department care.[62] Overall, transmission of the vaccine-derived attenuated virus to contacts is rare.

Consideration for in-hospital administration

To avoid missed opportunities for immunization in high-risk neonates, in-hospital administration should be considered (**Table 3**). Observational studies show tolerance of vaccination among NICU recipients without an increase in health care–associated transmission of RV-associated gastroenteritis.[63,64] Two hospital-based studies both found no evidence for transmission of RV to nearby unvaccinated infants using polymerase chain reaction–based detection of RV in stool samples.[65,66] In 1 study of 1192 stool samples, RV was detected in 13 samples (1.1%), 12 vaccine strains from vaccinated infants, and 1 native RV from an unvaccinated infant. Infection prevention practices such as hand hygiene and the use of gloves to handle biologically contaminated items effectively reduces opportunities for transmission.

Based on the high risk of RV gastroenteritis in premature infants and the low risk of in-hospital transmission, recommendations for RV vaccination in hospitalized infants are being reevaluated (see **Table 3**). Age-directed vaccination offers early protection against native RV-associated gastroenteritis, minimizes the risk of intussusception, and prevents infants from becoming age ineligible for RV immunization. These recommendations have been endorsed by advisory committees and pediatric infectious disease societies from several countries.

SPECIAL CONSIDERATIONS FOR IMMUNIZATIONS IN THE NEONATAL INTENSIVE CARE UNIT

Vaccines Are Immunogenic in Premature Infants

Studies evaluating the immune response of premature infants, from 24 weeks' GA and older, support vaccination at chronologic age, with the exception of HBV vaccine, which is commonly deferred from birth to 1 month of age to allow greater

Table 3	
In-hospital rotavirus vaccination: benefits, risks, and potential strategies	
Benefits	• Emphasizes the risk of severe RV gastroenteritis in unvaccinated age-eligible infants • Premature infants at higher risk of severe RV gastroenteritis and hospitalization • Younger age of first dose is associated with lower risk of intussusception • Recent studies document no in-hospital transmission with usual infection control practices • Transmission of attenuated vaccine strain, if it occurs, is more likely to result in asymptomatic immunity with seroconversion
Risks	• Theoretic risk of inadvertent, in-hospital transmission to critically ill or immunocompromised patients • Infants who remain hospitalized beyond 104 d of age become age ineligible and remain at risk for native RV infection
Vaccine strategies for age-eligible infants who remain hospitalized at ≥2 mo of age	• Administer at hospital discharge acknowledging that infants who remain hospitalized beyond 104 d of age are ineligible for vaccination and remain at risk for RV infection throughout childhood • Administer with routine 2-mo immunizations to provide early protection, decrease risk of intussusception, and promote timely vaccinations. Transmission risk is minimal and attenuated virus has minimal clinical impact. RV outbreaks among unvaccinated children have been associated with severe illness and even death

seroconversion. Their antibody response to initial doses is often lower than in term infants, but protective concentrations are typically achieved and memory is induced. Using the typical 2-month, 4-month, and 6-month CDC schedule, similar proportions of very premature (<29 weeks' GA and <1000 g) and term vaccinated infants reach protective antibody levels for Hib, pertussis, and polio.[67–70] In a recent review of 10 clinical studies, hexavalent combined DTaP, HBV, IPV, and Hib conjugate vaccine administered to 414 premature infants as young as 24 weeks' GA led to 92% seropositivity to all vaccine antigens after completion of the 3-dose primary vaccination series.[71] GA and BW were associated with lower magnitudes of initial antibody responses and geometric mean titers, although seropositivity greater than a protective cutoff was similar among very preterm and more mature infants. Booster vaccination of very premature infants induced a marked increase in titers, suggesting an effective initial response. Safety and efficacy of RV immunization has been shown in age-appropriate vaccinated premature infants at 25 weeks' GA.[5,37,72]

Immunodeficiency, Corticosteroid Exposure, and Critical Illness

The 2013 Infectious Disease Society of America, CDC, and AAP joint statement outlines vaccination recommendations for people with specific immunocompromised conditions, including both primary immunodeficiencies, such as severe combined immunodeficiency, and secondary immunocompromising conditions related to chemotherapy, immunosuppression after organ transplant, and corticosteroid exposure.[73] With regard to corticosteroids, high-level immunosuppression is assumed in patients exposed to high-dose prolonged therapy, defined as more than 2 mg/kg/d for more than 14 days.

Extremely premature infants often receive corticosteroids for adrenal insufficiency or evolving chronic lung disease. The impact of prior or concurrent corticosteroids on vaccine response has not been fully evaluated. In small case series, dexamethasone-exposed very premature infants had reduced antibody titers after vaccination with DTaP and Hib; however, protective antibody titers for diphtheria and tetanus toxoid were still achieved after a 3-dose series.[74,75] The most common corticosteroid exposures, physiologic replacement of hydrocortisone, or a 10-day course of dexamethasone does not typically meet the definition for high-level immunosuppression. In general, immunizations are still able to elicit response after a short course of low-potency to medium-potency corticosteroids.

Immunizations may be delayed in infants with critical illness, such as infants requiring cardiopulmonary bypass or extracorporeal membrane oxygenation. Intramuscular injections are often avoided in those with poor perfusion, such as infants treated with therapeutic hypothermia. These infants can be vaccinated as soon as they recover. There are no exceptions for administration of HBV vaccine to infants born to HBsAg-positive women, because hepatitis B vaccine optimally prevents transmission in this high-risk situation.

Safety and Tolerability in Premature Infants

The vaccine safety profiles of the newborn and infant immunization series are excellent. Common side effects include redness or pain at the injection site and increased temperature, which are expected given the immunogenic nature of vaccines. The risk of anaphylaxis is exceedingly low, particularly for newborns and infants, occurring in 1 in more than 1 million vaccinated patients overall.[76] There is no evidence of associations between infant vaccines and infection, autoimmune disease, malignancy, neurologic disease, autism, or sudden infant death syndrome.[23,77–79]

In premature infants, it is difficult to distinguish adverse events intrinsic to prematurity from a vaccine-related adverse event. During their NICU hospitalizations, very premature infants frequently have periods of clinical instability that manifest as inadequate thermoregulation, inconsistent oral feeding tolerance, and apneic and bradycardic events. When very premature infants approach 2 months of age, they are often weaning from their respiratory support and discontinuing stabilizing medications such as caffeine or diuretics. Uncontrolled studies document varying rates of postvaccination adverse events, but these studies cannot assess causation.

In uncontrolled studies, transient, postvaccination cardiorespiratory events occur in 10% to 20% of premature infants and a smaller number require increased respiratory support.[71,80] In 1 large retrospective study of 497 preterm infants, apnea occurred in 5% of infants in the 24-hours before vaccination and 13% in the 48-hours after vaccination.[80] Preexisting apnea was the strongest risk factor for postvaccination events. In a prospective, observational study of 239 premature infants in the NICU, 16% had cardiorespiratory events within 48-hours of vaccination.[81] Another study showed an increased incidence of sepsis evaluations (although not confirmed infections) and increased respiratory support after routine immunization, particularly among the most premature infants (ie, those born at 23–24 weeks' gestation) who were immunized at a younger corrected age when cardiopulmonary events and changes in respiratory support may be attributed to prematurity.[35] The occurrence of events is similar among infants receiving individual vaccines (DTaP, IPV, PCV13, Hib) or combination vaccines.[35,81] It is important to remember that these events are infrequent, typically transient, and can be managed with ongoing medical support present in the NICU setting.

Importantly, there is 1 multicenter, randomized controlled trial that assessed cardiopulmonary events after vaccination with DTaP in 191 infants born at mean GA of

27 weeks, BW 900 g, many of whom had chronic lung disease and history of intraventricular hemorrhage.[82] Event frequency and severity were determined by physiologic recordings of cardiopulmonary events 48 hours before and after either vaccination (treatment group) or control phase (control group, who were subsequently immunized after the control phase ended). In this study, 16% of infants receiving DTaP had at least 1 prolonged apnea event compared with 20% of control infants. At least 1 prolonged bradycardic event occurred in most infants: 58% of immunized and 56% of control infants. The frequency of episodes was not different between groups, with an average of 0.5 episodes of apnea and 2.6 episodes of bradycardia.[82] There was no difference in apnea, bradycardia, or severe events in the 48 hours after vaccination in premature infants (mean GA, 26.9 weeks) who received DTaP at mean age of 57 days compared with a control group of comparable premature infants who were not vaccinated.[82]

Improving Vaccination Rates in the Neonatal Intensive Care Unit

Despite the risk of vaccine-preventable diseases and the established immunogenicity and effectiveness of vaccines in premature infants, many are undervaccinated at the time of NICU discharge, with this status persisting into early childhood.[83,84] Significant variation in immunization practices has also been reported across NICUs.[85]

Factors contributing to delayed vaccination

Various factors contribute to delayed vaccination and undervaccination in the NICU; the most common is concern for adverse events,[86] followed by liability issues, and limited understanding of vaccine efficacy and safety.[84] Both parents and clinicians may be hesitant to administer vaccines to premature infants who are either clinically unstable or were previously unstable and now recovered. Although premature infants have higher rates of fever and cardiopulmonary events postvaccination compared with term infants, most do not experience events or clinical changes, and, if they do, they are usually transient and mild. An understanding of the efficacy, safety, and potential adverse effects of neonatal immunization may (1) inform discussions with parents to manage expectations, (2) provide reassurance to both parents and clinicians, and (3) guide management for postimmunization changes in clinical status. Delaying immunizations contributes to an increased risk of morbidity and mortality from vaccine-preventable diseases. Providing vaccine education in the NICU and discharging infants who have received age-appropriate vaccinations promotes immunization compliance through early childhood.

Talking to families/caregivers in the neonatal intensive care unit about vaccines

The NICU can be a stressful place for families and caregivers. Early presentation of the safety and efficacy of vaccines as a neonate approaches age eligibility facilitates ongoing discussion. Neonatal team members should align information and make time to have open, honest, and informative discussions with caregivers about vaccines. Emphasizing the shared goal of optimal outcomes for the infant may open the discussion.[87] Caregiver concerns should be validated and education and reassurance should be provided for each concern,[87] recognizing the sincerity of questions from family members as involvement in their infant's care.

Strategies to improve neonatal intensive care unit vaccination rates

Quality improvement initiatives have shown success in increasing immunization rates in NICUs, particularly in tertiary and quaternary units that care for infants with prolonged hospitalizations (**Table 4**).[83,90] Strategies used include evidence-based education for both physicians and nurses; multidisciplinary involvement; and electronic

Table 4
Strategies to improve neonatal intensive care unit vaccination rates

Authors	Setting	Strategies	Outcome Definition	Preintervention Vaccination Rate and Definition	Postintervention Vaccination Rate
Stetson et al,[83] 2019	26-bed level IV NICU	• Quality checklist for tracking immunization status and notifying providers when due • Readily accessible resource on immunization schedule • Intranet resource on communication method for vaccine hesitancy	Fully immunized rate at the time of NICU discharge or transfer	56% (419 out of 754)	94% (145 out of 155)
Cuna and Winter[88] 2017	120-bed level IV NICU	• Evidence-based education (didactic lectures, informational posters, emails, staff meetings) • Timely feedback (posters and emails with data on vaccination rate) • Recall system using electronic medical record (mandatory section for physicians to document vaccinations with monthly chart reviews and email reminders to ensure completion) • Standardized protocol for informed consent	Rate of medically eligible infants who received vaccinations within 2 wk of the recommended schedule	36% (26 out of 72)	82% (63 out of 77)
Ernst[89] 2017	Level IV NICU (bec # not reported); focused on infants born <2 kg who remained hospitalized until at least 58 d of age	• Electronic alert developed to remind doctors and nurses immunizations due	Rate of infants who received scheduled 2-mo immunizations (RV not included) by day 90 or discharge if sooner	71% (86 out of 121)	94% (132 out of 140)

(continued on next page)

Table 4
(continued)

Authors	Setting	Strategies	Outcome Definition	Preintervention Vaccination Rate and Definition	Postintervention Vaccination Rate
Milet et al,[90] 2018	98-bed level IV NICU; focused on premature infants with chronic lung disease	• Inpatient immunization record review • Email reminder when vaccines due • Weekly multidisciplinary eligibility discussion • Updated rounding tool	Rate of admitted patients who were immunized within 14-d from the due date	44% (numbers not reported)	75% (numbers not reported)
Schniepp, Cassidy, and Godfrey[91] 2019	18-bed pediatric cardiac care unit; focused on infants with congenital heart disease	• Education programs for staff nurses and medical providers	Rate of infants with immunizations up to date at discharge	60% (12 out of 33)	88% (7 out of 21)

medical record reminders, alerts, and resource access (see **Table 4**). Importantly, initiation of vaccination for premature infants in the NICU setting is associated with compliance with future immunization recommendations during early childhood.[92]

SUMMARY

Optimizing maternal, caregiver, and neonatal vaccination is of paramount importance to prevent vaccine-preventable diseases in young infants. The decision to administer a vaccine is based on balancing the risk of developing severe vaccine-preventable disease from the native pathogen or, rarely, a vaccine adverse effect. Vaccine-preventable diseases, serious bacterial infections, such as pneumonia, meningitis, and pertussis; and viral gastroenteritis remain relevant even in resource-advantaged communities. Premature infants, particularly those born before 32 weeks, remain especially vulnerable to serious disease. Quality improvement efforts can help to ensure that infants receive age-appropriate vaccinations during their NICU hospitalizations.

DISCLOSURE

All authors report there are no commercial or financial conflicts of interest to disclose.

REFERENCES

1. Baxter D. Impaired functioning of immune defences to infection in premature and term infants and their implications for vaccination. Hum Vaccin 2010;6(6): 494–505.
2. Baxter D. Vaccine responsiveness in premature infants. Hum Vaccin 2010;6(6): 506–11.
3. Marshall H, Clarke M, Rasiah K, et al. Predictors of disease severity in children hospitalized for pertussis during an epidemic. Pediatr Infect Dis J 2015;34(4): 339–45.
4. Ford-Jones EL, Wang E, Petric M, et al. Hospitalization for community-acquired, rotavirus-associated diarrhea: a prospective, longitudinal, population-based study during the seasonal outbreak. Arch Pediatr Adolesc Med 2000;154(6): 578–85.
5. Goveia MG, Rodriguez ZM, Dallas MJ, et al. Safety and efficacy of the pentavalent human-bovine (WC3) reassortant rotavirus vaccine in healthy premature infants. Pediatr Infect Dis J 2007;26(12):1099–104.
6. Kent A, Makwana A, Sheppard CL, et al. Invasive pneumococcal disease in UK children <1 Year of age in the post–13-valent pneumococcal conjugate vaccine era: what are the risks now? Clin Infect Dis 2019;69(1):84–90.
7. Vaccines before pregnancy. CDC. Available at: https://www.cdc.gov/vaccines/pregnancy/vacc-before.html. Accessed December 8, 2020.
8. Swamy GK, Heine RP. Vaccinations for pregnant women. Obstet Gynecol 2015; 125(1):212–26.
9. Vaccines During and after pregnancy | CDC. Available at: https://www.cdc.gov/vaccines/pregnancy/vacc-during-after.html. Accessed December 8, 2020.
10. Getahun D, Fassett MJ, Peltier MR, et al. Association between seasonal influenza vaccination with pre- and postnatal outcomes. Vaccine 2019;37(13):1785–91.
11. Cuningham W, Geard N, Fielding JE, et al. Optimal timing of influenza vaccine during pregnancy: a systematic review and meta-analysis. Influenza Other Respi Viruses 2019;13(5):438–52.

12. Thompson MG, Kwong JC, Regan AK, et al. Influenza vaccine effectiveness in preventing influenza-associated hospitalizations during pregnancy: a multi-country retrospective test negative design study, 2010–2016. Clin Infect Dis 2019;68(9):1444–53.

13. Zaman K, Roy E, Arifeen SE, et al. Effectiveness of maternal influenza immunization in mothers and infants. N Engl J Med 2008;359(15):1555–64.

14. Madhi SA, Cutland CL, Kuwanda L, et al. Influenza vaccination of pregnant women and protection of their infants. N Engl J Med 2014;371(10):918–31.

15. Skoff TH, Blain AE, Watt J, et al. Impact of the US maternal tetanus, diphtheria, and acellular pertussis vaccination program on preventing pertussis in infants <2 months of age: a case-control evaluation. Clin Infect Dis 2017;65(12): 1977–83.

16. Switzer C, D'Heilly C, Macina D. Immunological and clinical benefits of maternal immunization against pertussis: a systematic review. Infect Dis Ther 2019;8(4): 499–541.

17. Vaccinations | breastfeeding | CDC. Available at: https://www.cdc.gov/breastfeeding/breastfeeding-special-circumstances/vaccinations-medications-drugs/vaccinations.html. Accessed December 28, 2020.

18. Vaccines for family and caregivers | CDC. Available at: https://www.cdc.gov/vaccines/pregnancy/family-caregivers.html. Accessed December 9, 2020.

19. Jacobs K, Posa M, Spellicy W, et al. Adult caregiver influenza vaccination through administration in pediatric outpatient clinics: a cocooning healthcare improvement project. Pediatr Infect Dis J 2018;37(9):939–42.

20. Shah SI, Caprio M, Hendricks-Munoz K. Administration of inactivated trivalent influenza vaccine to parents of high-risk infants in the neonatal intensive care unit. Pediatrics 2007;120(3).

21. Shah S, Caprio M, Mally P, et al. Rationale for the administration of acellular pertussis vaccine to parents of infants in the neonatal intensive care unit. J Perinatol 2007;27(1):1–3.

22. Schillie S, Vellozzi C, Reingold A, et al. Prevention of hepatitis B virus infection in the United States: recommendations of the advisory committee on immunization practices. MMWR Recomm Rep 2018;67(1):1–31.

23. Hepatitis B | Red Book® 2018 | red book online | AAP point-of-care-Solutions. Available at: https://redbook.solutions.aap.org/chapter.aspx?sectionid=189640104&bookid=2205. Accessed November 24, 2020.

24. Mansoor OD, Salama P. Should hepatitis B vaccine be used for infants? Expert Rev Vaccin 2007;6(1):29–33.

25. Edmunds WJ, Medley GF, Nokes DJ, et al. The influence of age on the development of the hepatitis B carrier state. Proc R Soc B Biol Sci 1993;253(1337): 197–201.

26. Fitzgerald B, Kenzie WR Mac, Rasmussen SA, et al. Morbidity and mortality weekly report prevention of hepatitis B virus infection in the United States: recommendations of the advisory committee on immunization practices recommendations and reports centers for disease control and prevention MMWR Recomm Rep 2018;67(1):1-31. Available at: https://www.cdc.gov/mmwr/volumes/67/rr/pdfs/rr6701-H.PDF.

27. Recommended Child and Adolescent Immunization Schedule for ages 18 years or younger, United States, 2021. Centers for Disease Control. Available at: https://www.cdc.gov/vaccines/schedules/hcp/imz/child-adolescent.html. Accessed April 13, 2021.

28. Watterberg K, Benitz W, Hand I, et al. Elimination of perinatal hepatitis B: providing the first vaccine dose within 24 hours of birth. Pediatrics 2017; 140(3):e20171870.

29. Beasley RP, Chin-Yun Lee G, Roan CH, et al. Prevention of perinatally transmitted hepatitis B virus infections with hepatitis B immune globulin and hepatitis B vaccine. Lancet 1983;322(8359):1099–102.

30. Nelson NP, Easterbrook PJ, McMahon BJ. Epidemiology of hepatitis B virus infection and impact of vaccination on disease. Clin Liver Dis 2016;20(4):607–28.

31. Asian Pacific Journal of Cancer Prevention. Available at: http://journal.waocp.org/?sid=Entrez:PubMed&id=pmid:18990029&key=2008.9.3.507. Accessed December 28, 2020.

32. Wexler DL. Hepatitis B vaccine at birth saves lives!. Available at: www.immunize.org/protect-newborns. Accessed December 3, 2020.

33. Vaccine for Flu (influenza) | CDC. Available at: https://www.cdc.gov/vaccines/parents/diseases/flu.html. Accessed December 11, 2020.

34. GlaxoSmithKline Biologicals. Pediarix®. Diphtheria and tetanus toxoids and acellular pertussis adsorbed, hepatitis B (recombinant) and inactivated poliovirus vaccine. Package insert. Available at: https://www.fda.gov/media/79830/download. Accessed December 18, 2020.

35. DeMeo SD, Raman SR, Hornik CP, et al. Adverse events after routine immunization of extremely low-birth-weight infants. JAMA Pediatr 2015;169(8):740–5.

36. GlaxoSmithKline Rotarix®, package insert. Available at: https://www.gsksource.com/pharma/content/dam/GlaxoSmithKline/US/en/Prescribing_Information/Rotarix/pdf/ROTARIX-PI-PIL.PDF. Accessed December 18, 2020.

37. Omenaca F, Sarlangue J, Szenborn L, et al. Safety, reactogenicity and immunogenicity of the human rotavirus vaccine in preterm European infants: a randomized phase IIIb study. Pediatr Infect Dis J 2012;31(5):487–93.

38. RotaTeq®, Merck package insert. Available at: https://www.merck.com/product/usa/pi_circulars/r/rotateq/rotateq_pi.pdf. Accessed December 18, 2020.

39. Rha B, Tate JE, Payne DC, et al. Effectiveness and impact of rotavirus vaccines in the United States-2006-2012. Expert Rev Vaccin 2014;13(3):365–76.

40. Karafillakis E, Hassounah S, Atchison C. Effectiveness and impact of rotavirus vaccines in Europe, 2006-2014. Vaccine 2015;33(18):2097–107.

41. Prelog M, Gorth P, Zwazl I, et al. Universal mass vaccination against rotavirus: Indirect effects on rotavirus infections in neonates and unvaccinated young infants not eligible for vaccination. J Infect Dis 2016;214(4):546–55.

42. Mona Eng P, Mast TC, Loughlin J, et al. Incidence of intussusception among infants in a large commercially insured population in the United States. Pediatr Infect Dis J 2012;31(3):287–91.

43. Gadroen K, Kemmeren JM, Bruijning-Verhagen PC, et al. Baseline incidence of intussusception in early childhood before rotavirus vaccine introduction, The Netherlands, January 2008 to December 2012. Eurosurveillance 2017;22(25): 30556.

44. Folorunso OS, Sebolai OM. Overview of the development, impacts, and challenges of live-attenuated oral rotavirus vaccines. Vaccines 2020;8(3):1 64.

45. Murphy BR, Morens DM, Simonsen L, et al. Reappraisal of the association of intussusception with the licensed live rotavirus vaccine challenges initial conclusions. J Infect Dis 2003;187(8):1301–8.

46. Vesikari T, Matson DO, Dennehy P, et al. Safety and efficacy of a pentavalent human–bovine (WC3) reassortant rotavirus vaccine. N Engl J Med 2006;354(1): 23–33.

47. Ruiz-Palacios GM, Pérez-Schael I, Velázquez FR, et al. Safety and efficacy of an attenuated vaccine against severe rotavirus gastroenteritis. N Engl J Med 2006; 354(1):11–22.

48. Soares-Weiser K, Bergman H, Henschke N, et al. Vaccines for preventing rotavirus diarrhoea: vaccines in use. Cochrane Database Syst Rev 2019;2019(3): CD008521.

49. Haber P, Patel M, Pan Y, et al. Intussusception after rotavirus vaccines reported to US VAERS, 2006-2012. Pediatrics 2013;131(6):1042–9.

50. Oberle D, Hoffelner M, Pavel J, et al. Retrospective multicenter matched case–control study on the risk factors for intussusception in infants less than 1 year of age with a special focus on rotavirus vaccines – the German Intussusception Study. Hum Vaccin Immunother 2020;16(10):2481–94.

51. Vesikari T, Van Damme P, Giaquinto C, et al. European society for paediatric infectious diseases consensus recommendations for rotavirus vaccination in Europe: update 2014. Pediatr Infect Dis J 2015;34(6):635–43.

52. Dahl RM, Curns AT, Tate JE, et al. Effect of rotavirus vaccination on acute diarrheal hospitalizations among low and very low birth weight US infants, 2001-2015. Pediatr Infect Dis J 2018;37(8):817–22.

53. Javid PJ, Sanchez SE, Jacob S, et al. The safety and immunogenicity of rotavirus vaccination in infants with intestinal failure. J Pediatr Infect Dis Soc 2014;3(1): 57–65.

54. McGrath EJ, Thomas R, Duggan C, et al. Pentavalent rotavirus vaccine in infants with surgical gastrointestinal disease. J Pediatr Gastroenterol Nutr 2014; 59(1):44–8.

55. ACIP special situations Guidelines for immunization | recommendations | CDC. Available at: https://www.cdc.gov/vaccines/hcp/acip-recs/general-recs/special-situations.html. Accessed December 28, 2020.

56. Stumpf KA, Thompson T, Sánchez PJ. Rotavirus vaccination of very low birth weight infants at discharge from the NICU. Pediatrics 2013;132(3):e662–5.

57. Burke RM, Tate JE, Han GS, et al. Rotavirus vaccination coverage during a rotavirus outbreak resulting in a fatality at a subacute care facility. J Pediatr Infect Dis Soc 2020;9(3):287–92.

58. Shane AL, Weinberg GA. Can we further increase protection against rotavirus by reducing 2 barriers to immunization, inpatient hospitalization and older age? J Pediatr Infect Dis Soc 2019;2019:1–3.

59. Anderson EJ. Rotavirus vaccines: viral shedding and risk of transmission. Lancet Infect Dis 2008;8(10):642–9.

60. Rivera L, Peña LM, Stainier I, et al. Horizontal transmission of a human rotavirus vaccine strain-A randomized, placebo-controlled study in twins. Vaccine 2011; 29(51):9508–13.

61. Hemming M, Vesikari T. Vaccine-derived human-bovine double reassortant rotavirus in infants with acute gastroenteritis. Pediatr Infect Dis J 2012;31(9):992–4.

62. Payne DC, Edwards KM, Bowen MD, et al. Sibling transmission of vaccine-derived rotavirus (RotaTeq) associated with rotavirus gastroenteritis. Pediatrics 2010;125(2):e438–41.

63. Thrall S, Doll MK, Nhan C, et al. Evaluation of pentavalent rotavirus vaccination in neonatal intensive care units. Vaccine 2015;33(39):5095–102.

64. Monk HM, Motsney AJ, Wade KC. Safety of rotavirus vaccine in the NICU. Pediatrics 2014;133(6):e1555–60.

65. Hiramatsu H, Suzuki R, Nagatani A, et al. Rotavirus vaccination can be performed without viral dissemination in the neonatal intensive care unit. J Infect Dis 2018; 217(4):589–96.
66. Hofstetter AM, Lacombe K, Klein EJ, et al. Risk of rotavirus nosocomial spread after inpatient pentavalent rotavirus vaccination. Pediatrics 2018;141(1): e20171110.
67. D'Angio CT, Maniscalco WM, Pichichero ME. Immunologic response of extremely premature infants to tetanus, Haemophilus influenzae, and polio immunizations. Pediatrics 1995;96(1):18–22.
68. Kirmani KI, Lofthus G, Pichichero ME, et al. Seven-year follow-up of vaccine response in extremely premature infants. Pediatrics 2002;109(3):498–504.
69. Vázquez L, Garcia F, Rüttimann R, et al. Immunogenicity and reactogenicity of DTPa-HBV-IPV/Hib vaccine as primary and booster vaccination in low-birth-weight premature infants. Acta Paediatr Int J Paediatr 2008;97(9):1243–9.
70. Gagneur A, Pinquier D, Quach C. Immunization of preterm infants. Hum Vaccin Immunother 2015;11(11):2556–63.
71. Omeñaca F, Vázquez L, Garcia-Corbeira P, et al. Immunization of preterm infants with GSK's hexavalent combined diphtheria-tetanus-acellular pertussis-hepatitis B-inactivated poliovirus-Haemophilus influenzae type b conjugate vaccine: a review of safety and immunogenicity. Vaccine 2018;36(7):986–96.
72. Roué JM, Nowak E, Le Gal G, et al. Impact of rotavirus vaccine on premature infants. Clin Vaccin Immunol 2014;21(10):1404–9.
73. Rubin LG, Levin MJ, Ljungman P, et al. 2013 IDSA clinical practice guideline for vaccination of the immunocompromised host. Clin Infect Dis 2014;58(3):e44–100.
74. Slack MH, Schapira D, Thwaites RJ, et al. Acellular pertussis vaccine given by accelerated schedule: response of preterm infants. Arch Dis Child Fetal Neonatal Ed 2004;89(1):F57–60.
75. Robinson MJ, Heal C, Gardener E, et al. Antibody response to diphtheria-tetanus-pertussis immunization in preterm infants who receive dexamethasone for chronic lung disease. Pediatrics 2004;113(4 I):733–7.
76. McNeil MM, Weintraub ES, Duffy J, et al. Risk of anaphylaxis after vaccination in children and adults. J Allergy Clin Immunol 2016;137(3):868–78.
77. Lewis E, Shinefield HR, Woodruff BA, et al. Safety of neonatal hepatitis B vaccine administration. Pediatr Infect Dis J 2001;20(11):1049–54.
78. Maglione MA, Das L, Raaen L, et al. Safety of vaccines used for routine immunization of US children: a systematic review. Pediatrics 2014;134(2):325–37.
79. Friksen EM, Perlman JA, Miller A, et al. Lack of association between hepatitis B birth immunization and neonatal death: a population-based study from the Vaccine Safety Datalink Project. Pediatr Infect Dis J 2004;23(7):656–61.
80. Klein NP, Massolo ML, Greene J, et al. Risk factors for developing apnea after immunization in the neonatal intensive care unit. Pediatrics 2008;121(3):463–9.
81. Pourcyrous M, Korones SB, Arheart KL, et al. Primary immunization of premature infants with gestational age <35 Weeks: cardiorespiratory complications and C-Reactive protein responses associated with administration of single and multiple Separate vaccines Simultaneously. J Pediatr 2007;151(2):167–72.
82. Carbone T, McEntire B, Kissin D, et al. Absence of an increase in cardiorespiratory events after diphtheria-tetanus-acellular pertussis immunization in preterm infants: a randomized, multicenter study. Pediatrics 2008;121(5):e1085–90.
83. Stetson RC, Fang JL, Colby CE, et al. Improving infant vaccination status in a Level IV neonatal intensive care unit. Pediatrics 2019;144(5).

84. Hofstetter AM, Jacobson EN, Patricia De Hart M, et al. Early childhood vaccination status of preterm infants. Pediatrics 2019;144(3):e20190337.
85. Gopal SH, Edwards KM, Creech B, et al. Variability in immunization practices for preterm infants. Am J Perinatol 2018;35(14):1394–8.
86. Davis RL, Rubanowice D, Shinefield HR, et al. Immunization levels among premature and low-birth-weight infants and risk factors for delayed up-to-date immunization status. J Am Med Assoc 1999;282(6):547–53.
87. Discenza D. Talking to NICU parents about vaccination. Neonatal Netw 2020; 39(4):238–40.
88. Milet B, Chuo J, Nilan K, et al. Increasing immunization rates in infants with severe chronic lung disease: a quality improvement initiative. Hosp Pediatr 2018;8(11): 693–8.
89. Denizot S, Fleury J, Caillaux G, et al. Hospital initiation of a vaccinal schedule improves the long-term vaccinal coverage of ex-preterm children. Vaccine 2011; 29(3):382–6.
90. Cuna A, Winter L. Quality improvement project to reduce delayed vaccinations in preterm infants. Adv Neonatal Care 2017;17(4):245–9.
91. Ernst KD. Electronic alerts improve immunization rates in two-month-old premature infants hospitalized in the neonatal intensive care unit. Appl Clin Inform 2017;8(1):206–13.
92. Schniepp HE, Cassidy B, Godfrey K. Infant immunizations in pediatric critical care: a quality improvement project. J Pediatr Heal Care 2019;33(2):195–200.

Infection Prevention in the Neonatal Intensive Care Unit

Julia Johnson, MD, PhD[a],*, Ibukunoluwa C. Akinboyo, MD[b],
Joshua K. Schaffzin, MD, PhD[c,d]

KEYWORDS

- Health care–associated infections • Central line–associated bloodstream infections
- Low- and middle-income countries • Environmental cleaning • Disinfection

KEY POINTS

- Neonatal health care–associated infections (HAIs) are associated with significant morbidity and mortality.
- The neonatal intensive care unit (NICU) poses unique infection prevention and control (IPC) challenges due to its specialized population, equipment, and environment.
- IPC in the NICU requires a collaborative relationship between unit-based staff and the hospital's IPC program as well as local, state, and federal resources.
- Innovative strategies are needed to reduce HAI risk in limited-resource settings.

INTRODUCTION

Hospitalized neonates are uniquely vulnerable to health care–associated infections (HAIs), which are associated with increased mortality, increased length of stay, and health care costs, and risk of neurodevelopmental disability among survivors.[1–3] In the United States, incidence of neonatal central line–associated bloodstream infections (CLABSIs) declined significantly from 2007 to 2012, although rates have plateaued recently.[4,5] Global estimates suggest a significantly higher burden of HAI among hospitalized neonates in low-income and middle-income countries (LMICs).[6,7] Infection prevention and control (IPC) strategies that address both patients and their environment are therefore of utmost importance in neonatal care settings, especially in the neonatal intensive care unit (NICU).[8]

---

[a] Division of Neonatology, Department of Pediatrics, Johns Hopkins University School of Medicine, Johns Hopkins Children's Center, 1800 Orleans Street, Suite 8534, Baltimore, MD 21287, USA; [b] Department of Pediatrics, Division of Pediatric Infectious Diseases, Duke University, 2301 Erwin Road, DUMC 3499, Durham, NC 27710, USA; [c] Division of Infectious Diseases, Cincinnati Children's Hospital Medical Center, 3333 Burnet Avenue, Cincinnati, OH 45299-3033, USA; [d] Department of Pediatrics, University of Cincinnati College of Medicine, Cincinnati, OH, USA
* Corresponding author.
E-mail address: jjohn245@jhmi.edu

Clin Perinatol 48 (2021) 413–429
https://doi.org/10.1016/j.clp.2021.03.011
0095-5108/21/© 2021 Elsevier Inc. All rights reserved.

HEALTHCARE-ASSOCIATED INFECTIONS IN THE NEONATE
Central Line–Associated Bloodstream Infections

CLABSIs are associated with substantial morbidity and mortality, as well as increased health care costs and prolonged length of stay.[4,5,9] In the United States, gram-positive pathogens account for most neonatal CLABSIs. *Staphylococcus aureus* and coagulase-negative staphylococci account for nearly half of NICU CLABSI events.[10] Among gram-negative pathogens, *Escherichia coli* and *Klebsiella* spp are responsible for the greatest number of infections. *Candida albicans* remains an important fungal etiology, especially among extremely preterm neonates. Patient factors that contribute to CLABSI risk include prematurity, low birth weight, mucosal barrier injury, and critical illness.[11]

Catheter-Associated Urinary Tract Infection, Surgical Site Infection, and Ventilator-Associated Event

Due to limited use of indwelling urinary catheters in the NICU, reported catheter-associated urinary tract infection (CAUTI) rates have remained low. Despite this, standardized catheter insertion and maintenance bundles should be prioritized as part of effective infection prevention practices. Surgical site infections (SSIs) are associated with considerable morbidity, and hospital-wide prevention efforts often include the NICU. SSI surveillance may be performed locally or as part of a network for high-risk procedures common in neonates, such as ventriculoperitoneal shunt insertion or congenital heart defect repair.[12] Lack of a standardized neonatal ventilator-associated event (VAE) definition hampers surveillance and prevention efforts. With the availability of revised 2015 pediatric VAE guidelines, some units have opted to identify VAE using standard guidelines.[13] Incorporating changes in the fraction of inspired oxygen and mean airway pressure into surveillance definitions used by NICUs could standardize VAE reporting.

INFECTION PREVENTION AND CONTROL INFRASTRUCTURE AND HEALTH CARE–ASSOCIATED INFECTION SURVEILLANCE IN THE NEONATAL INTENSIVE CARE UNIT
Overview of Infection Prevention and Control Infrastructure and Linkage to the Neonatal Intensive Care Unit

In the United States, federal regulations require an infection control officer who is qualified to oversee a facility's plan for surveillance, prevention, and control of HAIs. IPC programs typically have a staff of infection preventionists (IPs) and may be governed by an Infection Control Committee composed of representatives from clinical units, hospital administration, infectious diseases, and other specialties. IPs support target areas through data dissemination, staff education, and implementation of policies and prevention activities. IPC programs will often assign a lead IP to be a liaison to the NICU and its specialized population. Annual risk assessments in the NICU inform identification of opportunities for improvement in key domains (**Table 1**). By collaborating within and between hospital networks, infections can be prevented, harm reduced, and health care costs saved.[2,20]

Surveillance and Reporting Requirements

HAI surveillance in the NICU is a key aspect of performance improvement. The Centers for Disease Control and Prevention (CDC) National Healthcare Safety Network (NHSN) is a surveillance system that provides data collection and reporting capabilities to identify IPC issues, benchmark progress, and comply with public reporting mandates.[14] Use of standardized definitions for HAIs creates a mechanism

Table 1
Key infection prevention and control domains and special considerations in the neonatal population

IPC Domain	Special Considerations in Neonates
HAI surveillance	NHSN reporting required for CLABSI, stratified by birth weight[14] NHSN CLABSI definition provides exclusion for neonatal infections (eg, GBS, NEC)
MDRO colonization	Innovative strategies to reduce transmission (eg, parental decolonization)[15]
HH	Potential role for wearing gloves after HH in high-risk populations[16]
Central line insertion and maintenance	Use of umbilical catheters
Topical antisepsis	Povidone-iodine systemic absorption rarely linked to hypothyroidism[17] Chlorhexidine use may be restricted by age and weight to reduce potential adverse effects in very preterm neonates[18]
Medication and IV fluid preparation and administration	Small doses used in neonates may make consistent use of SDV impractical
Cleaning and disinfection of reused medical equipment	Specialized equipment used in neonates may be difficult to clean
Structure, water, and air	Multibed pods pose additional HAI risk due to less physical distancing between patients
Environmental cleaning	Avoidance of phenol in the NICU due to risk of hyperbilirubinemia[19]
Families and visitor policies	Family-centered care and promotion of breastfeeding and human milk feeding Sibling visitation Vaccination policies for family
Employee health	No restrictions are necessary for health care workers in the NICU who receive routine immunizations
Exposures	High risk given critically ill patient population without or incomplete immunization against high-risk pathogens
IPC bundles and multimodal improvement strategies	IPC bundles linked to CLABSI risk reduction in the NICU CUSP successfully adapted to the NICU

Abbreviations: CLABSI, central line–associated bloodstream infection; CUSP, Comprehensive Unit-based Safety Program; GBS, group B *Streptococcus*; HAI, healthcare-associated infection; HH, hand hygiene; IPC, infection prevention and control; IV, intravenous; MDRO, multi-drug resistant organism; MRSA, methicillin-resistant *Staphylococcus aureus*; NEC, necrotizing enterocolitis; NHSN, National Healthcare Safety Network (NHSN); NICU, neonatal intensive care unit; SDV, single-dose vial.

for comparison across health care facilities nationally. NHSN requirements for NICUs include reporting of CLABSI events, device days, and patient days. Definitions attempt to account for neonatal infections that may not be catheter-associated (see **Table 1**).

NHSN reporting for SSIs, CAUTIs, and VAEs is not required, but these are often tracked locally. When an HAI event or near-miss is identified, root cause analysis (a systematic evaluation of the factors contributing to the event) is beneficial in identifying opportunities for improvement.[21]

Colonization with Resistant Organisms

Prospective surveillance for multidrug-resistant organism (MDRO) colonization is limited in the NICU setting and rates of resistant infections are typically lower than in other pediatric units.[22] Available MDRO data within US NICUs largely focus on methicillin-resistant *S aureus* (MRSA). The recent decline in the prevalence of MRSA colonization and infection in the NICU is likely due to effective IPC measures such as decolonization, cohorting, and use of personal protective equipment (PPE), as well as enhanced antimicrobial stewardship.[15,23] However, reports of infections with other resistant pathogens such as *Candida auris* and carbapenem-resistant Enterobacteriaceae are increasing among neonates, especially in LMICs.[24,25]

Outbreaks

Recognition of an outbreak requires vigilance by frontline staff and the IPC team; a cluster of infections with a known neonatal pathogen, increasing incidence above baseline, or the emergence of an unusual pathogen may signify an outbreak.[26] Recognition that a point source may not be identified should inform broad strategies to improve general IPC practices to contain the outbreak. In some instances, partial or complete unit closure is necessary to contain an outbreak.[27]

GENERAL INFECTION PREVENTION AND CONTROL CONCEPTS AND CONSIDERATIONS IN THE NEONATE
Hand Hygiene

Hand hygiene (HH) is the foundation of IPC in any health care setting, including the NICU. The World Health Organization (WHO) recognizes 5 moments of HH (**Box 1**).[28] Although WHO guidelines recommend use of alcohol-based hand rub (ABHR) for 20 to 30 seconds or use of soap and water for 40 to 60 seconds, CDC guidelines for HH in health care settings recommend a shorter duration of 20 seconds and 15 seconds, respectively.[29,30] Use of ABHR rather than antimicrobial soap has been associated with increased compliance.[31] Factors that may impede effective HH include limited access to clean water or ABHR and the wearing of artificial nails.[32] Direct observation or electronic devices are typically used to monitor HH compliance. Only direct observation can properly capture HH compliance by moment and by health care worker role; monitoring may be strengthened through routine observations over time or using "secret shoppers" to reduce bias.[33]

Box 1
Moments of hand hygiene

Before patient contact

Before aseptic task

After body fluid exposure

After patient contact

After contact with patient surroundings

Central Line Insertion and Maintenance

Preterm and critically ill neonates commonly require placement of central venous catheters (CVCs) and arterial catheters for provision of parenteral nutrition, medication administration, and hemodynamic monitoring. Umbilical venous and arterial catheters require attention due to their associated increased risk of infection. Recommendations for CLABSI prevention include standardized processes for insertion and maintenance (**Box 2**).[36] Topical antimicrobial ointments at the insertion site, systemic antibiotic prophylaxis, and antibiotic lock prophylaxis are not recommended. Prompt removal of central lines when no longer required is essential. Prolonged CVC presence and increased duration of parenteral nutrition has been associated with increased CLABSI risk in neonates.[3,37] Potential facilitators of early line removal include daily discussion of line necessity during rounds, documentation of line necessity in the medical record, and early introduction of enteral feeds.

Topical Antisepsis in the Neonate

Selection of the appropriate topical antiseptic agent in the NICU must carefully consider patient factors (eg, gestational age, birth weight, skin integrity) as well as intended use. Agents used for topical antisepsis in the NICU include isopropyl alcohol, povidone-iodine, and chlorhexidine. Povidone-iodine is routinely used for skin preparation before obtaining blood cultures and before performing surgical procedures. Associated harms include rare reports of systemic absorption with associated hypothyroidism in neonates.[38] Chlorhexidine is increasingly used in the NICU, for skin preparation before procedures, *Staphylococcus aureus* decolonization, and bathing for CLABSI prevention.[18,39,40] Burns and contact dermatitis have been reported, primarily with use of alcohol-based preparations and in young preterm neonates or those with nonintact skin.[41] Trace systemic absorption may occur, although clinical significance is uncertain.[42] Age-based and weight-based guidelines are commonly applied to avoid potential side effects.[18]

Box 2
Central line insertion and maintenance

Central line insertion
    Use of insertion checklist
    Dedicated procedure cart
    Hand hygiene
    Skin antisepsis
    Use of maximal barrier precautions
    Sterile occlusive dressing over peripherally inserted central catheter (PICC) and tunneled catheter sites
    Dedicated staff for insertion of PICCs[34]

Central line maintenance
    Daily assessment of dressing integrity
    Dressing changes weekly and as needed
    Prevention of insertion site bleeding
    Scrubbing the hub with an appropriate antiseptic before access
    Regular tubing changes
    Reduced access frequency
    Daily assessment of need and early catheter removal
    • Replacement of emergently placed catheters as soon as possible in a controlled setting
    • Replacement of umbilical venous catheters with PICCs within the first week of life
    Dedicated line maintenance team[35]

Medication and Intravenous Fluid Preparation and Administration

Antibiotics, anti-epileptic drugs, and analgesics or sedatives may be stored in the NICU to facilitate timely administration. Injections should be prepared using aseptic technique and following recommended procedures (**Box 3**). Multidose vials (MDVs) should be avoided when possible. When used, MDVs should be stored appropriately, dated when first opened, and discarded within 28 days unless otherwise specified by the manufacturer. If MDVs enter the immediate patient care area, their content should be reserved for a single patient. Single-dose vials (SDVs) should never be reused. Intravenous (IV) fluid solution bags should be used only for a single patient. IV tubing should be changed regularly, between every 96 hours and every 7 days, except for tubing used to administer blood products or fat emulsions, which should be changed within 24 hours of the infusion or according to hospital policy.[36]

Cleaning and Disinfection of Reused Medical Equipment

Levels of disinfection required for reused devices are based on intended use, and are summarized in **Table 2**.[44] A risk assessment should be conducted to ensure proper levels of disinfection for all devices used in the NICU. Noncritical devices and surfaces (eg, bed rails, computer keyboards, thermometers) are a potential nidus for transmission and must be cleaned regularly.[45] Similarly, hand-held equipment used by ophthalmologists on multiple patients (such as during retinopathy of prematurity examinations) must be properly disinfected between use to prevent potential pathogen transmission.[43] Due to its greater complexity and risk, facilities may centralize high-level disinfection (HLD) to ensure patient safety and regulatory compliance.[46,47] Outbreaks have been associated with airway and gastrointestinal devices due to defective design, improper reprocessing, and automated process failure.[48,49] Single-use devices should never be reprocessed or reused. During an emergency, federal regulatory guidance should be consulted before single-use items are reprocessed.[44] In LMICs, devices are more difficult to procure; reuse may be common, and proper HLD can be challenging.[50] WHO guidelines recommend against single-use item reuse but also provide a recommended framework to ensure proper decontamination, cleaning, drying, and storage when reuse is necessary.[47]

Environment

Structure, water, and air

The structure and design of a NICU may influence HAI risk. For example, transmission risk for *S aureus* was noted to be higher among infants in multibed pods compared with those in single bed rooms.[51] However, single occupancy room design is often

---

Box 3
Injection safety

Preparation in area separate from immediate patient care

Aseptic technique/proper cleansing of vials before drawing up medication

No reuse of needles and syringes

No needles left in the septum for access

Vials discarded if visible holes in septum

Appropriate sharp disposal in puncture-resistant container accessible to health care workers

Scheduled emptying of sharps disposals containers

Table 2
Agents appropriate for low-level disinfection and concerns within neonatal intensive care units (NICUs)

Disinfecting Agents Hospital-Grade Approved Agents Should Be Used with Proper Contact Time	Device Examples	NICU-Specific Issues
Alcohol (ethyl or isopropyl) 70%–90%	Stethoscope	Not appropriate for protein-rich materials (remove residue with soap and water)
Hydrogen peroxide 3%–5% (nonactivated)	Ultrasound probe (only on intact skin)	Can be damaging to surfaces and metals
Hydrogen peroxide 0.5% (activated)	Blood pressure cuff scale	Can be damaging to surfaces and metals
Household bleach (5.25%) diluted 1:500 (100 ppm)	Temperature probe (intact skin) Horizontal surfaces in care area (eg, bed rails, bedside tables, keyboards, ventilators, pumps)	Can be damaging to surfaces and metals Can be damaging to sensitive electronics If diluting onsite need to mix daily Odor may be bothersome or irritating
Quaternary ammonium compounds	Monitor leads (multi-use)	Less damaging to surfaces (eg, electronics, ultrasound probes) When mixed with bleach can release chlorine gas, a respiratory irritant
Phenols/phenolics	Surfaces/floors	Not recommended for NICU (including floors) May cause hyperbilirubinemia when used on devices and bassinets[19] Irritating to skin: use on surfaces only
Hypochlorite bleach or saline solution	Ophthalmoscope, calipers, pincers for eye examinations	Can leave residue on lenses and limit use Rinsing with sterile water after cleansing can remove residue[43]

not feasible, particularly in LMICs. NICUs with multibed pods could address the increased risk of HAI transmission by screening and cohorting, limiting shared equipment, or placing physical barriers between patients to prevent the potential for cross-contamination.

Colonization of plumbing fixtures has been linked to NICU outbreaks, both through direct and indirect water exposure.[52] Risk mitigation, such as avoiding areas of decreased flow and ensuring proper disinfection, should be included in water protection programs.[53] Sinks should be designated for waste disposal only or HH only.[54] Sterile water for infant bathing or dry warmers for human milk should be used to avoid infections associated with tap water, if possible.[55] Facilities with untreated source water should install filtration or chemical disinfection at the intake point. Environmental sampling, in the absence of an ongoing outbreak, is of unclear significance, but may be part of an environmental risk assessment.[53,56,57] Understanding plumbing and building structure is important to prevent inadvertent introduction of pathogens, if a breach occurs due to a leak or renovation.[58]

Airflow and ventilation maintenance are guided by federal regulatory standards in the United States.[59] If windows open or ventilation is decentralized, ensuring adequate exchange and accounting for humidity and potential vector encroachment may be necessary.[60] Because a NICU room has fewer air changes per hour than an operating room, emergent bedside surgical procedures for clinically unstable infants may pose an HAI risk. Implementing environmental control protocols during these procedures may be beneficial. A NICU should have at least 1 airborne isolation room (AIIR) for managing infants and their essential caregivers while preventing exposure to airborne pathogens by other infants and staff.[61]

Environmental cleaning

Protocols for cleaning and disinfection at regular intervals and at patient discharge should be established to prevent HAI.[62,63] Bedside and environmental services (EVS) staff can share routine responsibilities, with clear delineation, to ensure regular cleaning. Routine closure of clinical areas can facilitate deep cleaning while not disrupting infant development, such as with bright lights and loud machinery.[64] Adherence monitoring with regular feedback and using dedicated EVS teams are strategies to support effective cleaning.[65,66]

HAIs and outbreaks due to contaminated equipment requiring humidification (eg, isolettes, ventilator drains) could result from water, environment, or clinician contamination.[67,68] Small size, need for user-specific training, and frequency of use may limit appropriate cleaning of NICU-specific equipment. Increasing device and disinfectant supply may ensure clean devices are available when needed.

MITIGATING RISK OF POTENTIAL EXPOSURES IN THE NEONATAL INTENSIVE CARE UNIT
Families and Visitors

To promote family-centered care, NICUs must balance visitation policies with limiting opportunities for infection transmission. There are reports of outbreaks introduced by visitors or caregivers, leading NICUs to opt for intermittent visitor restrictions, such as during respiratory viral season.[69,70] However, restrictions might cause parent/caregiver dissatisfaction and adversely affect infant care.[71] Restrictions might be avoided with strict HH adherence, shown to reduce respiratory virus transmission.[71,72] Regardless of season, screening should be conducted to exclude ill individuals.

Recent guidance prioritizes HH for visitors to limit MRSA transmission within the NICU.[73,74] More restrictive visitation policies may apply to young children, who may not be fully vaccinated and have difficulty complying with HH.[72,75] Compliance with standard vaccination recommendations among parents and visitors may provide additional protection. Offering influenza vaccine to parents can improve vaccination rates while preventing influenza transmission.[76] Ideally, visitors, in particular siblings, should show proof of proper vaccination. However, this may not be practical to implement.

Vaccines that contain inactivated organism components pose no risk of infection to NICU patients. Risk of transmission of live-attenuated vaccine virus strains is very low.[77] In infants, the rotavirus and live-attenuated influenza (LAIV) vaccines pose a theoretic risk of transmission of attenuated vaccine virus strains. Units may consider placing patients in precautions (eg, contact for rotavirus) following receipt of vaccine for up to 2 weeks.

Employees

The CDC provides regularly updated guidance for health care worker vaccinations, often overseen by a system's Employee Health/Occupational Health program.[78] Special consideration should be made for seasonal influenza vaccination, as studies show that facilities that mandate seasonal influenza immunization of employees have the highest levels of coverage.[79] This is especially important in settings such as the NICU where most patients are age ineligible to receive a seasonal influenza immunization. Receipt of approved live-attenuated vaccines is not contraindicated in health care workers caring for severely immunocompromised patients.[77,80] Care must be taken for recipients of varicella or zoster vaccine, as virus from vesicular lesions formed at the vaccination site or elsewhere may have the potential for transmission.[77] Units may consider standard screening for receipt of these vaccines during the previous 1 to 2 weeks, and to ask specifically about rash following receipt of varicella-zoster virus vaccine (VZV).[77,81] In addition, some recommend that LAIV recipients wait 1 to 2 weeks following immunization before caring for vulnerable patients.[81]

Presenteeism, the practice of coming to work despite symptoms of infectious illness, is a potential source of pathogen transmission to employees and patients alike.[82] Employee Health (EH) and IPC can collaboratively promote minimal employee penalties for absences due to illness.[83] Any condition preventing adequate HH should result in exclusion from care until HH may be performed. Employees with herpes zoster lesions in a single dermatome should be excluded from the care of varicella nonimmune patients in the NICU until their lesions have crusted.[84,85]

Exposures

Despite prevention efforts, breaches in IPC or exposures to infectious agents will occur requiring a coordinated response. NICUs should collaborate with IPC and EH to develop and enforce policies to manage exposures. Pathogens of concern include severe acute respiratory syndrome coronavirus 2 (SARS-CoV-2), measles, VZV, and pertussis. Preemptive contact and droplet isolation of exposed infants may be necessary in multibed settings, where they can be assessed for the development of symptoms during the incubation period.

VZV transmission from contact with a clinician or visitor with uncovered herpes zoster lesions and the subsequent development of acute infection in a nonimmune infant is rare in the postvaccine era. Exposed nonimmune infants should be moved to an AIIR during the incubation period and consideration should be given for administration of immune globulin.[61] Pertussis infections pose a significant risk to nonimmune neonates, and postexposure prophylaxis may be indicated, with consideration of the limited safety data available for recommended agents.[86,87] Assessing exposure events and notifying families of potential transmission risk is part of a comprehensive exposure plan recommended for NICUs.[88]

INFECTION PREVENTION AND CONTROL BUNDLES AND MULTIMODAL IMPROVEMENT STRATEGIES

The use of bundles to reduce HAI risk via implementation of a package of evidence-based practices is a mainstay of IPC. A 2018 systematic review and meta-analysis of 24 NICU-based studies demonstrated a 60% reduction in CLABSI rate with care bundle implementation.[89] Care bundle composition varied significantly; the most common element included use of a specific protocol for skin preparation, maximal barrier precautions, and daily assessment of catheter need. IPC bundles also have been used to target other HAIs in the NICU, including VAE, and in response to outbreaks.[26],[90] Antimicrobial stewardship interventions should be embedded in HAI prevention bundles to link the core concepts of infection prevention and stewardship to optimize neonatal outcomes.[91]

Multimodal IPC improvement strategies are included in WHO core components for IPC programs and consist of 5 elements: (1) system change, (2) training and education, (3) monitoring and feedback, (4) reminders and communication, and (5) culture change (**Fig. 1**).[92] Multimodal strategies to reduce HAI risk include the Comprehensive Unit-based Safety Program (CUSP), first implemented to reduce CLABSI risk in adult ICUs.[93] CUSP has been successfully adapted to the NICU setting, as part of a national quality collaborative.[94]

LIMITED-RESOURCE SETTINGS
Burden of Health Care–associated Infections in Low-Income and Middle-Income Country Neonatal Intensive Care Units

LMIC health care facilities increasingly care for preterm and ill neonates who are at risk for HAIs, especially due to multidrug-resistant gram-negative pathogens.[7] Given limited treatment options and increased morbidity and mortality associated with these infections, optimizing IPC practices to reduce HAI risk is a key strategy. Delivery of IPC best practices in LMIC health care facilities may be compromised by water supply,

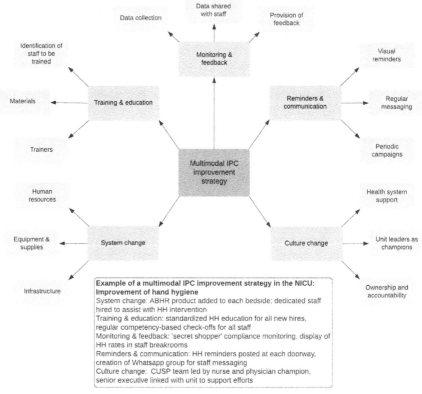

Fig. 1. The WHO multimodal infection prevention and control improvement strategy. The WHO multimodal IPC improvement strategy consists of 5 elements and is a core component of IPC programs.[92] ABHR, alcohol-based hand rub; CUSP, Comprehensive Unit-based Safety Program.

high patient-to-nurse ratios, facility overcrowding, PPE and HH supply shortages, reuse of single-use items, and high burden of antimicrobial-resistant colonization and infection, among other factors.[95]

Innovative Approaches to Preventing Health Care–associated Infections in Limited-Resource Settings

Kangaroo mother care, or provision of prolonged skin-to-skin contact and exclusive breastfeeding, was developed to support thermoregulation in low birth weight neonates in LMICs and is associated with decreased risk of sepsis and mortality.[96] In settings where omphalitis and associated sepsis is more common, use of topical antiseptics for cord care may be indicated to reduce risk. Chlorhexidine application to the cord has been shown to be effective in reduction of cord bacterial burden and resultant neonatal infections; data to support routine use in hospitalized neonates are scarce.[97,98] Topical emollient massage, a common practice in South Asia and other LMIC settings, has been demonstrated to improve skin integrity and reduce late-onset sepsis risk and mortality among hospitalized preterm neonates in LMICs.[99,100] Use of sunflower seed oil or coconut oil for topical emollient massage in hospitalized neonates with an HAI risk is a promising intervention, given its acceptance by caregivers and cost-effectiveness.[101]

SUMMARY

Numerous unique challenges exist within the NICU requiring innovative IPC strategies to deliver safe care to vulnerable neonates. Collaborative efforts to promote HH, standardize cleaning of specialized equipment, maintain environmental cleaning, perform HAI surveillance, and implement bundled interventions to prevent HAIs are integral to a NICU IPC program. Challenges of HAI prevention that exist in both resource advantaged and limited settings can be addressed through innovation and utilization of local expertise and resources.

CLINICS CARE POINTS

- Successful IPC programs in the NICU rely on a collaborative relationship between unit-based staff and the facility's IPC infrastructure.
- HAI surveillance and root cause analyses should inform performance improvement in the NICU.
- Disinfection and environmental cleaning in the NICU must consider the population, structure, and environment unique to the NICU.
- IPC bundles and multimodal improvement strategies are effective in reducing HAI risks in the NICU.

DISCLOSURES

J.J. receives support from the National Institutes of Health (K23HD100594). I.C.A. and J.K.S. have no disclosures.

REFERENCES

1. Stoll BJ, Hansen NI, Adams-Chapman I, et al. Neurodevelopmental and growth impairment among extremely low-birth-weight infants with neonatal infection. JAMA 2004;292(19):2357–65.

2. Donovan EF, Sparling K, Lake MR, et al. The investment case for preventing NICU-associated infections. Am J Perinatol 2013;30(3):179–84.

3. Stoll BJ, Hansen N, Fanaroff AA, et al. Late-onset sepsis in very low birth weight neonates: the experience of the NICHD Neonatal Research Network. Pediatrics 2002;110(2 Pt 1):285–91.

4. Patrick SW, Kawai AT, Kleinman K, et al. Health care-associated infections among critically ill children in the US, 2007-2012. Pediatrics 2014;134(4): 705–12.

5. Hsu HE, Mathew R, Wang R, et al. Health care-associated infections among critically ill children in the US, 2013-2018. JAMA Pediatr 2020.

6. Rosenthal VD, Lynch P, Jarvis WR, et al. Socioeconomic impact on device-associated infections in limited-resource neonatal intensive care units: findings of the INICC. Infection 2011;39(5):439–50.

7. Zaidi AK, Huskins WC, Thaver D, et al. Hospital-acquired neonatal infections in developing countries. Lancet 2005;365(9465):1175–88.

8. Suleyman G, Alangaden G, Bardossy AC. The role of environmental contamination in the transmission of nosocomial pathogens and healthcare-associated infections. Curr Infect Dis Rep 2018;20(6):12.

9. Snyder AN, Burjonrappa S. Central line associated blood stream infections in gastroschisis patients: a nationwide database analysis of risks, outcomes, and disparities. J Pediatr Surg 2020;55(2):286–91.

10. Weiner-Lastinger LM, Abner S, Benin AL, et al. Antimicrobial-resistant pathogens associated with pediatric healthcare-associated infections: summary of data reported to the National Healthcare Safety Network, 2015-2017. Infect Control Hosp Epidemiol 2020;41(1):19–30.

11. Dahan M, O'Donnell S, Hebert J, et al. CLABSI risk factors in the NICU: potential for prevention: a PICNIC study. Infect Control Hosp Epidemiol 2016;37(12): 1446–52.

12. Schaffzin JK, Harte L, Marquette S, et al. Surgical site infection reduction by the solutions for patient safety hospital Engagement network. Pediatrics 2015; 136(5):e1353–60.

13. Cocoros NM, Priebe GP, Logan LK, et al. A pediatric approach to ventilator-associated events surveillance. Infect Control Hosp Epidemiol 2017;38(3): 327–33.

14. Centers for Disease Control and Prevention. NHSN patient safety component manual 2020. Available at: https://www.cdc.gov/nhsn/pdfs/pscmanual/pcsmanual_current.pdf. Accessed December 13, 2020.

15. Milstone AM, Voskertchian A, Koontz DW, et al. Effect of treating parents colonized with *Staphylococcus aureus* on transmission to neonates in the intensive care unit: a randomized clinical trial. Jama 2020;323(4):319–28.

16. Kaufman DA, Blackman A, Conaway MR, et al. Nonsterile glove use in addition to hand hygiene to prevent late-onset infection in preterm infants: randomized clinical trial. JAMA Pediatr 2014;168(10):909–16.

17. Mitchell IM, Pollock JC, Jamieson MP, et al. Transcutaneous iodine absorption in infants undergoing cardiac operation. Ann Thorac Surg 1991;52(5):1138–40.

18. Johnson J, Bracken R, Tamma PD, et al. Trends in chlorhexidine use in US neonatal intensive care units: results from a follow-up national survey. Infect Control Hosp Epidemiol 2016;37(9):1116–8.

19. Doan HM, Keith L, Shennan AT. Phenol and neonatal jaundice. Pediatrics 1979; 64(3):324–5.

20. Wheeler DS, Giaccone MJ, Hutchinson N, et al. A hospital-wide quality-improvement collaborative to reduce catheter-associated bloodstream infections. Pediatrics 2011;128(4):e995–1004 [quiz e1004-1007].
21. Venier AG. Root cause analysis to support infection control in healthcare premises. J Hosp Infect 2015;89(4):331–4.
22. Lake JG, Weiner LM, Milstone AM, et al. . Pathogen distribution and antimicrobial resistance among pediatric healthcare-associated infections reported to the National Healthcare Safety Network, 2011-2014. Infect Control Hosp Epidemiol 2018;39(1):1–11.
23. Ericson JE, Popoola VO, Smith PB, et al. Burden of invasive *Staphylococcus aureus* infections in hospitalized infants. JAMA Pediatr 2015;169(12):1105–11.
24. Armstrong PA, Rivera SM, Escandon P, et al. Hospital-associated multicenter outbreak of emerging fungus *Candida auris*, Colombia, 2016. Emerg Infect Dis 2019;25(7):1339–46.
25. Johnson J, Robinson ML, Rajput UC, et al. High burden of bloodstream infections associated with antimicrobial resistance and mortality in the neonatal intensive care unit in Pune, India. Clin Infect Dis 2020.
26. Johnson J, Quach C. Outbreaks in the neonatal ICU: a review of the literature. Curr Opin Infect Dis 2017;30(4):395–403.
27. Gramatniece A, Silamikelis I, Zahare I, et al. Control of *Acinetobacter baumannii* outbreak in the neonatal intensive care unit in Latvia: whole-genome sequencing powered investigation and closure of the ward. Antimicrob Resist Infect Control 2019;8:84.
28. World Health Organization. Five moments for hand hygiene 2020. Available at: https://www.who.int/gpsc/tools/Five_moments/en/. Accessed December 13, 2020.
29. Boyce JM, Pittet D. Guideline for hand hygiene in health-care settings. Recommendations of the healthcare infection control practices advisory committee and the HICPAC/SHEA/APIC/IDSA hand hygiene task Force. Society for Healthcare Epidemiology of America/Association for Professionals in Infection Control/Infectious Diseases Society of America. MMWR Recomm Rep 2002;51(Rr-16): 1–45 [quiz CE41-44].
30. World Health Organization. Hand hygiene: why, how & when?. 2009. Available at: https://www.who.int/gpsc/5may/Hand_Hygiene_Why_How_and_When_Brochure. pdf. Accessed December 13, 2020.
31. Cohen B, Saiman L, Cimiotti J, et al. Factors associated with hand hygiene practices in two neonatal intensive care units. Pediatr Infect Dis J 2003;22(6):494–9.
32. Gupta A, Della-Latta P, Todd B, et al. Outbreak of extended-spectrum beta-lactamase-producing *Klebsiella pneumoniae* in a neonatal intensive care unit linked to artificial nails. Infect Control Hosp Epidemiol 2004;25(3):210–5.
33. Chen LF, Vander Weg MW, Hofmann DA, et al. The Hawthorne effect in infection prevention and epidemiology. Infect Control Hosp Epidemiol 2015;36(12): 1444–50.
34. Taylor T, Massaro A, Williams L, et al. Effect of a dedicated percutaneously inserted central catheter team on neonatal catheter-related bloodstream infection. Adv Neonatal Care 2011;11(2):122–8.
35. Holzmann-Pazgal G, Kubanda A, Davis K, et al. Utilizing a line maintenance team to reduce central-line-associated bloodstream infections in a neonatal intensive care unit. J Perinatol 2012;32(4):281–6.
36. O'Grady NP, Alexander M, Burns LA, et al. Guidelines for the prevention of intravascular catheter-related infections. Clin Infect Dis 2011;52(9):e162–93.

37. Sengupta A, Lehmann C, Diener-West M, et al. Catheter duration and risk of CLA-BSI in neonates with PICCs. Pediatrics 2010;125(4):648–53.
38. Linder N, Davidovitch N, Reichman B, et al. Topical iodine-containing antiseptics and subclinical hypothyroidism in preterm infants. J Pediatr 1997;131(3): 434–9.
39. McCord H, Fieldhouse E, El-Naggar W. Current practices of antiseptic use in Canadian neonatal intensive care units. Am J Perinatol 2019;36(2):141–7.
40. Quach C, Milstone AM, Perpête C, et al. Chlorhexidine bathing in a tertiary care neonatal intensive care unit: impact on central line-associated bloodstream infections. Infect Control Hosp Epidemiol 2014;35(2):158–63.
41. Vanzi V, Pitaro R. Skin injuries and chlorhexidine gluconate-based antisepsis in early premature infants: a case report and review of the literature. J Perinat Neonatal Nurs 2018;32(4):341–50.
42. Chapman AK, Aucott SW, Gilmore MM, et al. Absorption and tolerability of aqueous chlorhexidine gluconate used for skin antisepsis prior to catheter insertion in preterm neonates. J Perinatol 2013;33(10):768–71.
43. Sammons JS, Graf EH, Townsend S, et al. Outbreak of adenovirus in a neonatal intensive care unit: critical importance of equipment cleaning during inpatient ophthalmologic examinations. Ophthalmology 2019;126(1):137–43.
44. Rutala WA, the Healthcare Infection Control Practices Advisory Committee (HICPAC). Guideline for disinfection and sterilization in healthcare facilities 2008. Available at: https://www.cdc.gov/infectioncontrol/guidelines/disinfection/. Accessed December 13, 2020.
45. v Dijk Y, Bik EM, Hochstenbach-Vernooij S, et al. Management of an outbreak of Enterobacter cloacae in a neonatal unit using simple preventive measures. J Hosp Infect 2002;51(1):21–6.
46. Rutala WA, Weber DJ. Reprocessing semicritical items: outbreaks and current issues. Am J Infect Control 2019;47s:A79–89.
47. World Health Organization PAHO. Decontamination and reprocessing of medical devices for health-care facilities. 2016. Available at: https://www.who.int/infection-prevention/publications/decontamination/en/. Accessed December 13, 2020.
48. Kenters N, Huijskens EG, Meier C, et al. Infectious diseases linked to cross-contamination of flexible endoscopes. Endosc Int Open 2015;3(4):E259–65.
49. Weber DJ, Rutala WA. Lessons from outbreaks associated with bronchoscopy. Infect Control Hosp Epidemiol 2001;22(7):403–8.
50. Ogunsola FT, Mehtar S. Challenges regarding the control of environmental sources of contamination in healthcare settings in low-and middle-income countries - a narrative review. Antimicrob Resist Infect Control 2020;9(1):81.
51. Washam MC, Ankrum A, Haberman BE, et al. Risk factors for Staphylococcus aureus acquisition in the neonatal intensive care unit: a matched case-case-control study. Infect Control Hosp Epidemiol 2018;39(1):46–52.
52. Verweij PE, Meis JF, Christmann V, et al. Nosocomial outbreak of colonization and infection with Stenotrophomonas maltophilia in preterm infants associated with contaminated tap water. Epidemiol Infect 1998;120(3):251–6.
53. ANSI/ASHRAE. In: Legionellosis: risk management for building water systems, vol. 188-2018 2018.
54. Parkes LO, Hota SS. Sink-related outbreaks and mitigation strategies in healthcare facilities. Curr Infect Dis Rep 2018;20(10):42.
55. Molina-Cabrillana J, Artiles-Campelo F, Dorta-Hung E, et al. Outbreak of Pseudomonas aeruginosa infections in a neonatal care unit associated with feeding bottles heaters. Am J Infect Control 2013;41(2):e7–9.

56. Gamage SD, Kralovic SM, Roselle GA. The case for routine environmental testing for Legionella bacteria in healthcare facility water distribution systems-reconciling CDC position and guidance regarding risk. Clin Infect Dis 2015; 61(9):1487–8.

57. Demirjian A, Lucas CE, Garrison LE, et al. The importance of clinical surveillance in detecting legionnaires' disease outbreaks: a large outbreak in a hospital with a Legionella disinfection system-Pennsylvania, 2011-2012. Clin Infect Dis 2015;60(11):1596–602.

58. Bryce EA, Walker M, Scharf S, et al. An outbreak of cutaneous aspergillosis in a tertiary-care hospital. Infect Control Hosp Epidemiol 1996;17(3):170–2.

59. ANSI/ASHRAE/ASHE. In: Ventilation of health care facilities, vol. 170-2017 2017.

60. World Health Organization. Natural ventilation for infection control in health-care settings 2009. Available at: https://www.who.int/water_sanitation_health/publications/natural_ventilation.pdf. Accessed February 18, 2021.

61. Kimberlin DWBM, Jackson MA, Long SS. American Academy of Pediatrics, Committee on Infectious Diseases. In: Red book: 2018-2021 report of the Committee on Infectious Diseases. Elk Grove Village, IL: American Academy of Pediatrics; 2018.

62. Li QF, Xu H, Ni XP, et al. Impact of relocation and environmental cleaning on reducing the incidence of healthcare-associated infection in NICU. World J Pediatr 2017;13(3):217–21.

63. Schulster LM, Arduino MJ, Carpenter J, et al. Guidelines for environmental infection control in health-care facilities. In: Recommendations from the CDC and the Healthcare Infection Control Practices Advisory Committee (HICPAC). 2004. Available at: https://www.cdc.gov/infectioncontrol/pdf/guidelines/environmental/index.html. Accessed December 13, 2020.

64. Almadhoob A, Ohlsson A. Sound reduction management in the neonatal intensive care unit for preterm or very low birth weight infants. Cochrane Database Syst Rev 2020;1(1):Cd010333.

65. Deshpande A, Donskey CJ. Practical approaches for assessment of daily and post-discharge room disinfection in healthcare facilities. Curr Infect Dis Rep 2017;19(9):32.

66. Sitzlar B, Deshpande A, Fertelli D, et al. An environmental disinfection odyssey: evaluation of sequential interventions to improve disinfection of *Clostridium difficile* isolation rooms. Infect Control Hosp Epidemiol 2013;34(5):459–65.

67. Wenger PN, Tokars JI, Brennan P, et al. An outbreak of *Enterobacter hormaechei* infection and colonization in an intensive care nursery. Clin Infect Dis 1997; 24(6):1243–4.

68. Etienne KA, Subudhi CP, Chadwick PR, et al. Investigation of a cluster of cutaneous aspergillosis in a neonatal intensive care unit. J Hosp Infect 2011;79(4): 344–8.

69. Dunn GL, Tapson H, Davis J, et al. Outbreak of Piv-3 in a neonatal intensive care unit in England. Pediatr Infect Dis J 2017;36(3):344–5.

70. Popoola VO, Budd A, Wittig SM, et al. Methicillin-resistant *Staphylococcus aureus* transmission and infections in a neonatal intensive care unit despite active surveillance cultures and decolonization: challenges for infection prevention. Infect Control Hosp Epidemiol 2014;35(4):412–8.

71. Murray PD, Swanson JR. Visitation restrictions: is it right and how do we support families in the NICU during COVID-19? J Perinatol 2020;40(10):1576–81.

72. Linam WM, Marrero EM, Honeycutt MD, et al. Focusing on families and visitors reduces healthcare associated respiratory viral infections in a neonatal intensive care unit. Pediatr Qual Saf 2019;4(6):e242.

73. Goldstein ND, Eppes SC, Mackley A, et al. A network model of hand hygiene: how good is good enough to stop the spread of MRSA? Infect Control Hosp Epidemiol 2017;38(8):945–52.

74. Akinboyo IC, Zangwill KM, Berg WM, et al. SHEA neonatal intensive care unit (NICU) white paper series: practical approaches to *Staphylococcus aureus* disease prevention. Infect Control Hosp Epidemiol 2020;41(11):1251–7.

75. Shui JE, Messina M, Hill-Ricciuti AC, et al. Impact of respiratory viruses in the neonatal intensive care unit. J Perinatol 2018;38(11):1556–65.

76. Shah SI, Caprio M, Hendricks-Munoz K. Administration of inactivated trivalent influenza vaccine to parents of high-risk infants in the neonatal intensive care unit. Pediatrics 2007;120(3):e617–21.

77. Kamboj M, Sepkowitz KA. Risk of transmission associated with live attenuated vaccines given to healthy persons caring for or residing with an immunocompromised patient. Infect Control Hosp Epidemiol 2007;28(6):702–7.

78. Advisory Committee on Immunization Practices CfDCaP. Immunization of healthcare personnel: recommendations of the Advisory Committee on Immunization Practices (ACIP). MMWR Recomm Rep 2011;60(Rr-7):1–45.

79. Black CL, Yue X, Ball SW, et al. Influenza vaccination coverage among health care personnel - United States, 2016-17 influenza season. MMWR Morb Mortal Wkly Rep 2017;66(38):1009–15.

80. Shearer WT, Fleisher TA, Buckley RH, et al. Recommendations for live viral and bacterial vaccines in immunodeficient patients and their close contacts. J Allergy Clin Immunol 2014;133(4):961–6.

81. Grohskopf LA, Alyanak E, Broder KR, et al. Prevention and control of seasonal influenza with vaccines: recommendations of the Advisory Committee on Immunization Practices - United States, 2019-20 influenza season. MMWR Recomm Rep 2019;68(3):1–21.

82. Kuster SP, Böni J, Kouyos RD, et al. Absenteeism and presenteeism in healthcare workers due to respiratory illness. Infect Control Hosp Epidemiol 2020;1–6.

83. Szymczak JE, Smathers S, Hoegg C, et al. Reasons why physicians and advanced practice clinicians work while sick: a mixed-methods analysis. JAMA Pediatr 2015;169(9):815–21.

84. Gelber SE, Ratner AJ. Hospital-acquired viral pathogens in the neonatal intensive care unit. Semin Perinatol 2002;26(5):346–56.

85. Friedman CA, Temple DM, Robbins KK, et al. Outbreak and control of varicella in a neonatal intensive care unit. Pediatr Infect Dis J 1994;13(2):152–4.

86. Schaffzin JKCB. Pertussis. In: Kline MW, editor. Rudolph's pediatrics. 23rd edition. New York, New York: McGraw Hill Medical; 2018.

87. Tiwari T, Murphy TV, Moran J. Recommended antimicrobial agents for the treatment and postexposure prophylaxis of pertussis: 2005 CDC Guidelines. MMWR Recomm Rep 2005;54(Rr-14):1–16.

88. Kellie SM, Makvandi M, Muller ML. Management and outcome of a varicella exposure in a neonatal intensive care unit: lessons for the vaccine era. Am J Infect Control 2011;39(10):844–8.

89. Payne V, Hall M, Prieto J, et al. Care bundles to reduce central line-associated bloodstream infections in the neonatal unit: a systematic review and meta-analysis. Arch Dis Child Fetal Neonatal Ed 2018;103(5):F422–9.

90. Gokce IK, Kutman HGK, Uras N, et al. Successful implementation of a bundle strategy to prevent ventilator-associated pneumonia in a neonatal intensive care unit. J Trop Pediatr 2018;64(3):183–8.
91. Akinboyo IC, Gerber JS. Principles, policy and practice of antibiotic stewardship. Semin Perinatol 2020;151324.
92. World Health Organization. Guidelines on core components of infection prevention and control programmes at the national and acute health care facility level 2016. Available at: https://apps.who.int/iris/bitstream/handle/10665/251730/9789241549929-eng.pdf;jsessionid=1786EFF9B27E663EF00D501C4385053D?sequence=1. Accessed December 13, 2020.
93. Pronovost P, Needham D, Berenholtz S, et al. An intervention to decrease catheter-related bloodstream infections in the ICU. N Engl J Med 2006;355(26):2725–32.
94. Lin DM, Weeks K, Holzmueller CG, et al. Maintaining and sustaining the on the CUSP: stop BSI model in Hawaii. Jt Comm J Qual Patient Saf 2013;39(2):51–60.
95. Weinshel K, Dramowski A, Hajdu Á, et al. Gap analysis of infection control practices in low- and middle-income countries. Infect Control Hosp Epidemiol 2015;36(10):1208–14.
96. Boundy EO, Dastjerdi R, Spiegelman D, et al. Kangaroo mother care and neonatal outcomes: a meta-analysis. Pediatrics 2016;137(1).
97. Imdad A, Mullany LC, Baqui AH, et al. The effect of umbilical cord cleansing with chlorhexidine on omphalitis and neonatal mortality in community settings in developing countries: a meta-analysis. BMC Public Health 2013;13(Suppl 3):S15.
98. Sinha A, Sazawal S, Pradhan A, et al. Chlorhexidine skin or cord care for prevention of mortality and infections in neonates. Cochrane Database Syst Rev 2015;(3):Cd007835.
99. Darmstadt GL, Saha SK, Ahmed AS, et al. Effect of topical emollient treatment of preterm neonates in Bangladesh on invasion of pathogens into the bloodstream. Pediatr Res 2007;61(5 Pt 1):588–93.
100. Salam RA, Darmstadt GL, Bhutta ZA. Effect of emollient therapy on clinical outcomes in preterm neonates in Pakistan: a randomised controlled trial. Arch Dis Child Fetal Neonatal Ed 2015;100(3):F210–5.
101. LeFevre A, Shillcutt SD, Saha SK, et al. Cost-effectiveness of skin-barrier-enhancing emollients among preterm infants in Bangladesh. Bull World Health Organ 2010;88(2):104–12.

Moving?

Make sure your subscription moves with you!

To notify us of your new address, find your **Clinics Account Number** (located on your mailing label above your name), and contact customer service at:

Email: journalscustomerservice-usa@elsevier.com

800-654-2452 (subscribers in the U.S. & Canada)
314-447-8871 (subscribers outside of the U.S. & Canada)

Fax number: 314-447-8029

Elsevier Health Sciences Division
Subscription Customer Service
3251 Riverport Lane
Maryland Heights, MO 63043

*To ensure uninterrupted delivery of your subscription, please notify us at least 4 weeks in advance of move.

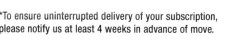

ELSEVIER

Printed and bound by CPI Group (UK) Ltd, Croydon, CR0 4YY

03/10/2024

01040406-0007